Praise for Myths of Menopause

Anita Bean. Nutritionist, Speaker and Author

"With so many myths and negative misconceptions around menopause it's no surprise that women are anxious about entering this phase of their life. This book will help women better understand what is happening in their bodies, take steps to overcome symptoms and gain more control over their health."

Peta Bee. Health and Fitness Journalist for *The Times*

"Dr Nicky Keay is an expert in the field of hormone study and unrivalled in her ability to distil complex scientific research into information that is understandable and useful to the general public. She's also a master at busting myths that swirl around on social media."

Martin MacDonald. CEO Mac-Nutrition Uni & Clinical Performance Nutritionist

"Dr Nicky Keay spoke at our Mac-Nutrition LIVE Conference on 'Supporting the Perimenopausal Period: Nutrition, Lifestyle & HRT Considerations' & her ability to bring the topic to life, linking the research effortlessly to real world application in an engaging & humorous way was second to none. With our commitment to only bringing in evidence-based speakers & tutors for our students, Nicky is one of our go to experts on all things menopause."

Dr Stephanie Potreck. Medical Doctor and Sports Nutritionist. AusDancersOverseas

"Dr Nicky Keay is such a positive influence on so many women's lives. With her expert knowledge, she always picks up her audiences where they are at in that particular moment, a trait that is invaluable in healthcare. Over the years, she has empowered and encouraged countless female athletes and dancers to take care of their health instead of listening to outdated and misleading messages from coaches and teachers, and now it must be the logical consequence to bust those myths for the other end of the spectrum, perimenopause and menopause. Nicky has created a treasure with this book, one that healthcare professionals and society will have to notice, for women are now meticulously informed about this transition in their lives."

Dr Stacy Sims. Female Physiologist and Nutritionist

"Menopause. A few years ago, no one was discussing it in open circles, now it seems to be water cooler and nightly news conversations. Unfortunately, misinformation has woven tightly into these conversations, creating noise and advice from social media influences. Dr Nicky Keay has done it again, with her new book Myths of Menopause, she expertly crafts scientific language into accessible, actionable points, based on the scientific research and expertise of colleagues in the space. This is a must have book for so many women looking for the truth."

Dr Izzy Smith. Australian Endocrinologist with expertise working with female athletes

"Witnessing the soar in women's involvement in exercise and endurance sports is incredible. There has never been a more important time for age group and masters' athletes to understand the impact of the menopause transition for health and performance.

Dr Nicky Keay's expertise and wisdom throughout this book will guide women to thrive for their full potential through the menopause transition and be empowered in decision making when it comes to their health, exercise and sporting goals."

Dr Mariza Snyder. National Bestselling Author

"Dr Nicky Keay is a go-to expert in the field of women's hormone health and she has provided a vital guide for all women navigating the menopause journey. Full of actionable information, it's a great resource for every woman approaching and enduring menopause."

Dr Mikki Williden. Registered Nutritionist, New Zealand

"Dr. Nicky Keay orchestrates a tour de force in hormone health, expertly clarifying complex research and empowering women to navigate menopause with confidence and science-backed knowledge."

Myths of Menopause

Every possible effort has been made to ensure that the information contained in this book is accurate at the time of going to press. The publishers and author(s) cannot accept responsibility for any errors and omissions, however caused. No responsibility for loss or damage occasioned to any person acting, or refraining from action, as a result of the material contained in this publication can be accepted by the editor, the publisher or the author. The views of the contributors are not necessarily those of the editor.

First published in 2024 by Sequoia Books

Apart from fair dealing for the purposes of research or private study, or criticism or review, as permitted under the Copyright, Designs and Patents act 1988, this publication may only be reproduced, stored or transmitted, in any form or by any means, with the prior permission in writing of the publisher, or in the case of reprographic reproduction in accordance with the terms and licenses issued by the CLA. Enquiries concerning reproduction outside these terms should be sent to the publisher using the details on the website www.sequoia-books.com

©Nicky Keay 2024

The right of Nicky Keay to be identified as editor of this work has been asserted in accordance with the Copyright, Designs and Patents act 1988.

ISBN
Print: 9781914110405
EPUB: 9781914110412

A CIP record for this book is available from the British Library

Library of Congress Cataloguing-In-Publication Data

Name: Nicky Keay
Title: Myths of Menopause
Description: 1st Edition, Sequoia Books UK 2024
Print: 9781914110405
EPUB: 9781914110412

Library of Congress Control Number: 2024919908

Print and Electronic production managed by Deanta Global

Myths of Menopause

Edited by Dr Nicky Keay

Editor Background

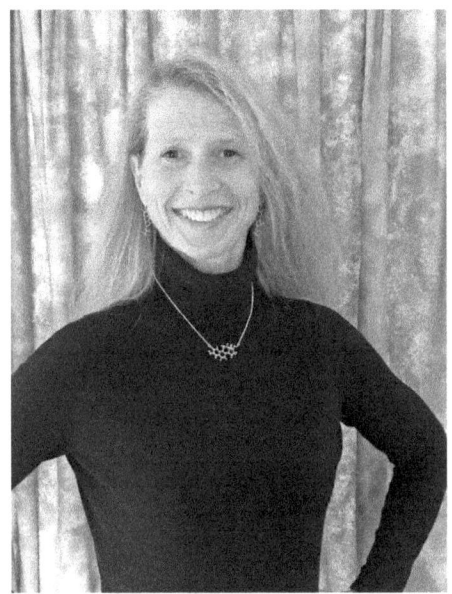

Dr Nicky Keay, BA, MA, MB, BChir (Cantab), MRCP Nicky is a medical doctor with specialist expertise in the field of exercise endocrinology. Her research into the impacts of lifestyle, nutrition and exercise on hormone networks has been published in peer-reviewed journals. She is the author of *Hormones, Health and Human Potential*. Nicky holds the position of Honorary Clinical Lecturer in the Division of Medicine, University College London. Nicky's clinical endocrine work is particularly with women experiencing perimenopause and menopause and all ages of exercisers, dancers and athletes, with a focus on relative energy deficiency in sport (REDs). Nicky's passion and objective is to provide a more personalised approach for female hormone health to optimise the overall health and performance of the individual. Nicky is the medical advisor to Scottish Ballet and a keen ballet dancer.

Nicky studied medicine at Cambridge University. After gaining Membership of the Royal College of Physicians, London, United Kingdom, Nicky worked as a Research Fellow at St Thomas' Hospital, London, where she was part of the international medical team that developed an anti-doping test for growth hormone. Nicky is a member of the British Menopause Society (BMS) and has completed the BMS Principles and Practice of Menopause Care training programme and the Management of Menopause certification. Nicky is currently working with colleagues at University College London, backed by leading women's health organisations, to develop an evidence-base UK menopause information and support programme InTune.

Thanks

Many thanks to all the brilliant contributors to this book for their insights and enthusiasm for this project. My thanks to my husband Gavin. Ever since we first met at St John's College, Cambridge, Gavin has been my steadfast support. This includes all the time and patience he has put in to help me with analysis and writing of research papers and now this book. Gavin has a clarity of expression that has been invaluable in shaping my ideas into something that I hope is both informative and engaging.

Thank you to Lucy Milligan who provided the artwork of Athena on the book cover to represent how wisdom, understanding and knowledge can reveal the truth behind the myths surrounding menopause.

Dedication

This book *Myths of Menopause* is dedicated to my sister Amanda Keay who died too young, so we could not share and enjoy the female hormone odyssey together.

Contents

Prelude — xv
Menopause as part of the female hormone odyssey
Dr Nicky Keay

Act 1 Misunderstandings around Menopause — 1
Distractions of social media Sirens

Scene 1 What is menopause? — 3
Dr Nicky Keay

Scene 2 Mythology in women's midlife – what's in a name? — 23
Professor Jerilynn Prior

Scene 3 What has progesterone got to do with menopause? — 31
Lara Briden

Act 2 Challenges of Menopause — 37
Pandora's box

Scene 1 Myths of menopausal 'symptoms' — 39
Dr Nicky Keay

Scene 2 "Sleep no more!?" — 51
Dr Zoe Schaedel

Scene 3 Myths of menopausal health — 63
Dr Nicky Keay

Scene 4 Don't let sticks, stones or falls break your bones!   67
Rebekah Rotstein

Scene 5 Menopause mix: metabolic and mental health   74
Dr Anne Latz

Act 3 Menopause, Sex and Pelvic Health   83

The metamorphosis of Aphrodite

Scene 1 No sex after menopause?!   85
Dr Shema Tariq

Scene 2 Goodbye to pelvic health after menopause?!   90
Dr Gillian Cambell and Christien Bird

Act 4 Mastering Menopause   111

"If we could give each individual just the right amount of nourishment and exercise, not too little and not too much, we would have found the safest way to health."

Hippocrates

How to navigate the female hormone odyssey?   112
Dr Nicky Keay

Scene 1 The menopause diet?   116
Renee McGregor

Scene 2 Where do I start with exercise?   126
Ally Atkins

Scene 3 Demystifying the myths of exercise   140
Dr Alyssa Olenick

Act 5 Treatment Options   159

Hormone replacement therapy (HRT)

Scylla and Charybdis   161
Dr Nicky Keay

Act 6 Active Women and the Hormone Dance — 181
Terpsichore

The hormone dance of life — 182
Dr Nicky Keay

Scene 1 Dancing through menopause — 185
Tiffany Stott

Scene 2 Gracefully ageing (we hope) forever swans — 194
Astrid Sherman

Scene 3 Menopause flamenco! — 197
Nikki Crane

Scene 4 Everybody leaks?! — 201
Dinah Hampson and Dr Brooke Winder

Act 7 Age Group Athletes — 223
Orpheus and Eurydice

Don't look back . . . — 224
Dr Nicky Keay

Scene 1 Relative energy deficiency in sport only happens in young exercisers?! — 225
Dr Nicky Keay

Scene 2 Can I maintain athletic effort and performance? — 236
Tenille Hoogland

Scene 3 Not always an injury?! — 247
Nicole Oh

Scene 4 Strength training for performance and health — 253
Dr Richard C Blagrove

Act 8 Experiencing Menopause — 295
Discord and harmony

Scene 1 Am I losing my mind? — 297
Professor Aimee Spector

Scene 2 Why do each of us experience menopause differently? — 304
Dr Helen Donovan, Professor Myra Hunter, Nora Bahhar, Professor Aimee Spector

Scene 3 Don't mention the 'M' word! — 322
Dr Meena Khatwa

Scene 4 Can we pass the baton from sport? — 341
Anna Allerton

Act 9 Towards Positive Ageing — 351
Collaboratively removing barriers for sustainable person-centred system support

Dr Marzena Nieroda, Dr Abdul Seckam, Dr Dania Posso, Dr Rodrigo Rodriguez-Fernandez, Dr Orlanda Allen, Professor André Coutinho, Thalia Anagnostopoulou, Professor Joyce Harper, Dr Nicky Keay

Coda — 373
The wisdom of Athena
Dr Nicky Keay
Dr Tamara Dragadze

Terpsichore and Menopause — 375
Dr Tamara Dragadze

Navigating Menopause Myths — 378

Contributor Backgrounds — 381

Prelude

Menopause as part of the female hormone odyssey

Dr Nicky Keay

"Nothing in life is to be feared, it is only to be understood. Now is the time to understand more so that we may fear less."

Marie Curie

Homer's epic poem, the Odyssey, describes Odysseus's long journey home after the Trojan War. Athena, the Ancient Greek goddess of wisdom, provides wise counsel, helping the Greek hero and his companions navigate the many challenges that threaten to throw them off course.

Over her lifetime, every woman experiences her body's ever-changing hormonal choreography, which is mythical in its beauty and complexity. She must navigate her own female hormone odyssey, according to her individual biological response to hormones and her unique personal background of life experiences and culture. One of the main challenges of the female hormone odyssey is the graduation to menopause and beyond.

The mythological, titaness, Themis, symbolised divine law, good counsel and justice. Sometimes depicted with a blindfold, she represented objectivity and balance. The menopause has been equally impartial throughout history. The production of hormones declines in the ovaries of all women, regardless of ethnicity, cultural background, religion or belief. Exploring the myths of menopause is relevant to women of all ages.

Although menopause is defined by the final menstrual period, from a hormone point of view, this is not an on-off event. The perimenopause describes the turbulent and unpredictable change in female hormone production in the graduation to menopause. The hormone symphony follows a score akin to Vivaldi's *The Four Seasons* in the lead-up to menopause and beyond, until the ovaries fully retire and menstrual cycle hormone levels settle to more static levels.

These turbulent changes in hormone choreography are reminiscent of those that occur around another waypoint in the female hormone odyssey: menarche, when periods start. The decline in ovarian hormones in perimenopause is the mirror image of the establishment of menstrual cycles during adolescence. Like menarche, menopause occurs alongside age-related flux in other hormones and changes in life, family and work. Negative connotations of menopause stem from the nature of these changes, which typically occur in middle age.

The word 'menopause' is derived from Ancient Greek "menos" meaning month and "pausos" meaning an ending. Ironically, due to shorter life expectancies, many women living in Ancient Greek times probably did not reach menopause. Women frequently died during or as a consequence of childbirth: the most perilous physical journey for both mother and baby. Today most women can expect to experience menopause and live up to a third of their lives in a menopausal state. Falling birth rates lead to a higher proportion of menopausal women in the population. It is helpful to have a positive, proactive outlook and to be as informed as possible to make decisions for your personal journey.

A lack of reliable information leaves an information vacuum that is often filled with myths. "Myths of Menopause" sets out to refute myths that are factually incorrect or misleading, while highlighting those that are genuine and based on evidence. This book draws on the expertise and experiences of a range of respected contributors, including medical doctors, healthcare professionals, clinical dieticians, physiotherapists, psychologists, psychotherapists, scientists, academics, coaches, athletes, dancers and writers. These female health champions provide you with the wisdom, understanding and strategies to navigate this stage of your personal female hormone odyssey.

The book is presented in the form of a performance, with a series of acts and scenes.

Act 1 Misunderstandings around Menopause discusses what menopause means and how a woman can understand and assess her progression through this transition. The symptoms and health consequences of menopause are covered in Act 2 Challenges of Menopause. The focus of Act 3 Menopause, Sex and Pelvic Health is sexual and pelvic health for menopausal women. The benefits of lifestyle adaptations are covered in Act 4 Mastering Menopause. The topic of Act 5 Treatment Options includes hormone replacement therapy (HRT). Drawing on the insights of dancers, Act 6 Active Women and the Hormone Dance aims to inspire women to remain active. The most up-to-date information relevant to the expanding group of female masters age group athletes is provided in Act 7 Age Group Athletes. Act 8 Experiencing Menopause addresses the issue of how cultural and social factors influence the way women experience menopause. In conclusion, Act 9 Towards Postive Ageing proposes a framework for positive ageing in society as a whole.

These are some of the top recurring myths of menopause explored in this book.

- Menopause is a physical/mental illness.
- Menopause is only about the capacity to reproduce.
- Menopause happens quickly.
- Menopause only happens in middle-aged women.
- Menopause is only about hot flushes.
- Weight gain is inevitable with menopause.

- Having sex is not possible after menopause.
- All women experience menopause in the same way.
- Menopause is a taboo topic and it is difficult to talk about.
- When the ovaries retire, it is time to retire from work and life.
- Menopause means you resign yourself to a poor quality of life and health: there is nothing you can do.
- There are specific "diets" and supplements for menopause.
- There is a particular exercise or type of exercise for menopause.
- HRT causes breast cancer.
- All women should take HRT.
- No woman needs HRT.
- Menopause means you can no longer be active.
- Menopause prevents athletes and dancers from training and performing.

Notes

Throughout this book, the terms "female" or "woman/women" refer to the biological sex of a person born with ovaries, and the terms "male" or "man/men" refer to the biological sex of a person born with testes, unless otherwise indicated by the contributor.

British spelling is used throughout this book. For example, the hormones oestradiol and oestrogen have American equivalents estradiol and estrogen. Hot flushes are also known as hot flashes.

The information in this book explains how hormones affect health. This should not be used for medical diagnostic purposes and is not a substitute for seeking medical advice. All hormone stories are fictitious, unless otherwise stated.

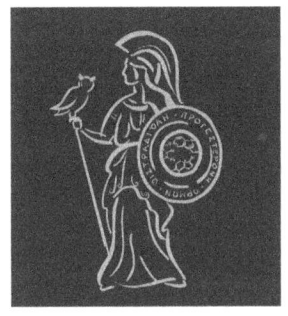

Act 1

Misunderstandings around Menopause

Distractions of social media Sirens

Act 1 Misunderstandings around Menopause
Distractions of social media Sirens

Dr Nicky Keay

Odysseus had to navigate many challenges on his epic 10-year journey home from the Trojan War. He had to resist the tempting, enchanting song of the Sirens, who lured sailors off course to shipwreck on the rocky shoreline. Odysseus ordered his sailors to lash him to the mast and to block their ears.

As women navigate the female hormone odyssey, alluring misinformation disseminated on social media can lead many astray. This act outlines the nature of the transition to menopause and beyond, seeking to dispel the misconceptions and misunderstandings that resonate around this stage of a woman's journey through life.

Scene 1 What is menopause?

Dr Nicky Keay

"Nothing in life is to be feared, it is only to be understood. Now is the time to understand more so that we may fear less."

Marie Curie

The female hormone odyssey is much older than Homer's epic poem. Throughout history, over the course of every woman's life, her hormone choreography changes. Although this is a recurring journey, every woman's experience is different, depending on her personal biological response to hormones and her unique background.

We start the female hormone odyssey in childhood when the production of hormones and the release of eggs by the ovaries is quiescent. During puberty the ovaries start to come online, marked by the start of menstrual periods (menarche) at an average age of 12. Once the intricate hormone choreography of the menstrual cycle is established, this repeats every 22 to 35 days, indicated by menstrual periods. There may be a temporary reversion to quiescent, childlike ovarian hormone levels and no periods (amenorrhoea), as a result of either hormonal contraception or unbalanced behaviours, such insufficient nutrition relative to activity levels. The cyclical production of ovarian hormones is suspended during pregnancy, when the placenta maintains high levels of these hormones. Menstrual cycles typically recommence after breastfeeding. The major waypoint of menopause usually occurs in middle age when the ovaries become unresponsive, causing periods to stop permanently. Perimenopause is the period of transition around menopause, when the ovaries gradually wind down in their production of hormones and release of eggs.

What controls the timing of the female hormone odyssey? The main hormones produced by the ovaries are the sex steroid hormones of oestradiol (most active form of oestrogen) and progesterone, together with some testosterone. The release of these hormones is orchestrated by the conductor of the endocrine (hormone) orchestra, the pituitary gland, which is nestled deep in the brain. The pituitary gland communicates with the ovaries by secreting the chemical messengers, follicle-stimulating hormone (FSH) and luteinising hormone (LH), which travel in the bloodstream. The pituitary gland itself is the subject of the master controller of many hormone axes: the hypothalamus. The hypothalamus is the top-level endocrine gland, physically located in the brain, just above the pituitary gland, masterminding the release of hormones from endocrine glands lower down in the chain of demand. The combination of the hypothalamus, pituitary and ovaries is known as the hypothalamic-pituitary-ovarian (HPO) axis. Over a lifetime, changes in the hormone signalling and feedback processes of the HPO axis determine the progression through the female hormone odyssey.

Figure 1.1.1 illustrates the characteristic patterns of hormone activity, within the HPO axis, at different stages of a woman's lifetime hormone journey[1]. The lower left corner represents childhood, when all hormones of the HPO axis are low, so no menstrual cycles occur. Adolescence marks the transition to centre stage, with the exquisite repeating hormone choreography of the menstrual cycle. In the top left, high levels of progesterone and oestradiol produced by the placenta during pregnancy feedback through the HPO axis, so that FSH and LH remain low. This is the precise opposite of the situation after menopause shown in the lower right, where reduced ovarian responsiveness results in low levels of ovarian hormones, in spite of pituitary hormones being high. Pregnancy and menopause are both times of physiological amenorrhoea, however underlying hormone patterns are diametrically different.

Although each of the states is relatively stable, the HPO axis has to recalibrate in order to transition between stages. The hypothalamus is also highly sensitive to external factors, including stressors, nutrition, physical activity and sleep. There's a lot of variability in the way that women experience the journey through the female hormone odyssey. This is particularly the case for the hormone changes that occur during the more extended transition of perimenopause.

Menopause represents a major, irreversible change in the HPO axis. It marks the endpoint of a gradual decline in the responsiveness of the ovaries to the stimulation of the pituitary's control hormones, FSH and LH, even at high concentrations. Eventually, the ovaries stop producing cyclical oestradiol and progesterone, and no longer release eggs. The permanent cessation of menstrual cycles leaves the HPO axis in a static pattern, with high levels of pituitary hormones and low levels of ovarian hormones.

Myth 1 Menstrual cycles are only for reproduction?

It is a common misconception that the only purpose of the menstrual cycle is reproduction. Although the menstrual cycle is an evolutionary requirement for reproduction, the actions of the ovarian hormones exert a multitude of positive effects on both physical and mental health.

Ovarian hormones are manifestations of Horme, the goddess of effort, energy and action. The clue is in the name of these mysterious, invisible and intangible molecules. The word "hormone" derives from Ancient Greek, meaning "setting in motion". Hormones are not simply chemical messengers circulating in our blood. When they reach the target cells, they set into motion a cascade of biochemical processes, causing the DNA in the cell nucleus to express selected genes to make specific proteins. Our hormones determine our health by ensuring that these proteins remain at optimal levels at the appropriate times. DNA is the blueprint for life, but hormones effectively bring DNA to life.

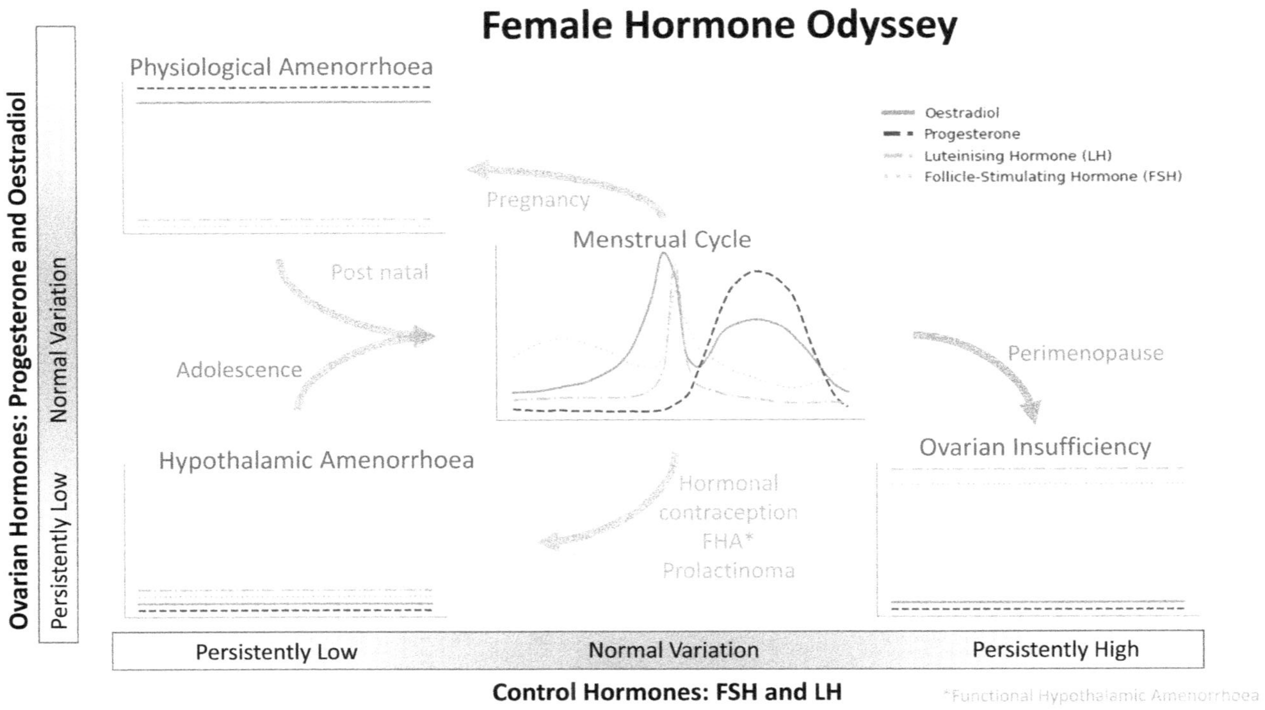

FIGURE 1.1.1 The characteristic patterns of female hormones at different stages of the Female Hormone Odyssey. Hormones, Health and Human Potential. Keay 2022 Sequoia books

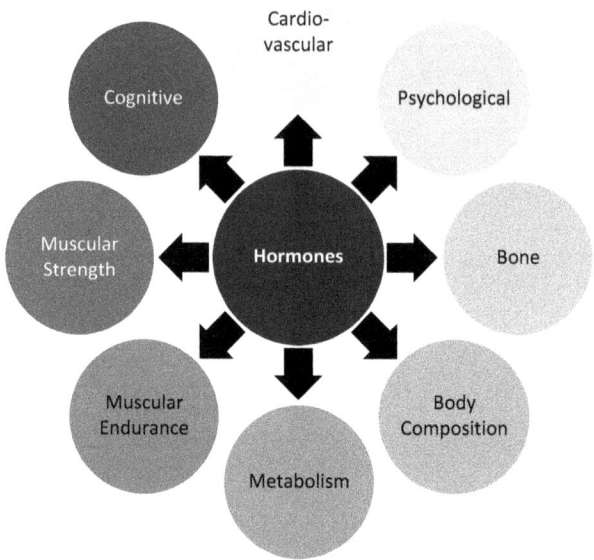

FIGURE 1.1.2 Ovarian hormones have many network effects. Hormones, Health and Human Potential. Keay 2022 Sequoia books

The main sex steroid ovarian hormones, oestradiol and progesterone, exert effects across all the systems in the body, by directing gene expression. Beyond the reproductive axis, these include the musculoskeletal, cardiovascular, metabolic, gastrointestinal and neurological systems. Figure 1.1.2 illustrates how these hormones impact many aspects of physical and mental health.

Myth 2 Menstrual cycle hormones and periods only cause problems?

Having periods can be viewed in a negative light, often originating in the teenage years as the hormone choreography of the menstrual cycles may take many dress rehearsals before settling into a rhythm. This state of hormone flux can produce physical and psychological challenges. However, establishing reasonably regular periods should be viewed positively as a barometer of internal healthy hormones, essentially a free monthly medical check. Periods are an indicator that the ovarian hormones of the menstrual cycle are at work securing health across many systems.

Musculoskeletal system

Oestradiol rules supreme when it comes to bone health. It is no coincidence that the trajectory of bone mineral density (BMD) over a woman's lifespan reflects that of oestradiol. Oestradiol is an anabolic (tissue-building) hormone for both bone and soft tissues like muscle, ligaments and tendons. The awakening of ovarian hormone production during puberty and the establishment of menstrual cycles is the main driver of the big increase in BMD associated with accrual of peak bone mass, attained by women in their early 20s. At menopause, with permanent cessation of menstruation and retirement of the ovaries, low ovarian hormones are associated with decline in BMD and increased risk of osteoporosis "brittle bones" and low trauma fractures. More details on bone health in menopause in Act 2.

Cardiovascular system and metabolic health

Oestradiol is cardioprotective. Up until menopause, the risk of cardiovascular disease is lower in women than men. After menopause, it rises to match men of similar age. Oestradiol plays an important role in maintaining a healthy lipid profile and supporting endothelial reactivity (the lining of artery walls). Oestradiol also supports metabolic health in terms of insulin sensitivity and maintaining a favourable body composition, limiting excessive deposition of visceral fat. Cardiometabolic health covers the interrelated factors of metabolic and cardiovascular health; united and supported by ovarian hormones, in particular oestradiol[2].

Neurological system

The ovarian hormones cross the blood-brain barrier and act as neurotransmitters: chemical connections between neurons. This allows ovarian hormones to interact with "feel good" neurotransmitters like serotonin and dopamine, making them important for mood, cognitive function and mental health[1]. Ovarian hormones are also important for neuromuscular function: the connection between brain and body, particularly muscle function. Evidence comes from studies of women with an imbalance in nutrition and exercise and subsequently experiencing functional hypothalamic amenorrhoea (FHA) with accompanying low levels of ovarian hormones. These women had slower reaction time and peak power production compared with their eumenorrhoeic (regular menstruating) peers[3].

Although menopause indicates a change in the ability to reproduce, we should not underestimate the powerful effect of the shift in ovarian hormone production on all aspects of our well-being and physical and mental health.

Definitions

British Menopause Society (BMS) and World Health Organisation (WHO)

> **Menopause** "is one point in a continuum of life stages for women and marks the end of their reproductive years"[4]. Menopause is the permanent cessation of menstruation as the ovaries stop their production of eggs and hormones. "Menopause is recognised to have occurred after 12 consecutive months of amenorrhoea for which no other obvious pathological or physiological cause is present. Menopause occurs with the final menstrual period and thus is known with certainty only in retrospect one year after the event"[5].
>
> **Perimenopause** is the stage of the female hormone odyssey around menopause, where there is a change in menstruation in terms of timing and menstrual flow. This is due to the underlying hormone choreography of the menstrual cycle, gradually changing towards more static hormone levels of the HPO axis. Typically, these changes can start from the age of 40 and perimenopause is defined as ending a year after the final menstrual period[5].
>
> **Postmenopause** is used to refer to as the time from the final menstrual period onwards[5]. During this time, the hormones of the HPO axis gradually settle and remain in a static pattern.

The word "menopause" is derived from Ancient Greek "menos" meaning month and "pausos" meaning an ending, while "peri" means around. Figure 1.1.3 shows the time course of events from the definitions above. Based on the definition of menopause being the final menstrual period, then it is only possible to pinpoint it retrospectively. Perimenopause typically begins about 6 years before menopause and extends for a year after the final period, when passage through menopause is confirmed. You might be

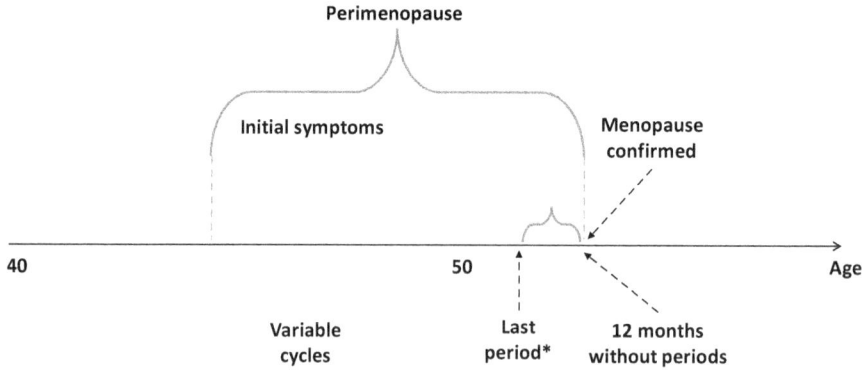

FIGURE 1.1.3 Perimenopause and menopause. *Age of menopause varies around an average of 51

wondering why it takes 12 months to confirm menopause. To be sure of the irreversible cessation of periods requires proving a negative. It takes time to be certain that the last period was the final one. There is a delay in aligning our epistemological knowledge with the ontological state of the world.

The average age of "natural" or physiological menopause is 51 years, with the range being 45–55 years. The term "postmenopause" considers menopause as an event in time, in the same way as postpartum and postnatal describe phases after birth. Nevertheless, the term "postmenopause" can have some negative connotations. Some prefer the adjectival use of menopause: being in a state of menopause or menopausal.

It is important to acknowledge that menopause is part of a continuum in a woman's hormone odyssey, as highlighted by WHO[4].

The definition used in National Institute for Health and Care Excellence[6] of "menopausal women" includes women in perimenopause and postmenopause. This is a solution that acknowledges the dynamic nature of this transition in the female hormone odyssey.

Why use menstrual periods as time points in the female hormone odyssey?

It can be argued that the temporal definition of menopause above might be problematic. These definitions are based on the clinical sign of menstrual periods: menstrual status at a time point. However, the underlying fluctuations of the female hormone odyssey, especially during times of transition from one stage to the next, do not follow a precise timetable. So why are these temporal definitions based on menstruation used?

Menstruation is an obvious clinical sign that can be readily reported and recorded without any cost implication. This is why menarche and menopause are defined in terms of age at the first menstrual period and age at the final menstrual period, respectively. Furthermore, between the age of menarche and menopause, the frequency of periods is used to classify menstrual status. Polymenorrhoea is where periods occur more frequently than every 22 days. Eumenorrhoea is where menstruation occurs every 22 to 35 days. Oligomenorrhoea is where there are fewer than 9 periods per year. Amenorrhoea may be either primary amenorrhoea (no periods by age 15 years) or secondary amenorrhoea (no periods for 3 months consecutively in a previously regular menstruating woman). In all these cases, menstrual pattern is a clinical sign, not a diagnosis. It is not possible to know the underlying hormone pattern based on menstruation alone.

Consider a woman with amenorrhoea (lack of periods). In the case of pregnancy, a lack of periods is entirely expected (physiological) and reversible, characterised by low levels of pituitary hormones FSH and LH, but high levels of oestradiol and progesterone. Otherwise, low-range levels of both the pituitary and ovarian hormones in the presence of non-elevated prolactin, would suggest an imbalance in behaviours causing adaptive, reversible FHA. In a woman who has experienced menopause, amenorrhoea is physiological and irreversible, with a hormone signature of high FSH and LH, and low levels of ovarian hormones. To identify the reason for amenorrhoea, a blood test based on levels of pituitary hormones FSH and LH can distinguish between a control centre issue in the hypothalamus or responsiveness issue in the ovaries[7]. To complicate matters further, it is possible to experience eumenorrhoea that belies an underlying subclinical ovulatory disturbance, lacking a robust luteal phase, with lower-than-expected levels and duration of progesterone rise[8].

Nevertheless, the menstrual period is useful in identifying waypoints in the female hormone odyssey. In addition to menarche and menopause, the menstrual period is used as a reference point in calculating the stage of pregnancy. The duration of pregnancy is based on the date of the last menstrual period (LMP) as this is an easy reference point, rather than trying to count from the date of fertilisation, which is impossible to know precisely.

Menstruation is important from a practical point of view as a timestamp to identify important stages of the female hormone odyssey, but it does not necessarily reveal the full detail of underlying female hormone patterns, or indeed individual responses to these hormonal fluctuations.

Myth 3 Does menopause happen quickly?

The menopause is defined as a point in time, a waypoint in the continuous female hormone odyssey. This does not mean that the ovaries suddenly retire like an on/off switch. Although there is a biological clock running on ovarian function, it does not have an alarm set for an exact time. In reality, the ovaries intermittently go part-time during perimenopause in the transition to menopause. In a similar way even after the waypoint of menopause has been passed, the ovaries might have a last flurry, a "rogue" period, which is why perimenopause is defined as running to a year after the last period. In terms of ovarian hormone production, typically, it might take up to 7 years after menopause for the HPO axis to settle and for the associated hormones to stay in a static pattern of postmenopause[9].

Why do I still not feel "myself" after menopause?

Although having a precise definition of menopause as a point in time might seem neat and tidy, this does not reflect the nature of hormone networks with complex timings, interactions and multiple effects throughout the body. Crucially, this is why women do not experience menopause in an on-off way as the definition of menopause might suggest. A menopausal woman experiences the effects of changes in female hormone choreography both in the lead-up to and after menopause, with variations in duration and intensity for the individual. This can add to misunderstanding and psychological challenges for women navigating this part of the female hormone odyssey[10].

Myth 4 Can I still get pregnant?

Although it is less likely, it is not impossible to fall pregnant even after menopause. For a year, even after the presumed final period, this is still officially a time of perimenopause. This is because, as described above, the ovaries might have a last flurry before fully retiring when the hormones of the menstrual cycle settle into a static pattern. For this reason, it is advised to use contraception if you do not wish to become pregnant after the final menstrual period for at least two years if under 50 and for one year if over 50[11].

Myth 5 What do puberty and perimenopause have in common?

Turbulent times of the female hormone odyssey

Puberty is a turbulent time as the hormones of the reproductive axis transition from low childhood levels to the intricate choreography of the menstrual cycle. Menarche is defined as a point in time when a young woman experiences her first menstrual period, in the later stage of puberty.

Although menarche is a waypoint in the female hormone odyssey, the full transition of menstrual cycle hormone activity takes time. For several years after menarche (postmenarche), there are many dress rehearsals of menstrual cycle hormone fluctuations before the hormone dance establishes itself. Early cycles may lack ovulation or a robust luteal phase characterised by sustained levels of progesterone. Oestradiol may be the dominant hormone resulting in heavy menstrual bleeding and short cycle lengths. This initial postmenarche time of menstrual cycle hormone turbulence is effectively a mirror image of perimenopause.

In the early stages of perimenopause, an initial indication may be a shortening cycle length, due to lower production of progesterone following ovulation and/or anovulation. Lower levels of progesterone put oestradiol in the driving seat so that menstruation can become heavier. Figure 1.1.4 shows how the time reversal of these changes makes the closing act of the menstrual cycle a reflection of the opening act.

Although postmenarche and perimenopause are times of hormone turbulence, the good news is that both lead to calmer, more consistent hormone activity. The young woman establishes regular menstrual cycles, while the more mature woman attains a more stable, static hormone pattern. For some mothers and daughters, these mirror images of hormone change coincide: Horme, the goddess of effort, energy and action expressing herself across the generations.

Myth 6 Menopause only occurs in "middle age"?

Although the majority of women experience menopause during middle age, menopause is not restricted to this age group.

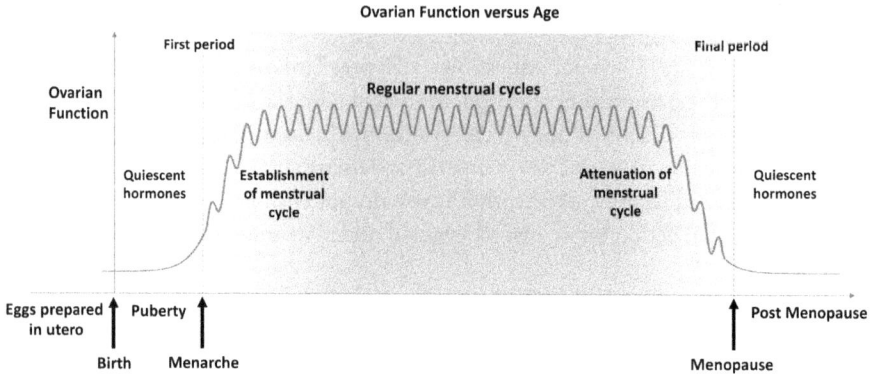

FIGURE 1.1.4 Reflections of menarche and menopause

Early menopause is when a woman experiences menopause between the ages of 40 and 45.
Premature ovarian insufficiency (POI) is reduced ovarian function before age 40.

As outlined above, the average age of "natural" physiological menopause is 51 years (range 45 to 55 years). However, about 5% of women experience early menopause between age 40–45 years. About 1% of women experience POI, which is more than two standard deviations below the average age of menopause in the Western World[12]. Prevalence of POI in women under the age 30 is estimated to be 0.1%.

As the name suggests, POI is an ovarian insufficiency (not "failure"). In the vast majority of cases, the cause is unknown. Since POI is not the total retirement of the ovaries, intermittent production of hormones and ovulation can still occur. It may take some time to reach the complete ovarian retirement of menopause. This is why women with POI may not experience the full range of typical menopausal symptoms and although reduced, there may be some possibility of conceiving. Nevertheless, hormone replacement therapy (HRT) is advised at least until the "natural" age of menopause for health reasons[13], in particular to support cardiovascular and bone health, where female hormones play a vital role as described above.

What determines the age of menopause?

The chronological age a woman reaches menopause is determined by a combination of genetic and environmental factors[1]. For example, poor nutrition during pregnancy and childhood is associated with an earlier menopause. Early puberty and no pregnancies can also be associated with an earlier menopause[5].

What are medical and surgical causes of reduction in ovarian function?

Reduction of ovarian function can be a result of a medical condition or medical or surgical interventions. Examples of medical conditions include the autoimmune disorder, Addison's disease, where autoantibodies impair the production of cortisol. Other associated autoimmune conditions include hypothyroidism, causing primary thyroid underproduction of thyroid hormones like thyroxine, and type 1 diabetes mellitus where there is reduced production of insulin. Medications typically include chemotherapy for malignancy as the germ cells in the gonads are very sensitive to chemotherapeutic agents. Ovarian function can also be specifically targeted with medication in the case of oestrogen-sensitive malignancies: typically, breast cancer.

A surgical cause of menopause is where both ovaries are removed (bilateral oophorectomy), resulting in an abrupt onset of menopause. When surgical menopause occurs before the physiological age of menopause, HRT is often advised at least until the "natural" age of menopause for health reasons. A higher dose of HRT may be required in these women experiencing an abrupt removal of female hormones, as opposed to the more gradual decline found in perimenopause leading to physiological menopause.

Myth 7 How do I know if I am in perimenopause?

Since we all like certainty, it is reasonable to ask if there is a test for perimenopause. The simple answer is "no", there is no "perimenopause test". In fact, all the leading professional bodies in women's health strongly advise against testing female hormones in women over 45 years for perimenopause[14]. Why?

Perimenopause is a time of great hormone turbulence. A snapshot test cannot provide a full picture of hormone health any better than a single frame taken from an action movie. Rather than offering certainty it adds more uncertainty. Even performing sequential tests can give misleading results and interpretations, because ovarian hormones are very labile and menstrual timing shows a lot of variation between individuals. Evidence comes from analysis of daily hormone "gold standard" blood levels of menstrual cycle hormones in women with regular cycles, who were ovulating[15].

Paradoxically, uncertainty is a sign of perimenopause. The most reliable indicator of early-stage perimenopause is variability in the nature of your personal menstrual cycle. If you can only ask one question, it would be *"has your cycle length shortened"*? This is because initially progesterone levels fall, causing a shortening of the cycle.

In contrast, blood testing would be appropriate for a woman younger than the expected age of entering perimenopause, presenting with irregular cycles or secondary amenorrhoea (lack of periods for 3 consecutive cycles). In this situation, checking hormone levels of the reproductive and thyroid axis is important to exclude causes of menstrual disruption, whether functional (e.g. imbalance in behaviours) or medical[1]. In this younger age group, having excluded pregnancy, levels of FSH and LH are used to determine whether there is a hypothalamic or ovarian cause for amenorrhoea. For example, to support the diagnosis of POI, both the European Society of Human Reproduction and Embryology and the BMS advise that in a woman under 40 years who has experienced amenorrhoea for 4 months or more, a blood test should be performed twice, 4 weeks apart, to ascertain if FSH is consistently raised.

Story of when blood testing is helpful

Kate and Katie were friends at a local running club, both 35 years of age. Although friends, they were also competitive and always vying for top place in races. They had heard that low body weight meant running faster, so there was another side competition to see who could be the lightest. Both women found that their periods stopped (amenorrhoea) and did not return after 4 months. Neither was taking hormonal contraception and neither was pregnant. Both wondered if they had a very early menopause. The only way to tell was to look carefully at blood test results. Kate had low-range levels of female hormones across the board (FSH, LH and oestradiol, with expected level of prolactin) plus low-range thyroid hormones: thyroid-stimulating hormone (TSH), thyroxine (T4) and triiodothyronine (T3) which indicated functional hypothalamic amenorrhoea (FHA) due to low energy availability. In contrast, Katie had high levels of FSH and LH and low oestradiol. Katie had her bloods repeated a month later and the pattern of hormones was the same, suggesting premature ovarian insufficiency (POI).

Both women needed advice and support. For Kate, this meant explaining why and how to restore energy availability to restore her menstrual cycles. Katie needed empathetic support to understand that POI meant she would not be able to restore her cycles and what to do next in terms of next steps, including HRT for health reasons.

Digital health: empowering or exploiting women?

There is an explosion in digital health. Digital health has the potential to offer inclusivity to women regardless of their background or where they live, including menopausal women. This is an exciting opportunity to provide reliable and evidence-based information to women to optimise their health and well-being. On the other hand, just because we now have the capability to measure an ever-expanding array of physiological, medical and genetic variables, should we? This vast "menu" of possible measurements and monitoring could produce a generation of the "worried well". It has been argued that we risk riding on a wave of interest in women's health, with an extensive, expanding array of offerings purporting to offer the ticket to longevity, health and happiness.

A problem with innovative monitoring systems is that they cannot be evaluated until large amounts of data have been collected. Some companies lure consumers into paying a fee to add their own personal data to the company's database, while offering nothing in exchange beyond bland, generic advice. Rather than deriving meaningful data and reliable information, this busy marketplace can leave women understandably confused and out of pocket at best and misled at worst[16].

Where a product or service measures a physiological variable, even if the medical data provided is accurate (regulation is focused on this aspect), the key is the clinical interpretation of this data in the clinical context for the individual. Even if a product is designed by a medical team, how this is marketed can lead to misunderstandings for the consumer. As outlined above, there is no such thing as a "perimenopause test", even if the medical data is accurate, because the menstrual cycle hormones measured are labile by definition. An isolated set of results could lead to an incorrect conclusion regarding ovarian function.

Providing women with good quality data, with correct clinical interpretation, in the clinical context for the individual is empowering. However, there is the potential for exploitation of women, if these clinical principles are not followed and information is not presented in this way.

Myth 8 How do I know if I have reached menopause if I don't have periods?

Hormonal contraception

Most forms of hormonal contraception alter the hormone networks of the menstrual cycle. This often means that menstrual periods, the barometer of internal menstrual cycle hormone health, are not available. So, you cannot know if you have reached menopause based on menstrual periods as these are not being experienced.

Inadmissible evidence: When cyclical bleeding is not a menstrual period

Depending on how the combined contraceptive pill (COCP) is taken, it typically produces a regular withdrawal bleed. Withdrawal bleeds, experienced by women taking the COCP, are artificially induced. They are not indicative of natural menstrual hormone choreography. The COCP suppresses ovulation and the production of all hormones of the reproductive axis. Since the artificially induced withdrawal bleed is not the result of internal hormonal variation, it is not a menstrual period. This means that a woman on this type of hormonal contraception cannot assess her progression to menopause based on menstruation patterns.

No cyclical bleeding

In contrast to the COCP, women using progestogen-only hormonal contraception typically do not experience cyclical bleeding, as the endometrial lining (lining of the uterus) is maintained at a "stable" thickness. Progestogen is the generic term that includes progesterone (with body identical molecular structure) and synthetic forms with slightly different molecular structures. It is the synthetic, non-body identical progestogens which are the type used in hormonal contraception. Depending on the type of progestogen-only contraception, ovulation and menstrual cycle hormone fluctuations may continue. A woman who has had a hysterectomy, with ovaries retained, is in a similar position. Her ovarian hormones fluctuate, but she has no bleeding. In the absence of menstruation, a woman lacks a barometer of internal hormones.

Figure 1.1.5 illustrates the various scenarios. Women whose cycles are driven by natural hormonal fluctuations have a barometer to assess their progression to menopause. The artificial monthly bleeds of women on the COCP mask the advance towards menopause. Women lacking cyclical menstrual bleeding have no tool to assess ovarian function. They fall into two categories: those with natural hormone cycles but no uterine response, or complete suppression of the female hormone network.

So how does a woman know if she is in perimenopause or has reached menopause in the absence of menstrual periods as the barometer of ovarian function?

In the absence of natural menstrual periods, menopausal symptoms are the key. Symptoms of low ovarian hormones are seen across a multitude of systems, including musculoskeletal, cardiovascular, gastrointestinal, psychological and sexual health. However, there is a problem: the symptoms of low ovarian hormones do not tell you the cause. Some causes are reversible, such as taking hormone-suppressing contraception or FHA. However, there is a symptom more specific to menopause. Hot flushes, formally known as vasomotor symptoms (VMS), occur in menopause. There is evidence that

Alterations of Cyclical Female Hormone Choreography and Bleeding Patterns

	Monthly bleed	No bleed
Natural hormone cycles	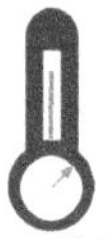 Menstruation: a Natural Barometer	Progestogen-releasing intrauterine coils Some progestogen-only pills *Hysterectomy with ovaries retained*
Supressed hormone cycles	**Combined Oral Contraceptive Pill** (COCP can artificially induce withdrawal bleeds)	**Progestogen injection and implant** **Progestogen-only pills** **Some progestogen-releasing intrauterine coils** *Oophorectomy (removal of ovaries)* Functional hypothalamic amenorrhoea

Hormonal contraception in bold
Medical procedures in italics
Other status in plain text

FIGURE 1.1.5 Alterations of cyclical female hormone choreography

VMS are linked to the permanent recalibration of the HPO axis in the brain, in the face of the irreversibly declining ovarian response that occurs at menopause.

Blood tests might also be useful to exclude other causes of symptoms, such as thyroid function and low vitamin D levels. An underactive thyroid (which is more common in women than in men) can give symptoms that are very similar to those of menopause in terms of general fatigue. In the case of hysterectomy, menopause with cessation of ovarian response can be deduced from elevated levels of FSH and LH in the context of age and any symptoms.

Menopausal story

Amy was 55 years of age. She had started taking the combined oral contraceptive pill (COCP) as a teenager, a couple of years after her periods had started, not so much for contraception but rather to "regulate periods", as many of her classmates were doing. Coincidentally, her mother, who was 51 at the time, seemed to be having heavy periods, headaches and emotional issues. As a teenager, Amy wanted to avoid all that "baggage" that seemed to come with having periods. In her late 40s, Amy was advised to switch from the COCP to a progestogen-only pill, so she was not experiencing any sort of bleeding. Recently, she had been experiencing night sweats and generally not feeling herself: issues similar to those she had seen her mother experience. What was going on with Amy?

The first point is that the COCP does not "regulate periods"; it switches off periods by suppressing the entire HPO axis. The bleeds Amy experienced, while taking the COCP, were withdrawal bleeds triggered by external synthetic hormones, not menstrual periods due to her own internal hormones. Most likely, Amy's mother was experiencing menopausal symptoms when Amy was a teenager, which put a negative spin on having menstrual cycles. Although Amy was not sexually active and did not have or want any children, she had continued taking hormonal contraception because she remembered how her mother had seemed to suffer from having periods. Like the COCP, the progestogen-only pill continued to mask changes in the menstrual cycle as an indicator of progressing through perimenopause and menopause. Nevertheless, in view of Amy's age and symptoms, most likely she had reached menopause.

Myth 9 Eggs run out at menopause

Although there is a decline in the number of eggs (follicles) in the ovaries over a woman's life, menopause is not caused by a shortage of eggs. Many millions of eggs are prepared while a woman is a foetus. However, these eggs are not renewable and effectively have a "shelf life". The biological clock is running for ovarian retirement from ovulation and hormone production. Blood tests can measure anti-Müllerian hormone (AMH) produced by the ovarian follicles. Although levels of AMH fall with increasing age, at present AMH is not used to predict the age of menopause in routine clinical practice[5].

The decline in ovarian responsiveness to pituitary hormones FSH and LH is the main reason that menopause occurs, not a shortage of eggs per se.

Myth 10 Menopause is only relevant for "old" women?

Menopause is something that all women experience during their lives. By its very nature, it is inclusive of all women, wherever they live and whatever their personal social, cultural, racial characteristics and backgrounds.

It is never too early to understand what happens at menopause. I often hear women saying that they felt totally unprepared for menopause and wish they had known about it before it happened. Being informed is being prepared. This book aims to dispel myths and provide reliable information for women (and men!) of all ages.

Myth 11 What about ageing?

Unlike male sperm, which are made continuously, all of a woman's eggs are prepared, in utero, before she is born. Incredibly, all the major organs in a foetus are made by week 12 of gestation, including the ovaries of a female foetus, where the egg cells are prepared by holding in suspended animation the halving of the chromosomes. This is the point at which the biological clock of a woman's egg cells starts ticking. The final packaging of a single chromosome into each egg cell is completed much later, after the female baby is born and she has reached menarche and only if and when that specific egg is selected for ovulation. If a woman becomes pregnant at 40, the egg cell from which her baby (male or female) develops is already just over 40 years old, compared with just days, for the sperm. So ageing does not suddenly start at menopause. Ageing is a lifelong process, with menopause a scene in the hormone odyssey of life.

> *"The golden age is before us, not behind us."*
> *William Shakespeare*

What about changes in other hormones?

Menopause typically occurs at a time of changes in other anabolic (tissue building) hormones, other than oestradiol. Figure 1.1.6 shows the decline of growth hormone (GH) and testosterone in women. Insulin-like growth factor 1 (IGF-1) is the specific active "offspring" of GH that plays an important role in maintaining a healthy body composition: favouring muscle mass over visceral fat deposition and supporting bone health. The ovaries also produce testosterone, so this anabolic hormone also declines with menopause. However, the big difference between men and women is in the extent of the reduction of their dominant anabolic sex steroid hormone. Women experience a drastic drop in oestradiol from their ovaries after menopause. In contrast, men see

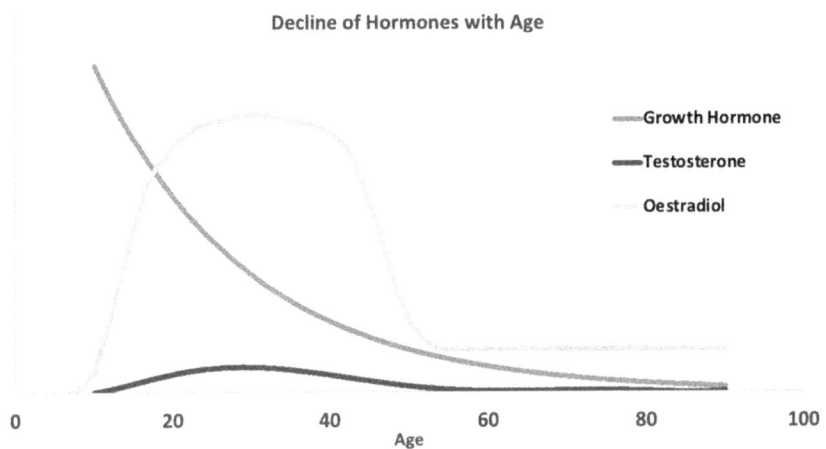

FIGURE 1.1.6 Decline of female anabolic hormones

a far less dramatic reduction in their testosterone levels after 50. So, although men and women share the same hormone profile with ageing in terms of GH, there is a very distinct difference when it comes to their respective dominant sex steroid anabolic hormones.

Myth 12 Over medicalisation of the menopause? Or lack of information?

A recent publication describes an empowerment model for managing menopause, which I think everyone can agree on[17]. However, it is also argued that 'over medicalisation' can lead to disempowerment with overtreatment and advocates that most women should navigate menopause without the need for treatment. The BMS points out that historically, there has been a lack of information about menopause and some women have found it hard to get the treatment they need.

Are women ready for menopause? Mind the information gap!

Various published surveys show strong evidence that most women under 40 feel they do not have enough information or understanding of menopause[18]. Unsurprisingly the same information gap was true for women over 40 in perimenopause[19]. Although accurate information from trusted sources is becoming more widely available, it has to compete against myths and other misinformation circulated broadly by unreliable sources.

The BMS raises the concern that the use of the word 'over medicalisation' could in fact lead to the disempowerment of women. If a woman obtains separate treatments for each menopausal symptom, she may end up with a cabinet full of many medications covering low mood, anxiety, lipid profile, fatigue, digestive issues, weight control, headaches, premenstrual issues as some examples. This can be avoided by recognising that the underlying unifying reason is a "natural", physiological process that occurs to every woman as part of her female hormone odyssey. Anecdotes suggest a predilection for prescribing antidepressants for menopausal women, despite advice from professional medical bodies that this should be limited to those with clinically diagnosed depression[20]. The BMS advises that a balanced approach is important, to ensure that the women who need support and treatment receive it[21].

Ultimately, the incisive quote from Professor Janice Rymer, former Vice President of the Royal College of Obstetrics and Gynaecologists, sums up the best approach: *"We need to treat women as individuals and not statistics"*[22].

Myth 13 (not unlucky!) All women experience menopause in the same way?

Individual women show great variation in their experiences of menopause. The timing and level of production of female hormones over the transition to menopause and beyond are unique for every woman. Furthermore, women differ widely in their personal biological responses to hormones. Prior experiences of premenstrual syndrome and/or postnatal mood issues may be indicators of elevated sensitivity to hormone fluctuations. It should come as no surprise that other external factors can have an important influence, such as changes in personal relationships or career roles.

Myth 14 Can I live a happy life through the female hormone odyssey?

We have the opportunity to make this journey through the female hormone odyssey as smooth and enjoyable as possible: to get the most out of life and reach our personal full potential. Over 2,000 years ago, Hippocrates wrote:

> *"If we could give each individual just the right amount of exercise and nourishment, not too little and not too much, we would have found the surest way to health."*
>
> Hippocrates

This is as true today as it was for the Ancient Greeks. Our lifestyle choices influence our hormone networks, which in turn impact all aspects of our mental and physical health. A key message of this book is that our hormone networks change as we progress through menopause. When our hormone networks change, we need to review and adjust our behaviours around nutrition, activity and exercise. This is discussed in detail in "Act 4 Mastering Menopause". The transition to menopause is both the end of one chapter and the beginning of a new one. Graduating to menopause offers positive aspects and the opportunity to refresh our lifestyle, which is something possible for all women at minimal cost.

References

1. Keay N. *Hormones, Health and Human Potential*. Act 1, Scene 5XX "Of Mice and Men . . . and Women." Sequoia Books, 2022.
2. British Menopause Society Consensus Statement. Primary prevention of coronary heart disease in women. https://thebms.org.uk/wp-content/uploads/2023/10/07-BMS-ConsensusStatement-Primary-prevention-of-coronary-heart-disease-in-women-SEPT2023-A.pdf. Accessed March 2024.
3. Tornberg Åsa B, Melin A, Koivula F et al. Reduced neuromuscular performance in amenorrhoeic elite endurance athletes. *Medicine & Science in Sports & Exercise* 2017; 49 (12): 2478–2485.
4. World Health Organization (WHO). Menopause. https://www.who.int/news-room/fact-sheets/detail/menopause. Accessed March 2024.
5. British Menopause Society. Chapter 1 Physiology and definitions. In Hilard T, Abernathy K, Manoda H, Shaw I, Everett M, Ayres J, Currie H (eds), *Management of the Menopause*, Sixth Edition. British Menopause Society.
6. National Institute for Health and Care Excellence. https://www.nice.org.uk/guidance/ng23/chapter/Recommendations#diagnosis-of-perimenopause-and-menopause. Accessed April 2024.
7. Keay N. *Hormones, Health and Human Potential*. Act 2, Scene 4 Young man and young woman. Sequoia Books, 2022.
8. Prior JC. Adaptive, reversible, hypothalamic reproductive suppression: More than functional hypothalamic amenorrhea. *Frontiers in Endocrinology* 2022; 13: 893889. doi: 10.3389/fendo.2022.893889.
9. British Menopause Society. What is the menopause? https://thebms.org.uk/wp-content/uploads/2023/08/17-BMS-TfC-What-is-the-menopause-AUGUST2023-A.pdf. Accessed April 2024.
10. Centre for Menstrual Cycle and Ovulation Research. Naming women's midlife. https://www.cemcor.ca/resources/naming-womens-midlife. Accessed March 2024.
11. British Menopause Society. *Management of the Menopause*, Sixth Edition. Chapter 6 Maintaining sexual health and contraception. British Menoause Society.
12. Nash Z, Davies M. Premature ovarian insufficiency. *British Medical Journal* 2024; 384: e077469.
13. British Menopause Society Consensus Statement. Premature ovarian insufficiency (POI). https://thebms.org.uk/wp-content/uploads/2023/10/05-BMS-ConsensusStatement-Premature-ovarian-insufficiency-POI-SEPT2023-A.pdf. Accessed March 2024.
14. British Menopause Society Menopause Practice Standards. https://thebms.org.uk/wp-content/uploads/2022/12/BMS-Menopause-Practice-Standards-DEC2022-A.pdf. Accessed April 2024.
15. Francis G, Keay N. Quantitative hormone analysis reveals sources of variability in the menstrual cycle. *Women in Sport and Physical Activity Journal* 2024; 32 (S1): wspaj.2023-0062. doi: 10.1123/wspaj.2023-0062.
16. Copp T, Pickles K, Smith J et al. Marketing empowerment: How corporations co-opt feminist narratives to promote non-evidence based health interventions *BMJ* 2024; 384: e076710. doi: 10.1136/bmj-2023-076710.
17. Hickey M, LaCroix A, Doust J et al. An empowerment model for managing menopause. *The Lancet* 2024. doi:10.1016/S0140-6736(23)02799-X.
18. Munn C, Vaughan L, Talaulikar V, Davies MC, Harper JC. Menopause knowledge and education in women under 40: Results from an online survey. *Women's Health* 2022; 18. doi: 10.1177/17455057221139660.

19 Harper JC, Phillips S, Biswakarma R et al. An online survey of perimenopausal women to determine their attitudes and knowledge of the menopause. *Women's Health* 2022; 18. doi: 10.1177/17455057221106890.
20 British Menopause Society. NICE: Menopause, diagnosis and management – from guideline to practice guideline summary. https://thebms.org.uk/wp-content/uploads/2022/12/09-BMS-TfC-NICE-Menopause-Diagnosis-and-Management-from-Guideline-to-Practice-Guideline-Summary-NOV2022-A.pdf. Accessed April 2024.
21 The British Menopause Society. Lancet series – Menopause 2024. https://thebms.org.uk/2024/03/lancet-series-menopause-2024/. Accessed March 2024.
22 Rymer J, Brian K, Regan L. HRT and breast cancer risk. We must prevent another setback in women's health. *BMJ* 2019; 367: l5928. doi: 10.1136/bmj.l5928.

Scene 2 Mythology in women's midlife – what's in a name?

Professor Jerilynn Prior

> "*If I call it a couch and you call it a chesterfield, but our mutual friend calls it a sofa, we are using different names for a common piece of living room furniture. We can easily figure what each of us means.*"
>
> "*It is much more complex and confusing, however, if we use* **same** *name to mean* **different** *things.*"

That is the "menopause" word situation today. (Note that I will put "menopause" in quotation marks unless it is the correct meaning). "Menopause" is commonly and confusingly used to indicate three aspects of women's normal lifecycle. Let's describe these different meanings first, and then I will tell you why I propose there is only one correct and scientific meaning for menopause. And what I see as the negative consequences of misuse of women's midlife naming.

If I were to ask a midlife woman (and she could be in urban India or Korea or Germany or Canada) what "menopause" means, she is likely to say, "*Oh, you know, all the changes and unwanted symptoms that start as we get older.*"

But, if I were to ask a physician**,** especially if they are a specialist in obstetrics and gynaecology (ob-gyn), what "menopause" means, they are likely to reply, "*Menopause is the last menstrual period*" (that is abbreviated LMP in gynae-speak). And everything after the last flow is called "postmenopause".

However, if I were to ask an epidemiologist who studies whole populations, or someone from the World Health Organization, to describe the meaning of the word, "menopause", they will reply, "*Natural menopause is deemed to have occurred after 12 consecutive months without menstruation for which there is no other physiological or pathological cause . . .*" https://www.who.int/news-room/fact-sheets/detail/menopause. This is what I consider as the only correct use of the word, menopause. Yet sometimes, confusingly, all three meanings are used within a single, supposedly scientific medical publication!

"How did we come up with the idea that menopause starts after no menstrual flow for a full year?"

The answer is, from a large and long study that started with undergraduate college women in the United States of America in the 1930s. The authors followed each of almost 5,000 women for about 40 years[1]. They found that 9 of every 10 women who was 45 years or older at what later turned out to be her last period, would have no further menstrual bleeding. They were well and truly menopausal. However, that also means that 10% of us will have an unexpected or rogue period in the two years after we initially thought we were menopausal. I did, although my original LMP was at the ripe old age (for menopause) of 56!

Did that extra period after one year without flow mean I had uterine cancer? It *could* have! But it was not an *asymptomatic bleed* which is the hallmark of endometrial cancer. I had been experiencing cramp-like lower abdominal pain that was beginning to worry me. Only after the flow started, did I also realise that my breasts were swollen and sore. Once the period began, I figured out that some lonely follicles still remaining in one or the other of my ovaries got poked and prodded by higher follicle-stimulating hormone (FSH) levels into making high oestrogen levels. These caused the mysterious cramping and breast tenderness as well as that bonus flow when I thought I was already in menopause. As soon as my extra period ended, those symptoms were gone.

You see, the year-long "menopause clock" is a statistical thing. So, I had to start my 1-year clock again and wait a further 12 months to celebrate being menopausal. I therefore graduated into menopause at the age of 57, not 56.

What about a woman who is younger than 45 at her last period? After a year without flow, she has only an 8 out of 10 likelihood that she won't bleed again (20% likelihood of a further, *symptomatic* period). She is twice as likely as someone older at their LMP to be troubled by further menstruation(s). And she, like all women with such a rogue period, needs to pay careful attention to this:

Did any clue indicate to you that you were going to get another period?

If the answer is **yes**, sigh; then shrug, and start your menopause clock again.

If the answer is **no**, make an appointment to see your healthcare provider!

Has that 1-year menopause calculation from an early study been confirmed in random, whole population research? The answer is yes[2]. Women at ages 45–55 years old from Denmark who gave the date of their last flow and were 1-year past it, were invited to keep a diary to record any and all further bleeding. Out of the whole group of women who were studied, 10.7% had another period (which is just over 1 of every 10). Most occurred within a year after they thought they were menopausal, but some occurred in year two and a very few in year three[2]. Unfortunately, the investigators did not ask participants if they knew that rogue period was coming. *That study still needs to be done.*

Does it really matter *what we mean* when we say "menopause"?

You bet it does!

Perimenopause (all the years of change before we've been that one year without flow) is *as different from* menopause *as* chalk *from* cheese. (*Seemed appropriate to use a British saying here!*) That is especially true for women who have a very symptomatic time during perimenopause, as I did. I had several episodes of flooding menstruation, over a decade of sore breasts, intermittent times of great sadness and many nights in which my sleep was disrupted by night sweats.

So, if I say perimenopause and menopause differ in their experiences or symptoms, what do I mean? First of all, we have information from a random population study from Melbourne, Australia, in women who started at age 45, were often in perimenopause and were followed for at least three years. Many more women reported not feeling well in perimenopause rather than in menopause[3]. Things like sore breasts, swelling, trouble concentrating or holding urine, tiredness and headaches decreased once they became menopausal[3]. Heavy flow and increased cramps also get totally better the closer to the end of perimenopause women are.

Those who brought us "postmenopause" and a retrospective, one-year-off way of deciding when a woman is "menopausal" have also long told us that "menopause" is a time of dropping and low oestrogen levels. True menopause is when levels of oestradiol (oestrogen) and progesterone are consistently low. But perimenopause goes through "estrogen's storm season" of higher and very variable oestrogen levels[4,5,6] before it eventually transitions into the lower levels in menopause.

However, the chaos of perimenopause is not just that oestrogen is unpredictably high and swinging. In total contrast to oestrogen, progesterone levels are gradually decreasing. Even if cycles are still ovulatory (meaning that they released an egg), fewer days of high progesterone are now present than are required for a successful pregnancy. So, while oestrogen is going up and bouncing about, progesterone is going down. Thus, oestrogen and progesterone are changing but in the opposite directions in perimenopause. I think that is one of the reasons that perimenopause causes so many disrupting experiences – it resembles the teen years more than it resembles menopause!

One of the biggest and most problematic midlife myths is that perimenopause and menopause are both about dropping oestrogen levels

Why would oestrogen levels become high before they become low? I think about it like this – we were all born with millions of egg-containing follicles stored in our ovaries. Each follicle can make oestrogen. It is generally a single follicle that becomes dominant and that provides most of the oestrogen and all of the progesterone for a given premenopausal menstrual cycle.

Therefore, we get into our late 30s and early 40s with *excess follicles* (since no one has millions of menstrual cycles during our 25–50 menstruating years). These additional and unneeded follicles need dealing with. The organisation that makes most babies come out solo (rather than part of a litter) has the hypothalamus and the pituitary paying attention to the directions of the ovarian staff that say it is time to stimulate, or to suppress signals to the ovary.

What if you lay off a bunch of administrators? *For those more scientifically inclined, this lack of reliable coordination occurs because a follicle-made protein called "Inhibin B" is produced in lower amounts or becomes absent.* So, the hypothalamus is increasingly doing its own thing. That means signals to the ovaries say to grow lots more follicles every cycle starting in our late 30s[7]. Since each follicle can make some oestrogen, and there is confusion about which follicle is that cycle's "boss" or dominant, oestrogen will become higher and start being unpredictable. One example is that there may be a second oestrogen peak during the middle of the time after ovulation[6] and just before the period (when oestrogen levels are usually dropping or low). Such chaos leads to heavy flow, and to few cycles with adequate coordination to release an egg. And even if an egg is released, it has less time to make progesterone. Or, when an approaching-perimenopause woman does become pregnant, she is more likely to have non-identical twins.

All of this allows women to get rid of those extra follicles, and to spare us menstruation in our 90s. In perimenopause, many follicles become oestrogen producers rather than just a dominant follicle as in premenopause. The rest just get absorbed.

The normal menstrual cycle has balanced actions of oestrogen and progesterone[8] which is optimal for our experiences and for pregnancy (if we choose). But the *im*balance of higher oestrogen and lower progesterone leads to heavy flow, sore breasts and shorter cycles *before they become irregular*. I think it is this hormonal incoordination that leads some women to have a peculiar dream, as I did when I was early in perimenopause, *that I was pregnant*. Interestingly, as diverse women as a !Kung hunter-gatherer and a sociology professor have reported such a perimenopausal pregnancy dream. (Given that I had a teenager and a grade-schooler at the time, my dream was closer to a nightmare!) But I am in awe at how smart our subconscious can be!

We've talked about the perimenopausal changes in oestrogen – increasing, and progesterone – decreasing, but another big change is also happening. Our stress hormones, like cortisol, from our adrenal glands, and norepinephrine, that is made in our brain as well as our adrenals, are both increasing. Why? Probably for two reasons, one of which has to do with culture and the other that is created by our bodies.

First of all, in perimenopause we are experiencing changes that are puzzling and uncomfortable and indicate to us that our culturally valued days of potential fertility and youth are coming to an end. (We've been taught that menopause is old and wrinkly). It is also stressful to no longer be able to predict, count on your period coming when you expect it or on having typical menstrual cycle experience changes. But also, and importantly, given that Western society values youth over old age, this is stressful, especially if we do not have the family we always wanted, or our concept of ourselves relies on a slim body, vibrant hair and a youthful face.

The second and physiological reason for higher stress hormone levels in perimenopause is that the huge drops in oestrogen levels (as all those eager follicles are absorbed) trigger stress hormone production as oestrogen levels inevitably also decrease. It is that down-swinging oestrogen, causing brain bursts of norepinephrine and every other stress and brain hormone we know how to measure, that causes night sweats and later hot flushes[9]. So, we experience the tiredness that goes with higher stress hormones and maybe some brain fog and difficulty concentrating, or perhaps migraines we haven't had since we were in puberty. Why? Because, the brain sees oestrogen down-swings as an emergency and releases norepinephrine, and triggers cortisol. The higher brain norepinephrine level changes the temperature at which we feel comfortable (called the thermoneutral zone). When oestrogen takes a dive, and we are not temperature resilient, we have a night sweat or a hot flush.

Thus, there are three major hormonal changes in perimenopause. Oestrogen becomes higher and unpredictable, progesterone becomes lower, even in cycles in which we release an egg and ovulate, and stress hormone levels also increase. These changes make the low levels of oestrogen and progesterone in menopause seem uninteresting, even boring. But they are major reasons *we should never confuse perimenopause with menopause.*

OK – so perimenopause and menopause differ in hormonal levels – why would we think that they were the same?

Someone, who expected oestrogen levels to be dropping, would not be able to see the higher levels in perimenopause[10]. Likewise, we have been taught that low oestrogen levels cause hot flushes and night sweats, although there is no *evidence* that they do[11]. If low oestrogen caused hot flushes, all children would have them!

These episodes of heat and sweating (together called "vasomotor symptoms") often start as night sweats during sleep in midlife women with regular cycles[12], and when they do, they tend to occur in the days before and during flow. Interestingly, this is often before daytime hot flushes have begun to be a problem! Thus, perimenopause and menopause share vasomotor symptoms. However, early in perimenopause women may experience a sense of dizziness, anxiety or even anger before the flush starts. And, for perimenopausal women, a hot flush may be acutely triggered by a sudden emotional or social stressor. Evidence more accurately says that vasomotor symptoms occur because the brain has got used to high levels of oestrogen and reacts when those levels drop. That can be an oestrogen decrease from a high to a normal level, or from a normal to a low level.

Ok, then, you say – why do hot flushes continue into the low oestrogen of menopause?

Good question – we're not really sure. But I think it is because someone who had them earlier continues to have the higher brain norepinephrine stress hormone level (maybe for other reasons now than diving oestrogens). This higher level keeps the VMS going, especially when the room is hot or we are stressed because normal life things happen.

I said at the start that the names matter. Maybe now you are starting to understand why perimenopause is so different from menopause. Perimenopause is a time of change that only some of us will find difficult. We don't know for sure what percentage of us that is, from large random population-based studies – but we currently guess that it is 15–30 of every hundred women.

What we do know, absolutely, is that both perimenopause and menopause are normal parts of our lives. We can't decide to skip either

I find "postmenopause" a confusing designation. Why? Because it is referring to something that won't happen for an, as yet, unknown period of time. Women's cycles are not a perpetual motion machine – they are, by definition, adaptive and responsive to changes in the environment, our feelings, our nutrition and the maturation of our whole reproductive system. No one knows which of our cycles are actually final – the only way to almost know, is to go a year without and see. Another reason is that, if you believe, as I do, that menopause lasts for the rest of our lives. Then *post*menopause *means* dead!

The confusion of the LMP with true menopause means that the last year of perimenopause could also be the first year of postmenopause.

OK – are there practical reasons why it is important for us and for our healthcare providers to know whether we are in perimenopause or menopause?

Yes. First of all, to allow us to make sense of our experiences. But an even more important reason is this – to know how to effectively and safely *treat* us.

The current guidelines created by multiple professional organisations worldwide (from UK to Korea, Europe to USA and Canada) universally recommend that a woman with problematic hot flushes and night sweats who is under age 60 (or not more than 10 years into menopause that usually occurs in the early 50s) take Menopausal Hormone Therapy (MHT). Arguably, for this age group, this is misleadingly called Hormone *Replacement* Therapy or HRT.

What is MHT? It is always some form of oestrogen, usually with a lower dose of synthetic progestin or progesterone

It is a very good idea to treat women whose hot flushes and night sweats are bothering them. And, we know from large USA studies of hormones, that MHT is safer if women are younger. But wait a minute – perimenopausal women may have problematic hot flushes and night sweats. And by definition, since natural menopause occurs before age 60, these younger women could be in *peri*menopause.

Now we have to ask about MHT in perimenopause:

Does it make sense to give women whose own oestrogen levels are often high and out of administrative control, more oestrogen?

Do we know that exogenous oestrogen wouldn't just add on top of the high oestrogen levels in early perimenopause.

Do we know that MHT is effective in treating early *perimenopausal* hot flushes and night sweats?

Then – why do the guidelines all say to treat perimenopausal VMS with MHT? Only if we consider perimenopause and menopause to be the same do we have the necessary treatment results.

So, all of that is likely to leave you saying – well, if MHT is not effective for night sweats and hot flushes in *peri*menopause, how can we treat problematic VMS in women who are still menstruating? Until June 2023, we did not have an answer to that. However, we at CeMCOR have known the answer since March 2018, when we presented our trial results at the Endocrine Society. (It took us five years and three months to get the first-ever large placebo-controlled trial only for *perimenopausal* night sweats and hot flushes to be accepted and published – it was rejected a dozen times, most often without review.)

Thanks to the volunteer time of 189 women across Canada (most of whom participated remotely), half of whom were randomised to an identical but inactive medicine, *we now know that oral micronised progesterone (300 mg daily) at bedtime significantly decreases night sweats*, improves sleep problems and makes perimenopause interfere 40% less with our daily lives[13]. This trial also showed that progesterone was safe over three months compared with placebo. Progesterone's major side effect is a blessed benefit – it improves deep sleep and decreases sleep interruptions. Progesterone also did not increase depression and surprisingly, did not change women's periods[13] (another evidence of the strength of higher perimenopausal oestrogen levels).

Since we now have something effective for symptomatic perimenopause, I propose it is time for women to claim perimenopause, and to take oestrogen-based therapy when they are a year without flow. When they are menopausal they may choose to take progesterone which we, 10 years ago, proved effective for *menopausal* VMS and sleep problems, as well as being safe[14].

Each of us, as a woman, enters the unknown when in midlife she first becomes aware that her period-related experiences and other things are changing. But perimenopause, although long and sometimes miserable, ends for all of us (who are privileged to live that long) in a calmer and more pleasant menopause. We are finally, for the first time since puberty, free from the demands of our ovaries!

References

1. Wallace RB, Sherman BM, Bean JA et al. Probability of menopause with increasing duration of amenorrhea in middle-aged women. *American Journal of Obstetrics and Gynecology* 1979; 135 (8): 1021–1024.
2. Astrup K, Olivarius Nde F. Frequency of spontaneously occurring postmenopausal bleeding in the general population. *Acta Obstetricia et Gynecologica Scandinavica* 2004; 83 (2): 203–207. doi: 10.1111/j.0001-6349.2004.00400.x.
3. Dennerstein L, Dudley EC, Hopper JL et al. A prospective population-based study of menopausal symptoms. *Obstetrics & Gynecology* 2000; 96: 351–358.
4. Santoro N, Rosenberg J, Adel T et al. Characterization of reproductive hormonal dynamics in the perimenopause. *Journal of Clinical Endocrinology & Metabolism* 1996; 81 (4): 1495–501.
5. Prior JC. Perimenopause: The complex endocrinology of the menopausal transition. *Endocrine Reviews* 1998; 19: 397–428.
6. Hale GE, Hughes CL, Burger HG et al. Atypical estradiol secretion and ovulation patterns caused by luteal out-of-phase (LOOP) events underlying irregular ovulatory menstrual cycles in the menopausal transition. *Menopause* 2009; 16 (1): 50–59.
7. Richardson SJ, Senikas V, Nelson JF. Follicular depletion during the menopausal transition: Evidence for accelerated loss and ultimate exhaustion. *Journal of Clinical Endocrinology & Metabolism* 1987; 65: 1231.
8. Prior JC. Balanced actions of estradiol and progesterone—A new paradigm of women's reproductive health. *Drug Discovery Today: Disease Models* 2020; 32: 27–29. doi: 10.1016/j.ddmod.2020.11.007.
9. Freedman RR. Menopausal hot flashes: Mechanisms, endocrinology, treatment. *Journal of Steroid Biochemistry and Molecular Biology* 2014; 142: 115–120.
10. Prior JC, Barr SI, Vigna YM. The controversial endocrinology of the menopausal transition (letter). *Journal of Clinical Endocrinology & Metabolism* 1996; 81: 3127–3128.
11. Gangar KF, Cust MP, Whitehead MI. Symptoms of oestrogen deficiency associated with supraphysiological plasma estradiol concentrations in women with oestradiol implants. *BMJ* 1993; 299: 601–602.
12. Hale GE, Hitchcock CL, Williams LA et al. Cyclicity of breast tenderness and night-time vasomotor symptoms in mid-life women: Information collected using the Daily Perimenopause Diary. *Climacteric* 2003; 6 (2): 128–139.
13. Prior JC, Cameron A, Fung M et al. Oral micronized progesterone for perimenopausal night sweats and hot flushes a Phase III Canada-wide randomized placebo-controlled 4 month trial. *Scientific Reports* 2023; 13 (1): 9082. https://www.nature.com/articles/s41598-023-35826-w [published Online First: 20230605].
14. Hitchcock CL, Prior JC. Oral micronized progesterone for vasomotor symptoms in healthy postmenopausal women–A placebo-controlled randomized trial. *Menopause* 2012; 19: 886–893.

Scene 3 What has progesterone got to do with menopause?

Lara Briden

Progesterone is the hormone made after ovulation (egg release), but only with natural 'ovulatory' menstrual cycles or 'cycles in which ovulation occurs'. That's because progesterone at significant levels is made by a temporary ovarian endocrine gland (corpus luteum) that is created every month after ovulation. Progesterone at low levels is made continuously by the ovaries, adrenal glands and nervous system.

Progesterone has many health benefits, which we're about to explore, but first, let's consider why progesterone has been the forgotten hormone or unsung heroine.

Progesterone was discovered second, and that made all the difference

Progesterone has always played second fiddle to oestrogen, thanks, in large part, to the simple accident of having been discovered second. Oestrogen was discovered in 1929. Progesterone was discovered only five years later, in 1934, but those five years were enough to designate oestrogen as '*the*' hormone for women.

Progesterone had another problem. Unlike oestrogen, progesterone was not (at first) an effective oral medication and therefore missed out on the hormonal 'gold rush' of the 1940s and 1950s. In the words of Professor Jerilynn Prior, the *"oestrogen-discovering scientists, oestrogen-treating clinicians, and oestrogen-making pharmaceutical manufacturers" were simply not interested in progesterone*[1]. By the time progesterone *could* be made into an effective pill (with the invention of oral micronised progesterone; see below), oestrogen had become established as the women's hormone just as testosterone was men's. Progesterone was left behind.

Enter progestins

In the days before progesterone could be made into a convenient medication, scientists invented synthetic analogues of progesterone called progestins, which many doctors, journalists and even scientists started mistakenly referring to as "progesterone". Crucially, *progestins are not progesterone,* and that's because progesterone is not a generic term. It's a little confusing because oestrogen *is* a generic term, so can legitimately describe any oestrogenic molecule, including oestradiol (our main ovarian oestrogen), estrone (another common oestrogen) and even ethinyloestradiol, the synthetic oestrogen used in hormonal birth control. The term "progesterone", on the other hand, refers *only* to a specific hormone that is made in small quantity by the adrenal glands and nervous system, and in large quantity by the ovary after ovulation or the placenta during pregnancy. Progesterone is also available as a type of hormone therapy called body-identical progesterone, which we'll come to shortly.

Definition: body-identical

Body-identical hormone therapy uses hormones, such as oestradiol and progesterone, that are molecularly identical to human oestradiol and/or progesterone.

Consider the difference between the following molecules of progesterone and the progestin, levonorgestrel, which is used in many oral contraceptives, implants, hormonal IUDs and the morning-after pill (Figure 1.3.1).

They're somewhat similar but also quite different. That's why levonorgestrel can mimic *some* of progesterone's effects – such as thinning the uterine lining and lightening menstrual flow – but not all of progesterone's effects. Specifically, progestins like levonorgestrel can have vastly different effects compared to progesterone in the breasts, brain, bones and hair follicles. As an example, consider the fact that the high progesterone of pregnancy famously promotes healthy hair growth. Conversely, levonorgestrel is known to cause male-pattern hair loss because it's derived from testosterone and is (in many ways) more similar to testosterone than it is to progesterone (Figure 1.3.2).

Tip: *Other "testosterone-like" effects of levonorgestrel and other androgenic (testosterone-like) progestins include acne and weight gain.*

Progestins are a motley crew

There are at least 30 different progestins, and they all have different effects. For example, some progestins (like levonorgestrel) are testosterone-like, while others (like drospirenone) can have *anti*-testosterone effects.

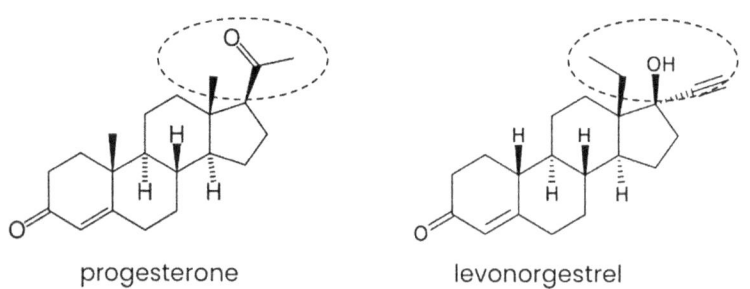

FIGURE 1.3.1 Differences in molecular structure of progestogens

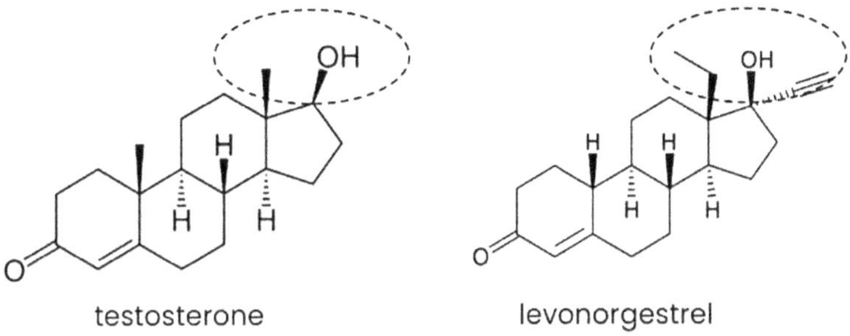

FIGURE 1.3.2 Similarities in molecular structure between testosterone and synthetic progestogens

Importantly, *no* progestins are exactly like progesterone, and all have the potential to affect the brain and cause negative mood side effects. Additionally, all progestins slightly increase the risk of breast cancer – while progesterone does not seem to increase the risk and may even reduce it[2].

Progesterone got blamed

In all the confusion about progestins, progesterone got mistakenly blamed for many of the risks and side effects of progestins, including breast cancer, weight gain, hair loss and mood symptoms. For example, the fact that many progestins cause mood side effects has resulted in the general narrative that progesterone is "bad for mood". Yet, according to Professor Jerilynn Prior's studies into progesterone treatment for the mood symptoms of both perimenopause[3] and menopause[4] body-identical treatment actually improve sleep and mood symptoms.

Progesterone and mood

Progesterone's mood-enhancing effects come from a metabolite called *allopregnanolone*, which acts on the brain's GABA system. (GABA or gamma-aminobutyric acid is the brain's primary calming or inhibitory neurotransmitter). Progesterone's calming GABA effect is why women tend to feel drowsy during pregnancy, a time of very high progesterone. It's also why body-identical progesterone capsules can produce drowsiness, so should be taken only at bedtime. Of course, *losing* progesterone's calming effect at the end of the cycle may contribute to premenstrual mood symptoms.

Tip: *Progestins do not convert to allopregnanolone, so they cannot soothe mood the way progesterone can.*

Special topic: Progesterone sensitivity

Although most women find progesterone calming or sleep-promoting, some women seem to find it anxiety-provoking, particularly in the presence of high, fluctuating oestrogen. If such a paradoxical anxiety-promoting progesterone effect does exist, it may stem from a problem with GABA receptors that renders them less able to adapt to the normal monthly ups and downs of progesterone and allopregnanolone[5].

Sensitivity to progesterone because of altered GABA receptors may play a role in *premenstrual dysphoric disorder (PMDD)*, which is a medical condition characterised by significant premenstrual mood symptoms.

Benefits of progesterone for general health

Progesterone's primary job is to mature the uterine lining and prepare it for pregnancy. As we just saw, progesterone can also help to maintain healthy breast tissue and calm the nervous system. Beyond that, progesterone works together with oestrogen to build long-term health. For example, progesterone supports bone health by stimulating osteoblasts, which are the cells responsible for bone formation. Progesterone also improves cardiovascular (heart) health by maintaining the elasticity of blood vessels, supporting normal blood pressure and may reduce the risk of heart attack[6]. Finally, progesterone can have an anti-inflammatory, immune-modulating effect. That's why regular ovulatory menstrual cycles (and good levels of progesterone) may be able to reduce the risk of autoimmune diseases such as Hashimoto's thyroid disease[7]. Progesterone therapy can also increase thyroid hormone[8].

With perimenopause, you'll lose progesterone years before you lose oestrogen

As we see in Professor Prior's section, progesterone is the first hormone to drop away during the perimenopause transition. You can see that illustrated in the following diagram of hormones across the lifespan (Figure 1.3.3).

Image credit: Hormones through the lifespan, adapted from JC Prior, "Perimenopause lost – reframing the end of menstruation"[9].

With the onset of perimenopause, oestrogen starts to fluctuate, but during the earliest phases of perimenopause, oestrogen actually goes *up*, not down. Progesterone, on the other hand, just goes down as less progesterone is produced during ovulatory cycles and no progesterone is produced during more frequent *anovulatory* cycles (cycles in which ovulation did not occur). In fact, a consistent drop in progesterone is essentially what defines the onset of perimenopause.

The combination of decreasing progesterone and higher, wildly swinging oestrogen can produce the perimenopausal symptoms of sleep disturbance, anxiety, night sweats, heavy periods, breast pain and an increased risk of migraines.

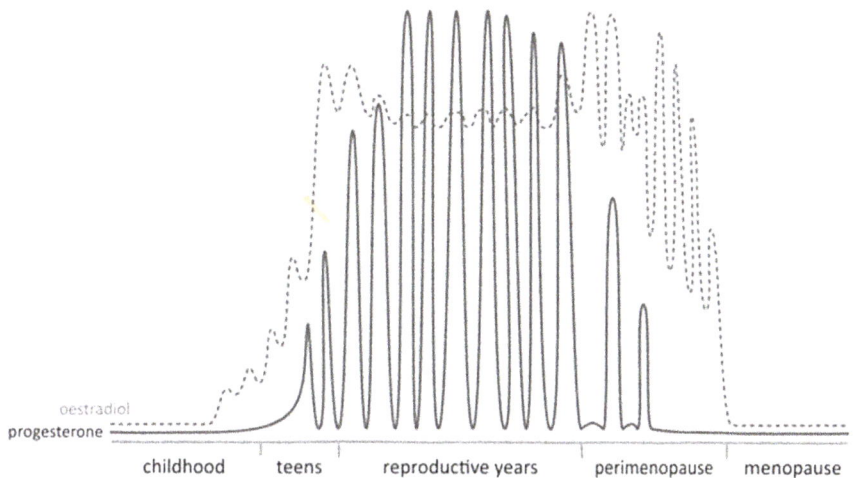

FIGURE 1.3.3 Changes in progesterone and oestradiol over the lifespan

It's possible to just take progesterone

As we'll see in the treatment section in Act 5, "oral micronised" progesterone is a preparation of body-identical progesterone that is micronised (made into tiny particles) to facilitate oral absorption. It can be used (together with oestrogen) as part of menopausal hormone therapy both as the 'protect the uterus' component of the treatment and for its own benefits for heavy flow, sleep, bones and breasts. Furthermore, as Professor Prior demonstrated in her clinical trial published in 2023[3] progesterone can also be used *on its own* to relieve perimenopausal neurological symptoms such as sleep problems and night sweats.

Takeaways

- Progestins are not progesterone.
- Progesterone works together with oestrogen to build long-term health.
- Progesterone can be used on its own to relieve symptoms of perimenopause.

References

1. Prior JC. Women's reproductive system as balanced estradiol and progesterone actions—A revolutionary, paradigm-shifting concept in women's health. *Drug Discovery Today: Disease Models* 2020; 32. doi: 10.1016/j.ddmod.2020.11.005.
2. Gompel A, Seifert-Klauss V, Simon JA et al. Lack of evidence that progesterone in ovulatory cycles causes breast cancer. *Climacteric* 2023 Dec; 26 (6): 634–637. doi: 10.1080/13697137.2023.2249813. Epub 2023 Sep 6.

3   Prior JC, Cameron A, Fung M et al. Oral micronized progesterone for perimenopausal night sweats and hot flushes a Phase III Canada-wide randomized placebo-controlled 4 month trial. *Scientific Reports* 2023 Jun 5; 13 (1): 9082. doi: 10.1038/s41598-023-35826-w.

4   Prior JC. Progesterone for treatment of symptomatic menopausal women. *Climacteric* 2018 Aug; 21 (4): 358–365. doi: 10.1080/13697137.2018.1472567.

5   Turkmen S, Backstrom T, Wahlstrom G et al. Tolerance to allopregnanolone with focus on the GABA-A receptor. *British Journal of Pharmacology* 2011 Jan; 162 (2): 311–327. doi: 10.1111/j.1476-5381.2010.01059.x.

6   Gorgels WJ, Graaf Y, Blankenstein MA et al. Urinary sex hormone excretions in premenopausal women and coronary heart disease risk: A nested case-referent study in the DOM-cohort. *Journal of Clinical Epidemiology* 1997; 50 (3): 275–281. doi: 10.1016/S0895-4356(96)00367.

7   Arduc A, Aycicek Dogan B, Bilmez S et al. High prevalence of Hashimoto's thyroiditis in patients with polycystic ovary syndrome: Does the imbalance between estradiol and progesterone play a role? *Endocrine Research* 2015; 40 (4): 204–210. doi: 10.3109/07435800.2015.1015730.

8   Sathi P, Kalyan S, Hitchcock CL et al. Progesterone therapy increases free thyroxine levels- data from a randomized placebo-controlled 12-week hot flush trial. *Clinical Endocrinology* 2013; 79: 282–287. doi: 10.1111/cen.12128. Epub 2013 May 6.

9   Prior JC. Perimenopause lost—reframing the end of menstruation. *Journal of Reproductive and Infant Psychology* 2006; 24 (4): 323–335. doi: 10.1080/02646830600974071.

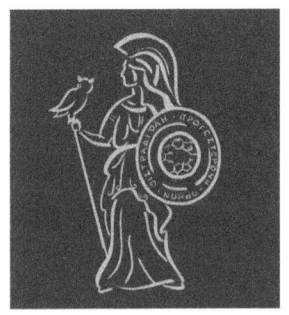

Act 2

Challenges of Menopause
Pandora's box

Act 2 Challenges of Menopause
Pandora's box

Dr Nicky Keay

When Pandora opened a box left in her care by the gods, it unleashed many negative things. However, hope remained in the box.

Approaching menopause can feel like opening Pandora's box, igniting a multitude of unrelated troublesome symptoms that can impact overall quality of life. The crucial thing to remember is menopause is not an illness or disease. Knowledge of the underlying cause provides a guide to the best way forward. Hope remains in Pandora's box, waiting to be engaged.

Scene 1 Myths of menopausal 'symptoms'

Dr Nicky Keay

Myth 1 Is menopause a medical condition?

Using the word "symptom" is problematic when discussing menopause, as symptoms are usually associated with a medical condition. Furthermore, the experiences of menopausal women can overlap with medical conditions. For example, feeling fatigued and sluggish could be an effect of the change in ovarian hormones around menopause or an underactive thyroid. Feeling hot could be a hot flush or the symptom of an infection. A racing heart rate at rest could be a menopausal symptom or a cardiac condition.

Menopause is definitely neither an illness nor a disease. It is a physiological event, an expected, natural part of the female hormone odyssey, when the ovaries retire from consistent production of hormones and eggs. "Indicators" of menopause might be a better word to avoid confusion. On the other hand, some of these indicators can impact quality of life and ultimately long-term health. The British Menopause Society (BMS) reports that 80–90% of women will have some menopausal symptoms, with 25% describing them as severe and debilitating[1].

The priority is to recognise that the graduation to menopause can come with a collection of symptoms, which can vary in range and severity for each individual. Although it is important to consider any underlying medical conditions, treating each symptom as a separate "medical" entity will lead to anxiety (*why am I "falling apart"?*) and unnecessary, potentially harmful polypharmacy.

Myth 2 "Menopause symptoms" only occur at this time point?

Although frequently described as "menopause symptoms" or "symptoms of menopause", in reality these symptoms can start in perimenopause and continue for some time after periods have stopped. Although the strict temporal definition of menopause is the point in time when the final period occurs, symptoms can extend over a number of years.

The reason why menopausal symptoms persist for so long is that the menstrual cycle has evolved to be resilient. The control systems in the brain keep trying to initiate a new cycle even as the ovaries become less and less responsive, a bit like someone who keeps trying to start a car over and again, until the battery eventually runs out of juice. The misfiring endocrine system has side effects in the form of biological responses that vary significantly between women.

Menopausal symptoms last on average more than 7 years. They can begin several years before menopause and continue afterwards, particularly in the first year after menopause as the ovaries become increasingly recalcitrant. It is estimated that more than a third of women experience long-term symptoms, which may continue for a number of years even beyond that[1].

Myth 3 Unrelated menopausal symptoms?

As ovarian hormones exert their effects throughout the body, a great variety of symptoms arise around the time of menopause. The levels and timing of release of these hormones go through a state of flux. The plethora of potential symptoms is shown in Figure 2.1.1. The apparently unrelated nature of these symptoms makes it hard to appreciate the common underlying cause. How could feeling anxious be related to dry skin? Treating each symptom in isolation simply leads to an overstocked medicine cabinet. In some cases, menopausal symptoms may be misattributed to an external event: *"I must be feeling anxious because I was delayed in traffic."* Some of the symptoms of menopause perpetuate each other. For example, hot flushes at night may lead to disturbed sleep, which affects mood and energy levels.

Myth 4 Full house of menopausal symptoms?

It is not necessary to experience a "full house" of symptoms to "qualify" as being menopausal. Each woman has her own unique pattern of ovarian hormone fluctuation that accompanies ovarian retirement. And each individual has her own personal biological response to these changing hormone patterns. Don't worry about statistical

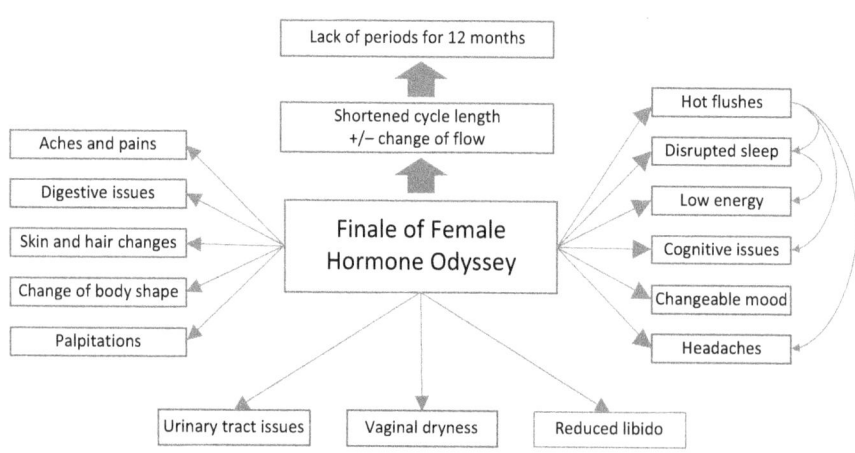

FIGURE 2.1.1 Multifaceted menopausal symptoms

significance on a population basis. Whatever your symptoms, the important point is that if they are impacting your quality of life, then they are significant for you.

To quote a former Vice President of the Royal College of Obstetrics and Gynaecologist: *"We need to treat women as individuals, not statistics."*

Perimenopausal symptom story

Amara was 47 years of age, working as a full-time teacher. She was a single parent with 2 teenage girls aged 14 and 16. Amara loved her job and her family, but recently she had been feeling overwhelmed and anxious and she wasn't sleeping well. She had been to see her GP, who thought that most likely her symptoms were due to the stresses of exam time at school, both for her pupils and her daughters, during a really hot summer. However, during the school holidays, she did not feel any better and wasn't able to keep up with her daughters playing tennis, as she had aching joints. Amara was concerned as her mother had rheumatoid arthritis.

Discussing with Amara, it transpired that her menstrual cycle length had become shorter. Usually, she had a period every 27 days, but these were now coming more frequently with some episodes of heavy periods. Given Amara's age and change in menstrual cycle, this all pointed towards the early stages of perimenopause, with variable ovarian hormone patterns as the underlying cause for her symptoms. Amara was relieved to have identified the underlying reason was not a medical condition.

Myth 5 What is the first clue of perimenopause?

Initially in perimenopause, the main symptom is a shortening of the menstrual cycle, due to a less robust luteal phase, with less sustained levels of progesterone and/or anovulation. This can leave oestradiol as the dominant sex steroid ovarian hormone and often results in heavier menstrual flow. With this initial shift in ovarian hormone patterns, new onset or worsening of premenstrual symptoms can often be experienced[2]. However, as discussed in Act 1, Scene 1, this clue is only relevant for women who are experiencing a menstrual cycle: in other words, those not taking any form of hormonal contraception and who have not had surgery to remove either the ovaries and/or uterus.

Myth 6 Hot flushes are the only menopausal symptom?

Hot flushes, technically known as vasomotor symptoms (VMS), are the most frequently reported menopausal symptom, experienced by 70–80% of women around menopause. However, hot flushes are certainly not the only menopausal symptom and appear to be linked with other symptoms. Nevertheless, VMS are specific to retirement of the ovaries. For a woman who is not experiencing menstruation as mentioned above (due to hormonal contraception or surgery), hot flushes can be a very important clue of perimenopause.

What happens during a hot flush?

Intense heat is felt in upper body, arms and face with flushing of the skin and sweating. This can be followed by chills and a feeling of anxiety. So, a hot flush will render you hot and bothered. If this sequence of events occurs at night, this can disrupt sleep. Although VMS are typically worse during the year after menopause and continue for about 5 years, about 42% of women in their 60s continue to experience hot flushes and night sweats.

What is the underlying reason for hot flushes?

VMS appear to be due to confusion and resetting in the centrally located brain "thermostat" in the hypothalamus, with a narrowing of the "thermoneutral zone". This is associated with changes in ovarian hormones and in neurotransmitters in the brain: hot flushes are worse during the year after menopause, when oestradiol levels are in consistent decline. However, there is no direct link between oestradiol levels and duration or severity of hot flushes. Most likely, this is because women have different biological sensitivity to female hormones. Other hormones and neurotransmitters might also play a part.

The big clue that hot flushes are not just related to oestradiol levels is that women whose periods stop (amenorrhoea) not due to menopause, but who also have low levels of oestradiol, do not experience hot flushes. Specifically, these are women with hypothalamic amenorrhoea (whether due to a suppressive form of hormonal contraception or unbalanced lifestyle choices around exercise and nutrition). Although women experiencing hypothalamic amenorrhoea experience symptoms associated with low oestradiol and progesterone (e.g. poor bone, cardiovascular and mental health), there is no alteration in the central thermostat associated with menopause and the permanent alteration of the HPO axis with accompanying irreversible amenorrhoea. This is why a new medication, detailed below, to combat VMS is directed at the short-range hormone communication between the hypothalamus and pituitary.

What can you do to alleviate hot flushes?

There is evidence that regular exercise can help mitigate the effects of VMS[3]. Getting hot during exercise can potentially help recalibrate the hypothalamic thermostat. This is good news for those experiencing hot flushes, as lifestyle changes can help. What about medication options? New neuroendocrine medications, neurokinin receptor antagonists acting in the hypothalamus-pituitary, have been shown to be helpful in combating VMS[4]. A recent study performed in Canada showed that taking micronised progesterone helped attenuate hot flushes and improved sleep[5]. This type of progesterone is already known to have a relaxing effect and help sleep, which is why it is prescribed to take in the evening. However, currently micronised progesterone is only routinely given as part of hormone replacement therapy (HRT) in clinical practice. As VMS are the most frequent symptom associated with menopause, in the future the combination of exercise and micronised progesterone might become an option.

Myth 7 "Brain fog" is a sign of senility?

"Brain fog" is the eloquent description of cognitive issues associated with menopause, due to decline in the ovarian hormones, which act as neurotransmitters and interact with other neurotransmitters in the brain. Neurotransmitters are short-range hormones that maintain the connectivity between neurones, which is important in mental processing and mood. With reduced brain neurone connectivity, thought processes feel sluggish, with poor memory: *What am I going to put on my list of things not to forget? What was the third point that I wanted to make in this presentation? What was that paragraph about that I just read?* There is interesting research emerging that links VMS with "brain fog". During a hot flush, blood gets diverted away from the brain to the skin. Alteration in blood flow to the brain can potentially impact brain function. So, improving VMS could potentially help cognitive function.

As shown in Figure 2.1.1, there is potentially a link between VMS and associated disrupted cerebral blood flow and other symptoms of cognitive issues, new-onset headaches and mood. Labile mood is a typical symptom associated with graduation to menopause and can include episodes of anxiety and low mood. There are also psychological factors at play at this stage of the female hormone odyssey, not limited to changes in hormones. This is often also a time of change in family, social and work dynamics, which will be discussed in depth in Act 8.

Myth 8 Is disturbed sleep a menopausal symptom?

"*Sleep is the chief nourisher in life's great feast,*" as quoted by Macbeth. Sleep is crucial for both mental and physical health. We all know how a poor night's sleep leaves us feeling sluggish both mentally and physically. Changes in ovarian hormone choreography alter sleep architecture. This can be aggravated by VMS with night sweats. In other words, the combination of symptoms, due to ovarian hormone changes, compounds the issue of poor sleep, both in quality and quantity, which in turn has a negative additive effect on other symptoms: a vicious cycle.

Furthermore, disrupted sleep patterns underlie circadian misalignment. Circadian misalignment is a mismatch between internal hormone biochronometers and the timing of behaviours, such as sleep patterns. Circadian misalignment is linked with metabolic syndrome: insulin resistance, hypertension, adverse lipid profile, which increases the risk of developing cardiovascular disease. This can be amplified by an increased risk of cardiometabolic health issues associated with a decline in anabolic hormones (tissue building) such as oestradiol and growth hormone occurring around natural menopause, discussed in Act 1. Poor sleep can also have a direct adverse effect on body composition:

bone loss and loss of muscle mass and function known as sarcopenia[6]. Being such an important topic, a later scene is dedicated to sleep.

Myth 9 Weight gain is inevitable at menopause? Where has my waist gone?

Although the changes in hormones associated with ageing and menopause favour change in body composition and potential weight gain, this is not an inevitable consequence.

Both men and women experience an age-related decline in the anabolic hormone (tissue building), growth hormone (GH). This hormone change favours the deposition of fat over the building of skeletal muscle. In women, an additional factor is the significant decline in another anabolic hormone, namely oestradiol, especially after menopause. This contrasts with men whose main anabolic hormone, testosterone, only decreases very slightly[7]. Reduced oestradiol favours visceral fat deposition. This type of fat is found around all the major organs in the abdominal cavity, such as the liver and kidneys. With menopause, there is a tendency to increase visceral fat deposition in an "android distribution" around the abdomen, which is why the waistline can expand. Decline in oestradiol with menopause also impacts metabolic health in terms of less effective blood glucose control, which can contribute to weight gain[8].

Story of menopausal weight gain

Polly was 52 years of age and had reached menopause, having had her final period over a year ago. Although she had not experienced any intrusive menopausal symptoms, she was really frustrated to find her clothes had become uncomfortably snug around the waistline and that the number on the weighing scales was creeping up. Polly had an important event coming up as her daughter was getting married and to her dismay, the dress that she intended on wearing was too tight around the waist. Polly decided to try one of the "menopause diets" she had seen advertised. This involved drastically reducing what she would normally eat, especially cutting carbohydrates like cereal, bread and pasta, plus a vast (and expensive) array of supplements, all claiming to ensure weight loss. Despite all these actions, she was really upset to see that after an initial modest weight loss, her weight had then increased to more than it was before and if anything, her dress was now even tighter.

Was Polly's weight gain an inevitable consequence of menopause? Why did going on a "diet" not work? As described above, the decline in anabolic hormones associated with increasing age and menopause makes it more challenging to maintain a healthy body weight and body composition. However, this does not mean that gaining both fat and weight is an inevitable outcome of menopause. The best strategy is to acknowledge and respect these hormone changes associated with menopause and modify your lifestyle choices around nutrition and exercise in step with changes in internal endocrine networks[9].

We all like a "quick fix" and reducing what you eat seems a logical approach to trying to lose weight. However crash diets, at any age, invariably backfire as severe calorie restriction causes an increase in the stress response hormone cortisol, which favours fat deposition. Furthermore, metabolic rate can slow to "save energy", which is counterproductive in weight loss[10]. Carbohydrates are not the villain of the weight management piece. Complex carbohydrates, such as wholemeal bread, pasta and cereals, are slow-release energy sources. Carbohydrates are the main substrate used to power high-quality exercise to maintain favourable body composition. Consuming insufficient carbohydrate to cover demand stimulates increased release of cortisol and the depletion of glycogen stores. Most likely, the initial modest weight loss Polly experienced was due to water loss as glycogen stores were broken down. Following a crash "menopause" diet had the exact opposite of the outcomes Polly was trying to achieve.

What is the solution? The good news is that adapting your lifestyle choices, in a sustainable way, to match the way your hormones change as you get older can mitigate changes in body composition and body weight. Regarding nutrition, this means maintaining regular eating patterns and including all the food groups but putting more of an emphasis on protein intake and being strategic in carbohydrate portion size. Protein intake is important to support reducing anabolic hormones in maintaining muscle mass[11].

Polly had just focused on reducing food intake and had not considered exercise as a synergistic tool to mitigate the effects of changing hormone networks[7]. As with nutrition including all the food groups, but with altered emphasis; similarly, this is the optimal strategy for exercise. It is important to cover all elements of fitness (cardiovascular, muscular strength, muscular endurance, flexibility and neuromuscular skills) with different exercise types, but with a particular emphasis on strength work. This type of exercise supports metabolic health, body weight and body composition[12]. High-quality exercise fuelled appropriately by carbohydrate (anabolic stimulus) together with appropriate refuelling with complex carbohydrates and protein has a synergistic effect on weight control and body composition. This focused approach, on the background of regular eating patterns and general activity, means that weight gain is not an inevitable outcome of ageing and menopause.

What about supplements? There are a plethora of supplements purported to produce weight loss, change in body composition and achieve many other outcomes. If you are including all the food groups in your nutrition, you do not need supplementation. The exception is vitamin D. You cannot gain enough vitamin D from diet alone. Vitamin D is a steroid hormone made by the action of sunlight on the skin and unless you are outside, living in a sunny country year-round, you cannot produce sufficient vitamin D, for optimal bone, muscle and immune health. Vitamin D supplementation is important across the lifespan, but in particular in this phase of the female hormone odyssey as sex steroid anabolic hormones work synergistically with vitamin D.

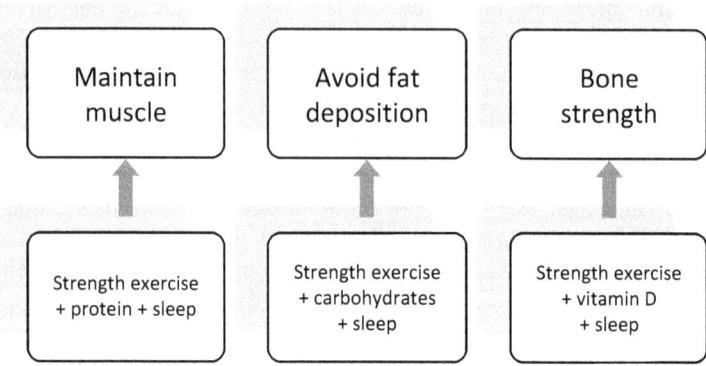

FIGURE 2.1.2 Adapting to declining anabolic hormones

Sleep is the other key ingredient. The key anabolic hormones, albeit at lower levels than in youth, come into action during sleep. You get fitter and control body weight and body composition when you are asleep! This happens if you have laid the groundwork with good nutrition and exercise during the day.

Figure 2.1.2 summarises how modifying lifestyle factors can help with weight management and body composition. These lifestyle strategies are discussed in further detail in Act 4 Mastering Menopause.

Myth 10 Have I developed arthritis?

Although autoimmune joint disease is more common in women, "aches and pains" are a recognised menopausal symptom. Sometimes these musculoskeletal issues can be mistaken for injury, as will be discussed in Act 7. Of course, it is important to exclude an underlying medical condition such as autoimmune arthritis. However, if this has been ruled out, you may be left wondering what is going on, unless you appreciate this could be part of the spectrum of menopausal symptoms. Fluctuating and ultimately dropping levels of oestradiol around menopause are a big contributing factor to a very frequently reported menopausal symptom of "aches and pains"[13].

Myth 11 Why has my skin become dry and itchy? And why is my hair thinning?

It is not a pleasant experience to be unable to sleep due to itchy skin or to notice that your hair is getting thinner. What is going on? The change and ultimate decline in oestradiol impacts production of the complex protein, collagen, which is the major component of ubiquitous connective tissue. Connective tissue is like a bandage found in many tissues such as skin, hair, ligaments, tendons and intervertebral discs[14]. Change in oestradiol production has a knock-on effect on the production and quality of collagen, as hormones direct gene expression in the production of specific proteins.

Myth 12 Is bloating a menopausal symptom?

The ovarian hormones, in particular oestradiol, are important players in gut health, both directly and indirectly via the gut microbiome. There is a fascinating bidirectional interaction between oestradiol and the gut microbiome. The gut microbiome includes a range of microbes, mainly in the large intestine. It may surprise you to hear that the amount of microbial genetic material in our body is greater than our own. Furthermore, the gut microbiota produce metabolites that are helpful locally for digestion and absorption of food, as well as for eating behaviours and mental health: the gut-brain axis[15]. Declining oestradiol levels around menopause mean that the helpful gut microbes "go hungry", which can lead to an imbalance in the types of gut microbiota and lack of diversity: dysbiosis[16]. The net result can be digestive symptoms such as bloating.

Figure 2.1.3 shows the interaction of oestrogen and a specific group of the gut microbiome called the oestrobolome. The gut microbiota of the oestrobolome have an enzyme called beta-glucuronidase. This enzyme "recycles" oestrogens which have been "deactivated" by the liver and sent to the gut via the enterohepatic circulation for excretion. If there is a healthy community of gut microbiota, including those that can rejuvenate conjugated oestrogen, then "re-activated" oestrogen is sent back to boost the systemic circulation. The oestrobiota can also extract oestrogen from dietary sources of phytooestrogen (found in plants). Crucially, the amount and function of the oestrobolome is dependent on circulating levels of oestrogen. So fluctuating and declining levels of

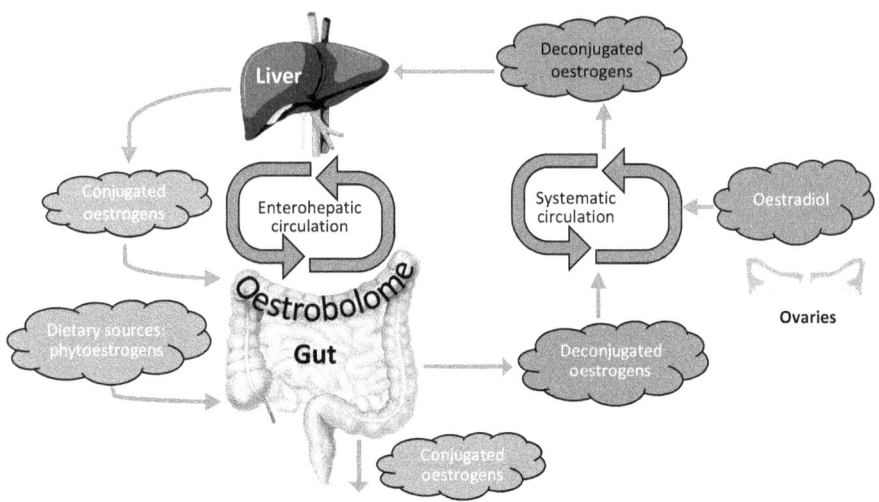

FIGURE 2.1.3 Actions of the oestrobolome

ovarian oestrogen cause a decline in the oestrobolome, which compounds reducing oestrogen levels and the symptoms associated with this. Based on this interaction between the oestrobolome and circulating oestrogens, there is emerging evidence that this could influence the response to HRT[17]. A corollary is that menopausal women could consider prebiotics and probiotics to support a gut microbiome favourable to supporting internal and/or external ovarian hormones and menopausal symptoms[18].

Myth 13 Racing heart?

Oestradiol has a cardioprotective effect. Changing oestradiol levels around menopause can be associated with a racing heart rate. Increased heart rate, not associated with exercise, can be experienced with hot flushes, when anxiety is felt with increased stress response hormones. However, as an irregular heartbeat could be due to underlying cardiovascular disease, it is advisable to see your GP to get recurring palpitations checked out.

Myth 14 Is being "caught short" a menopausal symptom only for women who have given birth?

Increased urgency and frequency of passing urine is a common menopausal symptom, regardless of whether you have given birth or not. This can feel like a urinary tract infection, with burning/stinging when urinating. Even if an infection is not present, there is an increased risk of urinary tract infections with menopause. The underlying reason is that the lower urinary tract (bladder and urethra) is in very close proximity to the lower reproductive tract (uterus, cervix, vagina, vulva) and the tissues of the urinogenital tract (urinary and reproductive systems combined) are sensitive to oestradiol[19]. Dropping levels of oestradiol around menopause is the underlying reason behind urinary symptoms. This is why these urogenital symptoms are more likely to occur after menopause. There can be a contributing factor from pelvic health, which is discussed in further detail in Act 3, Scene 2, "Goodbye to pelvic health after menopause?!" and also in Act 6, Scene 4, "Everybody leaks?!"

Myth 15 Some menopausal symptoms are difficult to discuss . . .

Vaginal dryness is not a topic that is easy to discuss, even with your GP. Dropping oestradiol levels mean that the tissues of the reproductive tract change, which can lead to vulval and vaginal dryness, as well as symptoms of external itchiness and painful intercourse. Recent research suggests that, as with the gut microbiome, the vaginal microbiome may be impacted by dropping oestradiol levels, which may contribute to and potentially exacerbate issues of dryness[20]. This important topic of sexual health will be discussed in detail in Act 3, Scene 1. "No sex after menopause?!"

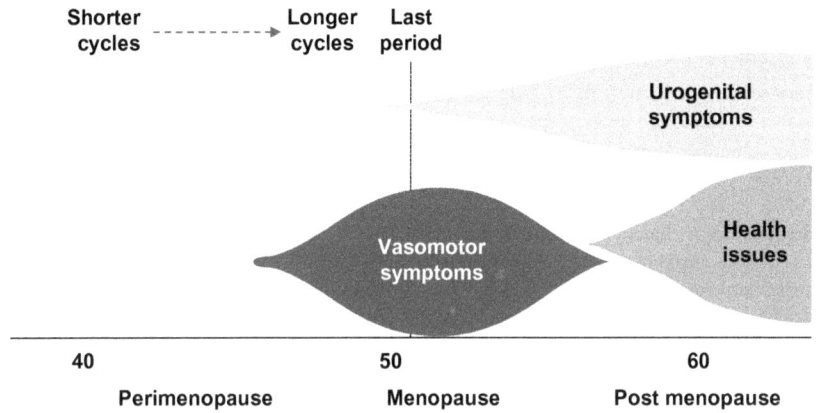

FIGURE 2.1.4 Typical timing of menopausal symptoms

Figure 2.1.4 shows the typical time course of symptoms around menopause. Initially, typically from age 40 onwards in early perimenopause, progesterone levels fall, resulting in shorter cycles and possibly heavier menstruation while oestradiol dominates. As oestradiol levels fall, longer cycles and skipped periods can occur. VMS are the most common symptom, peaking in the year after the last period (menopause). With continued low levels of oestradiol, the next symptoms to dominate are those associated with the urogenital system. More general age-related health issues start to emerge next due to the retirement of ovarian function in hormone production. These health issues will be discussed in detail in Scene 3 of this Act 2.

Mastering Pandora's box

Although it may seem overwhelming to have to deal with the multifaceted symptoms associated with this part of the female hormone odyssey, the lifestyle approaches that can help are discussed in detail in Act 4 Mastering Menopause. Treatment options, including hormone replacement therapy (HRT), are discussed in Act 5.

References

1. British Menopause Society. What is the menopause? https://thebms.org.uk/wp-content/uploads/2023/08/17-BMS-TfC-What-is-the-menopause-AUGUST2023-A.pdf. Accessed March 2024.
2. British Menopause Society. *Management of the Menopause*, Sixth Edition. Hilard T, Abernathy K, Manoda H, Shaw I, Everett M, Ayres J, Currie H. British Menopause Society, 2017.
3. Bailey T, Cable T, Aziz N et al. Exercise training reduces the acute physiological severity of post-menopausal hot flushes. *Journal of Physiology* 2016; 594 (3): 657–667. doi: 10.1113/JP271456.
4. British Menopause Society. https://thebms.org.uk/2023/12/new-treatment-for-vasomotor-symptoms-hot-flushes-and-night-sweats-licensed-by-the-mhra/. Accessed January 2024.

5. Prior J, Cameron A, Fung M et al. Oral micronized progesterone for perimenopausal night sweats and hot flushes a Phase III Canada-wide randomized placebo-controlled 4-month trial. *Scientific Reports* 2023. doi: 10.1038/s41598-023-35826-w.
6. Lucassen EA, de Mutsert R, le Cessie S et al. Poor sleep quality and later sleep timing are risk factors for osteopenia and sarcopenia in middle-aged men and women: The NEO study. *PLoS ONE* 2017; 12 (5): e0176685. doi: 10.1371/journal.pone.0176685.
7. Keay N. *Hormones, Health and Human Potential*. Act 2, Scene 5 "Middle Age". Sequoia Books, 2022.
8. Bermingham K, Linenberg I, Hall W et al. Menopause is associated with postprandial metabolism, metabolic health and lifestyle: The ZOE PREDICT study. *Preprint Lancet*. SSRN: https://ssrn.com/abstract4051462. doi: 10.2139/ssrn4051462.
9. Keay N. *Hormones Health and Human Potential*. Act 1 Scene 3 Harnessing Hormones. Sequoia Books, 2022.
10. Keay N. *Hormones Health and Human Potential*. Act 1 Scene 4 It's All in the Timing. Sequoia Books, 2022.
11. Denby N. Menopause: Nutrition and weight gain. *Post Reproductive Health* 2023; 29 (4): 232–234.
12. Mandrup C, Roland C, Egelund Jon et al. Effects of high-intensity exercise training on adipose tissue mass, glucose uptake and protein content in pre- and post-menopausal women. *Frontiers in Sports and Active Living* 2020; (2): 60. https://www.frontiersin.org/article/10.3389/fspor.2020.00060. doi: 10.3389/fspor.2020.00060.
13. Magliano M. Menopausal arthralgia: Fact or fiction. *Maturitas* 2010; 67 (1): 29–33. ISSN 0378-5122. doi: 10.1016/j.maturitas.2010.04.009.
14. Calleja-Agius J, Brincat M. The effect of menopause on the skin and other connective tissues. *Gynecological Endocrinology* 2012; 28 (4): 273–277. doi: 10.3109/09513590.2011.613970.
15. Keay N. *Hormones, Health and Human Potential*. Act 1, Scene 8 "Mind the Gut". Sequoia Books, 2022.
16. Gilbert J. Microbiome and menopause. British Menopause Society annual conference 2023.
17. Dothard MI, Allard SM, Gilbert JA. The effects of hormone replacement therapy on the microbiomes of postmenopausal women. *Climacteric* 2023; 26 (3): 182–192.
18. Barnard N, Kahleova H, Holtz DN et al. A dietary intervention for vasomotor symptoms of menopause: A randomized, controlled trial. *Menopause* 2023; 30 (1): 80–87.
19. British Menopause Society. Urogenital atrophy. https://thebms.org.uk/wp-content/uploads/2024/04/09-BMS-ConsensusStatement-Urogenital-atrophy-MARCH2024-A.pdf. Accessed April 2024.
20. Muhleisen AL, Herbst-Kralovetz MM. Menopause and the vaginal microbiome. *Maturitas* 2016; 91: 42–50.

Scene 2 "Sleep no more!?"

Dr Zoe Schaedel

Sleep during the menopause transition

If you are struggling with sleep during menopause, you are not alone. About 40–60% of women will experience some sleep issues during menopause, though the actual experience will vary hugely; everyone's sleep challenges are unique. Some of you will struggle to drift off when your head hits the pillow, and for many the mornings will start much too early as sleep becomes harder to come by as the night progresses. Then there is the all-too-familiar scenario of unwanted and sometimes frequent wakings during the night, with these interruptions affecting both the quality and quantity of sleep.

Why does sleep go wrong during the menopause transition?

There is a myriad of aspects of the menopause transition that have the potential to negatively affect our sleep. Firstly, there are the hormone changes. We know that both oestrogen and progesterone start to vary during the perimenopause phase. Oestrogen is released more chaotically and over time oestrogen levels will gradually fall until they become very low in the postmenopause phase. Before the perimenopause (if you are not taking a hormonal contraceptive), most menstrual cycles will include the release of an egg during ovulation. In the perimenopause, we experience fewer ovulations, which means less progesterone is being produced. Oestrogen and progesterone have multiple functions all over the body. They are important in reproduction, brain function, maintaining bone strength, metabolic function and in the genitourinary system, to name but a few. It turns out that they also have a role to play in maintaining healthy sleep too[1].

In addition to this background hormone chaos, there are notorious symptoms that it causes. Hot flushes and night sweats, also known as vasomotor symptoms, are big culprits when it comes to sleep issues during menopause. For natural sleep to occur, we rely on our core body temperature dropping and staying lower throughout the night, right up until we wake up when the temperature starts to rise to its pre-sleep level. It makes complete sense that if our internal thermostat becomes disrupted due to menopause, then the temperature stability that we rely on for sleep will disappear and our good continuous sleep might go with it. A number of other menopause symptoms can also affect sleep during this phase, and we will explore more about them (and more importantly, what you can do about them).

Why does sleep matter during menopause?

Most of us instinctively know that the amount of sleep we get is directly linked to how we feel the next day. After a night of very little sleep, we are more likely to feel tired, grumpy, struggle with our memory and to do everything we would like to do. Even one or two nights of disturbed sleep can contribute to low mood and increased anxiety. Good sleep helps us to feel empathy and to manage our relationships. Many women struggle with mood swings and feeling snappy and irritable during menopause and a lack of sleep definitely does not help with this[2].

Sleep science has progressed a long way in the last 30 years, and we are continually learning about how important sleep is to physical and mental health. In addition to how you feel, getting enough sleep of good enough quality is associated with lower cardiovascular risk, better cognitive function, improved immunity and better mental health.

So, if you are struggling with sleep during menopause, it makes sense to try to improve things, for your own energy, mood and quality of life, but also with an eye on your long-term health.

I would like to tell you about three women I have met in my clinic (with their permission). They each have a very different sleep story, but I hear versions of these repeatedly. After learning more about sleep and what can help, they have all found a way back to healthy sleep again. I hope that their stories may resonate with some of you, and their solutions may offer ideas and hope.

Sleep stories

Rebecca, age 48

Rebecca's sleep just had not been the same since she entered perimenopause. She struggled to fall asleep at night, sometimes tossing and turning for more than an hour before falling into a light sleep from which she was easily woken. The nights were punctured by wakings, sometimes to pass urine and other times for no good reason at all. She was feeling increasingly tired during the daytime and after a really bad night, she often took a short nap to keep her going. Along with mood swings and brain fog, she was not feeling like herself.

Sangeetha, age 52

Sangeetha's menopause symptoms started about 2 years ago, just before her last menstrual period and she is now postmenopausal. The most annoying of her symptoms were the hot flushes and night sweats she experienced. During the day she can just about cope with her 8 to 10 hot flushes, which were fairly short-lived, though embarrassing at work. But it was at night that things really went downhill. Sangeetha woke up up to five times each night. Once awake, she would feel generally hot, before experiencing a sense of extreme heat in her upper chest, which spreads to her neck and face. This inner heat was accompanied by sweating, sometimes a little, sometimes a lot. After this hot hell passed, Sangeetha was left either drenched, needing to change her bedclothes, or freezing cold and shivery, needing to dive further under the duvet to get comfortable. Sleep did usually return, but only until the next waking, which could be 1–2 hours later. With so much sleep disruption, Sangeetha was feeling fatigued and was too tired to do anything in the evenings, missing out on the dance classes she used to enjoy and meals out.

Caroline, age 54

Caroline's symptoms hit hard during perimenopause. At around age 47, she knew something was not right. Having never experienced anxiety before, she became very anxious about things that would not have previously been an issue. Sleep problems followed and Caroline would lie awake at night for hours, feeling completely "wired" and far from sleep. Hot flushes were not a problem for Caroline, but a combination of anxiety, sleep problems and an increase in headaches convinced Caroline to start HRT at age 49 during perimenopause. It helped hugely and Caroline felt like herself again. The anxiety settled, as did the headaches and all the other symptoms except for sleep. The sleep problems remained the same; despite trying different types and doses of HRT, they did not improve at all.

Myth: Hot flushes are the only sleep disrupter during menopause

About 75% of women will experience hot flushes and night sweats. If you do experience these symptoms at nighttime, they will commonly disrupt sleep, just as they did for Sangeetha. For some women, these disruptions will be brief and after a short waking, they can return to sleep easily. For others, these episodes are prolonged, and they have to get up out of bed to cool down and get changed, which can make it much harder to fall back to sleep again. A night's sleep can feel as though it has had big chunks nibbled out of it. That is why, for women experiencing these symptoms, it is important to treat them as effectively as possible.

However, it is not just vasomotor symptoms that can disrupt sleep; menopause is a time when there are increased rates of depression and anxiety, and these are both strongly linked to sleep disruptions[2]. Anxiety often occurs before the onset of sleep disruption, and like Caroline, many of my patients experience a racing mind when they get into bed. Feeling worried or fearful or having a racing mind will often get in the way of falling asleep.

Other menopause symptoms that can affect sleep include musculoskeletal aches and pains. Waking up to pass urine is more common postmenopause, due to the lack of oestrogen in the urinary tract and can lead to frequent wakings.

If you are struggling with your sleep and this seems to be related to other menopause symptoms, it is important to consider how best you can treat those symptoms. The most effective treatment available is Hormone Replacement Therapy (HRT). Sangeetha decided to try HRT after weighing up its benefits and risks, and she emailed 5 days later to let me know that her night sweats had almost gone. It is not uncommon for improvements like these to occur really quite quickly. Sangeetha felt huge relief. Without the night sweats, she was not waking through the night and after a month of treatment her sleep was completely back on track, her energy had improved and it was wonderful that she no longer needed to worry about hot flushes when at work.

Myth: Menopause symptoms are all about oestrogen

Oestrogen is an important hormone and is the major component of HRT. The changes in oestrogen levels that occur during the menopause transition can lead to numerous symptoms, including sleep problems. By smoothing out chaotic oestrogen levels in the perimenopause and boosting low levels postmenopause, HRT can help restore that premenopausal sleep regulation. It can also help with many other symptoms of menopause and has a number of other advantages for your health.

However, there is another hormone to be aware of that can also impact sleep: progesterone. Progesterone is released after ovulation during most menstrual cycles. Any woman using oestrogen in HRT, who still has a uterus, needs to also take progesterone or a synthetic hormone similar to progesterone (a progestin). This is in order to protect the lining of the uterus from becoming thickened during oestrogen treatment. If you are able to take HRT and do not have a medical reason not to, there are many different types of hormones that women can choose from to make up their HRT. For women who sleep poorly during menopause, it is worth considering a trial of natural micronised progesterone alongside their oestrogen. When these capsules are swallowed, they are broken down into a substance called allopregnanolone that helps to relax us and has been proven to help sleep for many women[3].

For Sangeetha, the improvement in her sleep came mostly from her night sweats being treated, but there are other ways that HRT can help sleep. For instance, some women will notice an improvement in mood and anxiety, and this can have a knock-on effect on improving their sleep[2]. Other women who feel generally better in themselves on HRT, perhaps with less joint pain and more energy, find themselves able to be more active during the day, with exercise or other enjoyable activities. Wearing yourself out by being active during the day, is another effective way to improve sleep![4]

What about for women who do not have other menopause symptoms but are struggling with sleep disruptions that are related to the menopause transition? Studies suggest that HRT can be helpful, even if poor sleep is your only symptom. The hormone stability can be helpful for sleep, even in the absence of hot flushes or mood changes. So, do discuss this option with your doctor if you would like to consider it.

Myth: Only systemic hormonal treatment can help with HRT

Sometimes local vaginal oestrogen can also play a part in helping to restore good sleep. Vaginal oestrogen is used to treat symptoms like vaginal dryness, soreness, pain during sex and bladder issues. Very little is absorbed into the system, so you may wonder how this treatment could help with sleep. Well, for many women that I see, their bladder function has become one of the many menopause experiences disrupting their sleep. If you find you are waking up frequently at night with the need to pass urine or are experiencing other genitourinary symptoms, you may find that vaginal oestrogen helps to replace oestrogen in the bladder and urethra and this can help reduce the frequency and urgency of urination, thereby reducing visits to the bathroom at night. I recommended this treatment for Rebecca, whose frequent wakings seemed to coincide with needing to urinate, and I think the regular vaginal oestrogen pessaries that she uses have played a small role, amongst a number of other targeted strategies, in restoring her good sleep.

Myth: Menopausal sleep problems are solely due to hormonal changes

As you have heard, many of the symptoms experienced by Sangeetha, Rebecca and Caroline are due to changes in hormones that occur over the menopause transition. But there are often other things going on in life that can lead to stress and worry. These can have an additive effect on sleep. Menopause can happen at almost any age, but is most often experienced in midlife, which is often when women's responsibilities and commitments can really ramp up. These may be related to caring responsibilities for children, teenagers or even unwell parents, and also demands at work and in other areas of life. It can be a time of high stress combined with limited opportunity for self-care and often little time for activities that promote relaxation and good mental health. Sometimes women that I see with sleep problems know that they have let their lifestyle slip in recent years, for many reasons. They may have let go of some of their healthier habits, and they see a negative impact on their sleep. Rebecca was in this position when I saw her. She was not keen on starting HRT initially, and she first wanted to see if changing her lifestyle could help her sleep and get her feeling more like herself again.

Myth: It helps to grab sleep when you can get it, take naps if you can

Short naps can be helpful for many people and provide benefits such as increased energy and improved memory and concentration. Unfortunately, naps are often not at all helpful for women who are struggling to sleep at night. On reviewing Rebecca's sleep, she was going to bed early due to sheer exhaustion, then spending much of the night awake before getting an hour or two of sleep when she could during the daytime. This type of pattern is confusing to the internal body clock (or "circadian rhythm"). Keeping regular sleep timings is one of the best ways to approach difficulty sleeping, and it can be particularly important to set a regular waking up time that you stick to, even on weekends. Rebecca set a wake time of 7 a.m. and tried to avoid very early nights and naps. This is a clever way of helping to build up something we call "sleep pressure" or "sleep drive". Sleep pressure starts building the moment you wake up, and you want this to reach really high levels by the time you go to bed, to help you fall asleep and stay asleep. The longer you are awake during the day, the higher the sleep pressure[5]. Naps and early nights can limit this. In addition to avoiding naps, Rebecca started incorporating more exercise into her routine – the activity is good for promoting sleep. Exercise also started to help her with anxiety and had a positive impact on her weight. It was difficult for her to make these changes due to feeling so tired, but the payoffs kept her going, and she could feel things gradually getting back on track. We discussed that the best approach is often to focus on small changes in a variety of areas of lifestyle – they all add up.

Myth: Anxiety is just a part of menopause; you just need to put up with it

Exercise helped to manage Rebecca's mood swings, but for Caroline, the changes she made to her lifestyle were not enough to help with her anxiety symptoms. Anxiety is important to think about when sleep is poor, as these two experiences are often linked to each other.

Anxiety is one of the biggest sleep disruptors and menopause can often throw this spanner in the works. It can help to understand why anxiety has such a significant impact on sleep. There are a variety of internal processes that regulate your sleep. These could all be working perfectly, but if your brain senses your body is under threat, you will not be able to fall asleep. This makes perfect sense, as when you are asleep you are vulnerable. Looking back in time, thousands of years ago, being asleep would mean that you could be eaten by a sabre-tooth tiger or attacked by an enemy tribe. Your body needs to feel safe in order to make the transition from wake to sleep. You have a sophisticated threat detection system to help decide if it is "safe" called the sympathetic nervous system. This system scans the environment for any signs of danger, and if it detects trouble, it kickstarts the body's fight or flight response. Anxiety, which often increases during menopause, triggers the sympathetic nervous system to activate, leading to the release of the hormones such as adrenaline and cortisol. These would be helpful if you needed to escape from a predator but are the opposite of helpful when you want to wind down to sleep. They can lead to an increase in heart rate and breathing rate, and increased sensations of threat or danger. This is what was happening to Caroline, and it became a vicious cycle. The more anxious she felt during perimenopause, the harder it became to sleep. The poor sleep only served to fuel the anxiety and it began to feel like a never-ending loop of stress and exhaustion.

If you feel this may be happening to you, please do seek support. There are lots of approaches that can help, in addition to exercise. Try relaxation techniques until you find one that suits you. Diaphragmatic breathing is popular, and an exercise called progressive muscular relaxation has been shown to help with both anxiety and sleep. There are plenty of videos explaining how to do this online. Introducing mindfulness or meditation can be helpful, particularly if you practise these during the day; in time, they can help you to calm an anxious mind and promote relaxation.

It is important to realise that some wind-down time is often needed to transition between the busy, active daytime mindset and the calm and relaxed mind we need for sleep. Creating a routine with dim lights and relaxing activities can help to set the scene for sleep.

There are many other approaches to help with anxiety during menopause; some women, like Caroline, find HRT helpful. There are other medications available as well as talking therapies. When sleep problems feel very linked to anxiety, a program called Cognitive Behavioural Therapy for Insomnia (CBT-I) can be particularly useful, and we will talk more about that later.

Myth: It does not matter what your bedroom is like – you should be able to sleep anywhere!

There is some truth in this one. Humans have been sleeping since the dawn of time. And very often this was not in temperature-controlled environments with satin sheets, memory foam pillows and double sprung mattresses! It was often in a cave with a comfortable rock for a pillow. However, our environment does matter, and during menopause, this may be a time when you need to reevaluate whether your bedroom is working for you and consider making some changes. Your bedroom should be both dark and cool. Light and temperature are both crucial factors in regulating sleep. The darkness helps encourage the release of melatonin, which is a hormone that helps your body to get ready to sleep. In order to fall asleep, your core body temperature drops and should remain low throughout the night, rising again at waking time. Rebecca found it really helpful to make some changes to her bedroom, investing in blackout blinds and starting the night with as cool a bedroom as she could manage.

If possible, the bedroom should be a place you like that feels welcoming and relaxing to you (rather than the war zone where you have a nightly battle). Your bed should only be where you sleep (and have sex), so if you are used to doing other things on your bed, such as working, chatting or relaxing during the day, find somewhere else for these activities. This is all so that you can train your brain to produce sleep when you get into bed. Menopause often brings with it aches, pains and temperature changes, so make sure your mattress is as comfortable as possible and choose bedding and nightwear that help you stay cool. There are all sorts of products available – cooling mats, moisture-wicking pajamas, sheets that you can wave up and come down cool. Set yourself up for success. Rebecca was not so concerned with cooling but wanted to feel cosy and warm. Like many of my patients, she found a weighted blanket helpful. There is limited data on the impact of weighted blankets on sleep disturbances, but they have been shown to have an anxiety-reducing effect, and I think that is often how they help with sleep also. I often encourage my patients to give them a try.

Myth: I can eat when and what I like during menopause, and it will not affect my sleep

What (and when) you consume during the day actually does matter to your sleep. There are two major sleep disruptors that are worth considering. Caffeinated drinks, if taken too close to bedtime, can block that "sleep pressure" that needs to be at high levels at sleep time. Caffeine can also impact other menopause symptoms such as anxiety and palpitations, so consider reducing your caffeine intake and limiting it to the mornings to ensure it does not get in the way of sleep. Alcohol is the next thing to consider. If you have poor sleep, you may find that alcohol actually helps you to fall asleep, and a glass of wine can creep into an evening routine. Unfortunately, after that initial drowsiness that assists with dropping off, alcohol is a strong disruptor of sleep, often causing tiny awakenings that you may or may not remember and leaving you feeling unrefreshed when you wake in the morning. Alcohol is definitely not something to use too regularly if you are struggling.

It would be great if there was a specific food or diet that would resolve sleep difficulties during menopause, but sadly there is not. When you eat maybe more important than what, and it can help to avoid eating too close to bedtime so there is plenty of time for food to be digested before sleep, avoiding acid reflux. I recommend leaving a minimum of 2–3 hours between eating and sleeping.

Myth: Insomnia is the only sleep disturbance during menopause

Insomnia is a condition where you experience difficulty falling asleep, staying asleep or waking early, to the point it causes a negative impact on daytime functioning. This sounds a lot like menopause for some women! However, there are other things that can go wrong with sleep during the menopause transition, and it is really worth being aware of them, so that you can take steps to resolve them.

Firstly, a condition called Restless Legs Syndrome, or RLS. This is where you experience an uncomfortable desire to move your legs around. If you have experienced this, you will know exactly what I am talking about, though if you have not, it can be difficult to imagine. It is not painful but still very unpleasant. RLS usually occurs in the evening before bed, and if it continues past bedtime, it can make it hard to fall asleep. Many women experience this during pregnancy, and it becomes more common again during the menopause transition. If this is something you experience, particularly if it is getting in the way of your sleep, please discuss this with your doctor. Low iron levels are a common cause, and so a blood test for iron stores called "ferritin" should be arranged for anyone with restless legs. Sometimes there is no cause to be found, but there are treatment options available in the form of different medications, so it is important to discuss with your doctor if your sleep is affected by RLS.

Obstructive Sleep Apnoea (OSA) is the next most common sleep disorder after insomnia and RLS. It is a condition where the upper airway closes off very briefly during sleep. Because the airway briefly closes, the oxygen supply to the brain drops momentarily, and this triggers you to wake up so that you can take a breath and restore the essential oxygen supply. The hormone changes of menopause can contribute to the upper airway having less tone and being more liable to close off. Weight gain is also a common trigger for sleep apnoea, and many women also gain weight during the menopause transition. Hormone changes and increased weight are probably the most important reasons that the incidence of sleep apnoea doubles at the time of menopause. In addition to causing multiple micro-wakings through the night – which can leave you exhausted and sleepy the next day – the condition also increases your risk of a number of serious illnesses later in life, including cardiovascular disease and diabetes. Therefore, it is very important to get a diagnosis of OSA so that it can be treated, usually by a combination of lifestyle changes and a mask that delivers pressurised air to keep the airway open overnight. It can be difficult to know if you have sleep apnoea, as you often will not be aware of the airway issues yourself. If your bed partner notices loud snoring or pauses in your breathing overnight, please see your doctor to request a sleep study. However, in women, the symptoms may not be so obvious as in men, and there are other more subtle signs to look out for, including morning headaches, nightmares, depression, insomnia and daytime sleepiness[6].

When Rebecca came to see me, I considered OSA as a possible cause of her sleep problems. She had noticed mood changes and reported intermittent morning headaches. She was sleepy during the day and told me that she avoided booking social activities in the afternoons as she would be at risk of falling asleep mid-conversation. She was also overweight, and her weight had increased over the last few years due to a combination of feeling too tired to exercise and finding high-carbohydrate foods comforting when feeling low. For these reasons, I referred her for a sleep study, where measurements are taken overnight (these are usually done in your own home nowadays but can be done in a hospital sleep centre also). The results of this test did not show signs of OSA, and Rebecca continued to make lifestyle changes that eventually resolved her sleep disturbance during perimenopause.

Myth: You must not use screens before bed

You may have heard advice to avoid screens before bedtime. This has been associated in part with the blue light that screens emit. Blue light can suppress melatonin (the hormone that prepares you for sleep). However, the impact of blue light on sleep is much smaller than the impact of what is happening on the screen itself. For instance, the use of social media can ramp up comparison, anxiety and FOMO "fear of missing out." These can all increase alertness; we call this "heightened arousal".

For this reason, I do not think a blanket ban on screens is needed. It is how you use screens that matters. If you find a television programme relaxing, then it may be a good segue from a busy day/mind to a more relaxing nighttime sleep.

However, what is almost always true is that using a phone or other device to "doom scroll", use social media or to check work emails, can all be harmful to the night that follows, making it harder to fall asleep. Even watching the news before bed has been shown to heighten arousal in an unhelpful way.

Think about making some rules for yourself. Rebecca decided to keep the phone out of the bedroom, which helped her feel much more relaxed at bedtime. Perhaps you could try this too?

Myth: Sleeping pills are the best solution for menopausal sleep problems

So, we know how Rebecca improved her sleep with lifestyle changes and for Sangeetha HRT made all the difference. But what about Caroline? With no success from hormones or healthy habits, should she consider sleeping pills as a solution for her insomnia?

Sleep difficulties during menopause can be incredibly challenging and have negative consequences on all aspects of life. Treatment is really important, and for some people, this may mean using prescribed medication. However, there is another approach that is often more effective and longer-lasting than the impact of medication. The most effective and longest-lasting treatment for insomnia is called Cognitive Behavioural Therapy for Insomnia (CBT-I). This is a programme that usually lasts for 4–6 weeks and helps to restore healthy sleep by changing habits, thinking patterns and behaviours around sleep. It can be done using online programmes or books, in groups or one-to-one with somebody specially trained, such as a psychologist. This is the treatment that Caroline embarked on for her menopausal sleep difficulties. Caroline had tried various lifestyle changes: she had cut out caffeinated drinks, was doing more exercise and her sleeping environment and habits were healthy. Starting HRT had improved most of the other symptoms of menopause. But her sleeplessness was stubborn. It was as if she had developed a habit of *not sleeping* and she felt as though she had forgotten how to sleep normally. I referred Caroline to a psychologist who specialises in CBT-I. It was not always easy, and one of the techniques meant she needed to go to bed much later than her usual bedtime, which was a challenge. Gradually, Caroline could see improvements in her sleep, and after 6 or 7 weeks, she was managing to sleep through the night with only one or two brief awakenings. Her daytime energy was improved, and she stopped worrying about her sleep completely. One of the benefits of CBT-I is that it teaches you strategies that you can use in the future if things should go offtrack. CBT-I is the first-line recommended treatment for insomnia by the National Institute for Health and Care

Excellence. Many studies show it can be effective for women during the menopause transition. I often recommend this to patients, especially if their menopause symptoms are otherwise well controlled[7].

Myth: You just need to find the right sleep hack to solve your sleep issues

Many of us would love to find the one top tip or hack that would quickly and painlessly lead to consistently good sleep. Unfortunately, I am not sure that this exists for many of us. Improving our sleep quality or quantity is usually a combination of small techniques and lifestyle tweaks, and lasting improvements take time. Everybody has a different journey to sleep problems and the route back to healthy sleep will not be the same for everyone.

It is a sad truth that, unlike other lifestyle pillars of movement and nutrition, when thinking about sleep, effort does not equal output. Trying hard to sleep is often the opposite of what is needed. It is not physically possible to force yourself asleep – the body has to do that on its own. All we can do is set up the conditions that make it most likely. As hard as it sounds, sometimes the best thing we can do is take the pressure off ourselves and take comfort in the fact that we will be able to cope with what life throws at us, even having had suboptimal sleep.

Too often, I see people who have decided to live with their sleep problems, despite the problems causing them real distress and impacting their day-to-day quality of life and functioning. Sometimes this is because it feels like there are no good treatment options. I hope this chapter has helped you to see there are actually many approaches that can help with sleep during menopause. Sometimes it requires a trial-and-error approach, and they almost take longer to work than you would like, but please do not suffer alone. You can seek support from your doctor and discuss some of these options.

Summary

- Sleep issues are common during the menopause transition: about 40–60% of women experience sleep disturbances during menopause, with huge variations in experiences.
- Sufficient, good-quality sleep is essential for physical and mental health, cognitive function, immunity and cardiovascular health.
- There are multiple causes of sleep problems, including hormonal changes, the impact of menopause symptoms such as anxiety and nocturia, as well as other life stresses.
- Other sleep disorders, such as Restless Legs Syndrome (RLS) and Obstructive Sleep Aponea (OSA), are common during menopause and may require medical attention.
- Hormonal treatments like HRT can alleviate sleep issues.

- Lifestyle changes, including exercise and avoiding caffeine and alcohol, can improve sleep.
- It can be helpful to adapt your sleep environment to ensure it is dark and cool, and weighted blankets can be helpful for some women.
- Anxiety can disrupt sleep, but relaxation techniques, mindfulness and therapy can help manage it effectively.
- Cognitive Behavioral Therapy for Insomnia (CBT-I) is an effective long-term solution for insomnia during menopause.
- There is no one-size-fits-all solution or universal sleep hack; improving sleep often requires a combination of strategies and time. Seek support if you are struggling with sleep during menopause.

References

1 Baker FC, Zambotti M de, Colrain IM et al. Sleep problems during the menopausal transition: Prevalence, impact, and management challenges. *Nature and Science of Sleep* 2018 Feb 9; 10: 73–95.
2 Schaedel Z, Holloway D, Bruce D et al. Management of sleep disorders in the menopausal transition. 2021 [Internet]. [cited 2022 Jun 3]. https://journals.sagepub.com/doi/full/10.1177/20533691211039151.
3 Pan Z, Wen S, Qiao X et al. Different regimens of menopausal hormone therapy for improving sleep quality: A systematic review and meta-analysis. *Menopause* 2022 Jan 31; 29 (5): 627–635.
4 Lowe H, Haddock G, Mulligan LD et al. Does exercise improve sleep for adults with insomnia? A systematic review with quality appraisal. *Clinical Psychology Review* 2019 Mar 1; 68: 1–12.
5 Borbély AA, Daan S, Wirz-Justice A, Deboer T. The two-process model of sleep regulation: a reappraisal. *Journal of Sleep Research* 2016 Apr; 25 (2): 131–143. doi: 10.1111/jsr.12371. Epub 2016 Jan 14. PMID: 26762182.
6 Wimms A, Woehrle H, Ketheeswaran S et al. Obstructive sleep apnea in women: Specific issues and interventions. *BioMed Research International* 2016; 2016: 1764837.
7 Tal JZ, Suh SA, Dowdle CL et al. Treatment of insomnia, insomnia symptoms, and obstructive sleep apnea during and after menopause: Therapeutic approaches. *Current Psychiatry Reviews* 2015; 11 (1): 63–83.

Scene 3 Myths of menopausal health

Dr Nicky Keay

The more general effects on health of hormones changing with age tend to occur at a later stage in the female hormone odyssey, some years after initial menopausal symptoms. The delay is due to a cascade of effects. Changes in hormone patterns modify gene expression and the balance of protein production. This affects the activity of physiological systems, with subsequent longer-term implications for various aspects of health. For example, although bones are dynamic, the recycling of the whole skeleton takes about 8–10 years. The cumulative hormone changes over menopause have effects on multiple facets of health, some of which are shown in Figure 2.3.1.

What are the most common potential health consequences of menopause?

Myth 1 Is breast cancer the most common cause of death in menopausal women?

When women are asked what they believe is the most common cause of death after menopause, the majority think it is breast cancer. In fact, it is cardiovascular disease (CVD). CVD includes blockage of coronary arteries: coronary heart disease (CHD), causing a "heart attack" and/or blockage of the cerebral arteries causing a stroke. CHD accounts for twice as many deaths in women as breast cancer[1]. Before the retirement of the ovaries, oestradiol has a cardioprotective effect, which is why before menopause, women have a lower risk of CVD than men[2].

There are other consequences of the decline in ovarian hormones that contribute towards an increased risk of CVD[3]. Evidence shows that metabolic health is impacted, specifically blood glucose control and lipid profile, which contribute to the risk of CVD[4]. Cardiometabolic health covers the combination of these interlinked aspects of health.

The good news is that lifestyle factors can help mitigate the effects of menopause on cardiometabolic health and the subsequent risks of CVD and metabolic disease such as type 2 diabetes mellitus. Being active, taking regular exercise, making good nutritional choices and avoiding smoking or high alcohol intake all play an important part in supporting good cardiometabolic health. These lifestyle factors will be discussed in detail in Act 4 Mastering Menopause. There is also an interesting interplay between metabolic and mental health, which will be explored in more detail shortly.

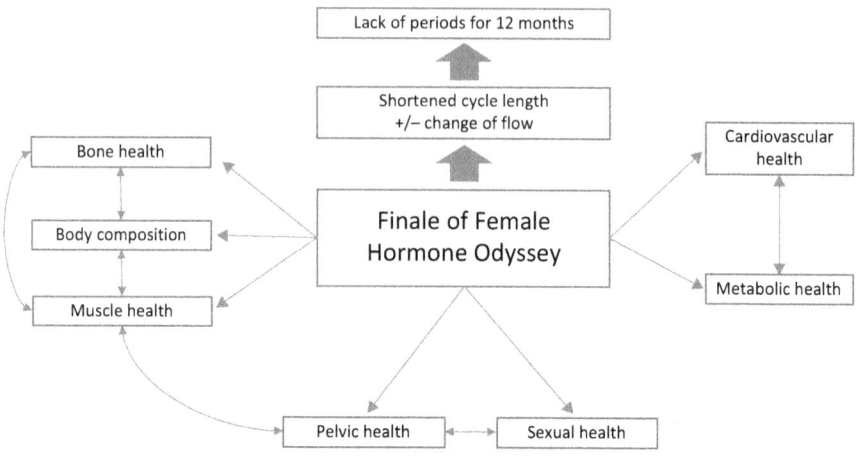

FIGURE 2.3.1 Multifaceted aspects of menopause health

Myth 2 What is the "silent killer" for menopausal women?

Unlike CVD, osteoporosis tends not to be fatal. Nevertheless, having brittle bones increases the risk of fracture, whether this is from a seemingly innocuous fall or the more insidious vertebral crush fractures of the spine. The consequences of weak bones have a massive impact on quality of life in terms of pain, difficulty moving safely, difficulty breathing with stooped posture and loss of height. Osteoporosis affects 1 in 3 older women and 1 in 5 older men[5]. Why are menopausal women at particular risk of this "silent killer"?

As described in Act 1, oestradiol rules supreme for bone health. The trajectory of bone mineral density (BMD) shown in Figure 2.3.2 matches the profile of oestradiol levels over the lifetime. There is a rapid increase during the teenage years associated with the start and establishment of menstrual cycles. This is mirrored by a permanent cessation of menstrual cycles with decline in oestradiol and BMD at menopause and beyond[6].

Bones are continuously being remodelled, effectively "recycled", with the whole skeleton being replaced every 10 years or so. Throughout life, there are two opposing processes happening in the skeleton: formation of bone, driven mainly by oestradiol and resorption or breakdown of bone. During the teenage years, as the reproductive axis comes to life, the balance sways greatly in favour of bone formation with rapid accrual of BMD to attain peak bone mass (PBM) in the early 20s in women. A balance between bone formation and resorption is maintained during the reproductive years, provided menstrual cycles remain regular. After the final period at menopause and decline in oestradiol, the balance swings in favour of bone resorption, as bone formation is attenuated in line with decreased oestradiol levels.

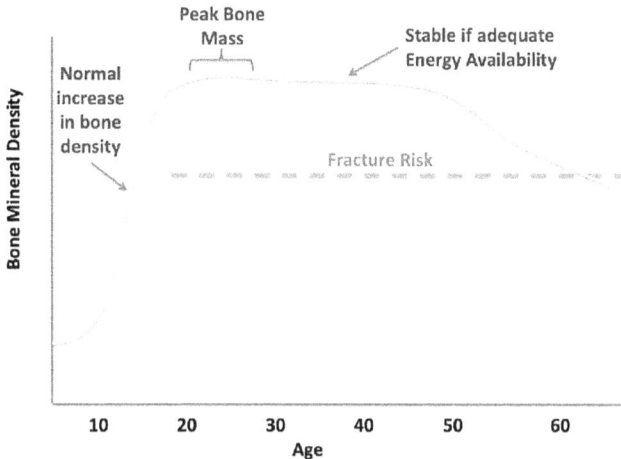

FIGURE 2.3.2 Change in bone mineral density with age. Hormones, Health and Human Potential. Keay 2022, Sequoia books

Why are men less at risk of developing osteoporosis than women? Men convert some of their testosterone to oestradiol for bone health. However, testosterone declines less dramatically in men after age 50 than oestradiol in women after menopause. The testes never fully retire like the ovaries. This means older men maintain a more consistent level of oestradiol compared with women.

This balance of power between bone formation and resorption with age is shown in Figure 2.3.3.

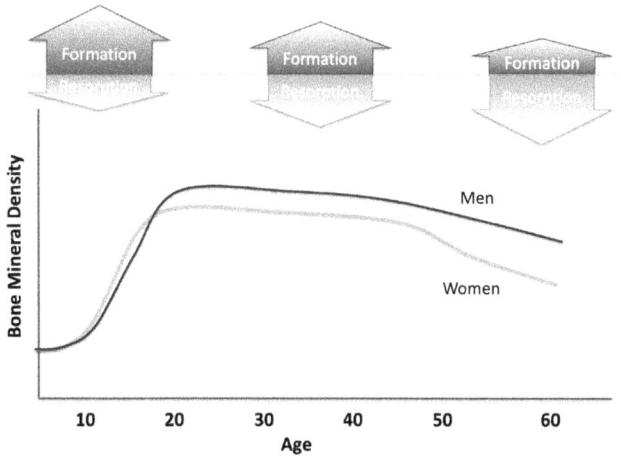

FIGURE 2.3.3 Bone turnover with age. Hormones, Health and Human Potential. Keay 2022 Sequoia books

The decline in other anabolic (tissue-building) hormones with age, such as growth hormone (GH), can also impact bone health both directly and indirectly. A decline in GH causes a change in body composition as there is decreased drive for skeletal muscle compared with fat deposition. The combination of loss in muscle mass and function (sarcopenia) and fat gain can potentially lead to a condition known as sarcopenic obesity. Furthermore, weaker muscles mean that there is less of a mechanical stimulus for bone formation.

The good news is that there are proactive steps you can take towards supporting bone health and mitigating fracture risk in terms of lifestyle, with exercise[7,8] and medication with hormone replacement therapy (HRT) being the mainstay[4]. Fractures are not an inevitable outcome of menopause.

References

1   British Menopause Society. Chapter 3 Long-term health conditions affecting postmenopausal health. In Hilard T, Abernathy K, Manoda H, Shaw I, Everett M, Ayres J, Currie H (eds), *Management of the Menopause*, Sixth Edition. British Menopause Society.
2   Stanhewicz AE, Wenner MM, Stachenfeld NS. Sex differences in endothelial function important to vascular health and overall cardiovascular disease risk across the lifespan. *The American Journal of Physiology-Heart and Circulatory Physiology* 2018; 315: H1569–H1588.
3   Ryczkowska K, Adach W, Janikowski K et al. Menopause and women's cardiovascular health: Is it really an obvious relationship? *Archives of Medical Science* 2022 Dec 10; 19 (2): 458–466. doi: 10.5114/aoms/157308. PMID: 37034510; PMCID: PMC10074318.
4   British Menopause Society Consensus Statement. Primary prevention of coronary heart disease in women. Accessed April 2024.
5   British Menopause Society Consensus Statement. Prevention and treatment of osteoporosis in post menopausal women. https://thebms.org.uk/wp-content/uploads/2023/10/06-BMS-ConsensusStatement-Prevention-and-treatment-of-osteoporosis-in-women-SEPT2023-A.pdf. Accessed April 2024.
6   Keay N. *Hormones, Health and Human Potential.* Act 1, Scene 7 Bare Bones. Sequoia Books, 2022.
7   Royal Osteoporosis Society. Strong, straight, steady. https://theros.org.uk/media/0o5h1l53/ros-strong-steady-straight-quick-guide-february-2019.pdf.
8   Watson S, Weeks B, Weis L et al. High-intensity resistance and impact training improves bone mineral density and physical function in postmenopausal women with osteopenia and osteoporosis: The LIFTMOR randomized controlled trial. *JBMR* 2018; 33 (2): 211–220. doi: 10.1002/jbmr.3284.

Scene 4 Don't let sticks, stones or falls break your bones!

Rebekah Rotstein

There are abundant visible and symptomatic changes we experience at menopause, but one of the most life-altering health shifts is a silent one that often goes unrecognised. The dramatic impact on bone health from loss of oestrogen is largely overshadowed by more immediately sensed disturbances like hot flushes, mood swings and vaginal irritation. We tend to triage the vasomotor and genitourinary symptoms, which in fact may dissipate over a number of years; yet decline in bone mass, which is all-too-often overlooked, never recovers on its own and can lead to devastating consequences in the future if not addressed.

This chapter is a call to action for bone health, a manifesto for movement and a reminder to take charge of your skeleton right now, to protect you and your independence for the years to come. Menopause is a time of major change, and it can also be a moment to revisit your beliefs and behaviours. Let's start with identifying several myths surrounding bone health and revealing the realities to see how you too could take action to avoid fractures.

Myth 1 Bone loss just affects older women

Most of us think of a skeleton as a static structure like what we see at Halloween. In reality our bones are living tissues, rich in nerve innervation, vascularised with blood supply and filled with cells that hold certain functions for the bone and other tissues of the body. As such, bones go through a metabolic process somewhat similar to an exfoliation during a facial. Think of it like a day spa for bones! Thanks to specific cells, old bone tissue is removed and replaced with new bone on an ongoing basis. This continuous process occurs throughout our lives, but the rate at which it occurs changes with age. When we're younger and culminating in our teenage years, we build more bone than we remove, which is what allows us to develop what is known as peak bone mass, a state we arrive at by our early 30s. At that point, we begin removing or destroying more bone cumulatively than we're developing. That's right – we all begin to lose bone mass in our 30s!

Around the time of menopause, this process takes a sharp turn, as the loss of oestrogen leads to much more bone removal than formation, sparking a dramatic decline in bone mass. It's estimated that we can lose up to 20% of our bone mass in the first 5–7 years after the menopause transition[1]. The rate of bone loss after that time levels off, but we continue to lose bone if there is no intervention to counteract it.

Bone loss is a natural part of ageing. But excessive bone loss is classified as osteoporosis. This is determined when bone mass drops to a specified marker, or when a fracture has occurred from a standing height or less.

Myth 2 Bone density is the only determinant of fracture risk

Let's first define osteoporosis and shed light on a missing piece that's often ignored. Many people think of osteoporosis as a disorder of low bone density, yet an early definition referenced by a 1994 World Health Organization report defined it as "a disease characterized by low bone mass **and microarchitectural deterioration** of bone tissue, leading to enhanced bone fragility and a consequent increase in fracture risk"[2]. In other words, bone density is part of the problem, but not the entire picture of osteoporosis.

Bone density is measured in terms of standard deviations below the mean of healthy young women around 30–35 years of age, provided in the form of a T-score. Most commonly performed through a test called a DEXA (dual energy X-ray absorptiometry), it's a *quantitative* measurement of mineralised tissue within a given area of the lower spine and hip (and sometimes forearm). Yet the DEXA has a number of shortcomings, including the fact that it's only a two-dimensional view, it can have variability among machines and technicians, it discriminates among those with small bones and can provide false readings in those with osteoarthritis in the measured areas.

Furthermore, the *qualitative* component of bone, including its microarchitecture and structural integrity, holds an important role that is not examined in the DEXA. This matters not only because the microarchitecture is part of that definition of osteoporosis, but because the majority of fractures occur in those with higher bone density in the range of osteopenia (the precursor to osteoporosis) rather than in osteoporosis itself[3].

For many years, qualitative measurements of bone have been restricted to research rather than used in clinical practice, but the last decade has given rise to greater availability of screening and diagnostic tools for assessing bone quality. While still not widely available as of 2024, they can be helpful in providing greater insight into the structure of the bone and its ability to withstand fracture.

A helpful assessment tool is the Fracture Risk Assessment Tool (FRAX), an algorithm anyone can access online using the hip bone mineral density score and other risk factors to calculate a 10-year probability of a fracture of the hip and also a major osteoporotic fracture. Bone turnover markers, measured in blood and urine testing, are also useful tools that a physician can order to identify metabolic activity of the bone. Used in conjunction with the DEXA, which is still the gold standard for bone density screening, these other tools and tests can paint a broader picture of the state of your bones.

Bone measurement story

When Maria first contacted me, she panicked that her previous DEXA classified her as having osteoporosis in her spine and borderline osteopenia in her hip. I looked closely at the DEXA report, beyond just the cover page, to examine the T-score at each vertebral level of the spine and different aspects of the hip. She was a 62-year-old woman with a small body frame, no fractures or loss of height, and I wondered if the size of her bones influenced the density reading. I recommended that at her next upcoming DEXA, she obtain a Trabecular Bone Score, which offers a qualitative measurement of the spine in conjunction with the DEXA. The results of this showed better bone quality with a higher score than her DEXA alone, indicating only osteopenia in her spine.

Myth 3 Having osteoporosis means you will fracture a bone

As we identified in Myth 2, the diagnosis of osteoporosis is usually based solely on your bone density, which at times can be misleading or not reflect the actual strength of your bones, which stems from more than just their mineralisation. Collagen plays a significant role in the tensile strength of bone tissue and ensures that bones that are hard are not also brittle. Yet like other qualitative elements of the bone, collagen is not depicted in a DEXA.

All this to say, that just because you have a diagnosis of osteoporosis does not mean you'll experience a fracture. As we also pointed out in Myth 2, more fractures occur in the higher bone density range of osteopenia than in that of osteoporosis. Does the diagnosis of osteoporosis matter? Yes. But you should also filter this through a wider lens and recognise action steps to take to improve your chances of remaining mobile and independent.

First, if you smoke, stop. Nicotine interferes with various bone-regulating activities from bone formation to calcium absorption. Next, identify key nutrients needed in your diet and ensure you're obtaining sufficient protein intake to meet the needs of muscle and bone maintenance or even growth. If possible, work with a nutritionist or dietitian to help you and determine if supplementation is appropriate. Next, engage in exercise and daily movement as a means of adding the necessary stress to your bones to fortify them and also to protect them against future fractures via strength and balance training. (More on this in the next myth!) Monitor your sleep and stress levels; a deficiency in the former and abundance of the latter can wreak havoc on your bones. Additionally, meet with a physician, or an endocrinologist specifically who is the most common type of specialist to treat osteoporosis, to rule out any underlying conditions via lab work. Have a discussion about hormone therapy to see if you're a candidate to preserve bone tissue and discuss whether treatment is appropriate for you.

Remember, osteoporosis isn't a death sentence. Unlike other pathologies, say cancer, it does not have a clear path. That said, it does require that you step in to change the course of your health. In my case, I was diagnosed with osteoporosis when I was 28 years old, thankfully without the occurrence of a fracture as a warning sign. While I'd prefer not to have had the experience of fear, anxiety and despair from that initial diagnosis 20 years ago, I am indeed grateful that it was a wake-up call to make change – and to change the path of my health.

Story of bone health anxiety

Leslie approached me as a 56-year-old, long-time Pilates teacher, who followed a healthy lifestyle but had been told by her physician that she had osteoporosis and warned that she might easily fracture. Terrified by this and by hearing that certain spinal motions of forward bending needed to be eliminated to avoid fracture, she moved with excessive caution and lived in a state of panic, expecting her bones to break when simply walking down the street. After learning her medical history and other risk factors, I framed the reality of her situation that the state of her bones was likely no different that week than the week prior, BEFORE she'd had the diagnosis when she'd lived freely and joyfully. The only difference was the knowledge of this diagnosis. While I adhered to safety precautions in movement with Leslie, mindful not to include exercises that might put her spine at risk, I reassured her not only verbally but through example that her body was indeed strong. She worked with a nutritionist to look at her diet, and in the last few years she met with a physician to run various tests, which identified an overactive parathyroid contributing to high bone turnover. She addressed this medically, and throughout our 15 years together, I progressively challenged her through a variety of skills. To this day, she's never had a fracture, and her confidence in her body is restored.

Myth 4 Heavy weightlifting is the only way to support bone health through exercise

Recent years have seen a proliferation of discussions about lifting heavy weights for women at perimenopause and after the menopause transition. Research has shown the importance of lifting heavy weights to maintain and build muscle mass, combat insulin resistance, boost metabolism, benefit brain and heart health and of course improve bone mass.

What does it mean to lift "heavy"? And how is weightlifting different from strength training? Strength training is a form of exercise to increase muscle strength using some form of resistance, mostly commonly seen with gravity, weights or resistance bands. A key principle of strength training is known as progressive overload, which identifies the importance of continuously increasing the stimulation over time to overcome adaptive musculoskeletal changes and sustain the challenge in order to avoid plateau.

Weight training is a form of strength training and enables the possibility of much higher loads from external weights than would be achievable with your body weight alone, or even with the use of bands. Lifting heavy refers to weightlifting at a high intensity that would only involve up to 5 or 6 repetitions of an exercise and perhaps up to 5 sets of those. A common example of performing 3 sets of 8–12 repetitions would be classified as moderate intensity[4].

In the bone health research, an important study known as the LIFTMOR trial was published in 2018, which found that heavy lifting could not only maintain but also increase bone density in postmenopausal women with osteoporosis and osteopenia with little adverse effects[5]. This was exciting news for many who had been previously warned against lifting weights more than 10–20 pounds for fear of inducing a fracture, and it's been empowering for many women to also discover strength gains they had no idea they were capable of.

The study, like others using weight training for this population, has excluded those with certain conditions, which obviously complicate the research, but at the same time may be a reality for many in the general population. And that includes those with localised back pain and those who've experienced a fracture in the last year, and sometimes longer. For these women, and others with various health conditions and other injuries, lifting heavy is not usually advised.

Access is an obstacle to heavy lifting that many cite. The research demanded supervision for this style of weightlifting, which not only requires a trainer but typically also gym membership, as it eventually requires higher loads than most people have access to at home in the absence of a home gym.

Newer research will be comparing the effects of moderate versus heavy lifting to identify any difference in bone density changes between the two. And while increasing bone density is ideal, maintaining it through exercise can be a respectable goal as well, since bone density can decline 1% per year without activity and other interventions.

Ultimately, our goal is not to increase bone density but to prevent fractures. And that includes training balance and agility for fall prevention, since falls remain the leading cause of fragility fractures. We may or may not feel unsteady in daily activities currently, but the challenge will only become greater as we age. A 2021 study called the Medex trial showed that improvements in muscle strength, balance and function could be achieved in a low-intensity setting for postmenopausal women with low bone mass[6].

The Royal Osteoporosis Society 2022 Consensus Statement, Osteoporosis Canada's 2023 Guidelines, the Bone Health and Osteoporosis Foundation (the United States) and Healthy Bones Australia all call for not only progressive muscle strengthening (including back extension exercises to strengthen the spine and prevent falls) but also impact exercises at varying degrees of intensity depending on fracture history to stimulate the bones, along with mobility, balance, posture and functional training for fall prevention and as part of a multimodal approach to bone health.

Ideally, we all should lift as heavy as we can. But for those who can't due to physical, socioeconomic, geographic or cultural reasons, or for personal preference choose not to, know that engaging in some form of exercise and physical activity that involve weight-bearing resistance training and impact, along with balance practice, mobility, agility and coordination are essential. For those who wish to learn to lift heavy, it's important to recognise that form is critical to prevent injury, and that progression is key.

Many of us in midlife also experience joint pain and have other conditions ranging from osteoarthritis to tendinopathies. This makes it essential to also address the fascia, the important yet greatly ignored connective tissue of the body. We need to hydrate it through motion and release restrictions that lead to stiffness, pain, misalignment and potential injury, while also integrating it within full body movement to enhance performance. Body conditioning as such improves health and longevity.

Story of exercise for fracture prevention

At age 50, Shania wanted to improve her exercise regimen in her plan to fight osteoporosis. But with a history of low back pain, hip tenderness and a previous frozen shoulder, she was concerned about how to start and worried about flare-ups. I ran her through a number of assessments and observed her movement patterns to identify fascial restrictions, deficiencies in mobility and strength and deficits of motor control (coordination and sequencing of muscle activation). Together we worked on her body mechanics and organisation with how she moved and coordinated different motions, improved the hydration of soft tissues and increased her joint range of motion in restricted areas. She developed better core control and then greater strength through exercises using bodyweight, resistance bands and weights by continuously increasing the challenge. She also consistently engaged in balance training, which progressively became harder with tasks and drills that also simulated real-life activities. Eventually, she added elements of speed, power training and high impact. Two years later, she is living pain-free, hiking every weekend and fearlessly lifting weights 2–3 times a week.

For the exercise averse and the adrenaline junkies alike, we can all find common ground in engaging in activities we enjoy. The most important physical activities we can do are those that we WILL do, and do consistently, with variety included. Don't be intimidated by exercise that is foreign to you. Partake in what's available to you, but also be curious to inquire about options you're unfamiliar with.

Myths surrounding bone health abound and we could tackle many more. But hopefully these examples illuminate several key misconceptions that frequently arise and provide answers to common questions. Fractures are not inevitable after menopause, and we can truly change the trajectory of our bone health.

References

1   Bone Health and Osteoporosis Foundation. https://www.bonehealthandosteoporosis.org/preventing-fractures/general-facts/what-women-need-to-know/. Accessed May 2024.
2   Assessment of fracture risk and its application to screening for postmenopausal osteoporosis. Report of a WHO Study Group. *World Health Organization Technical Report Series* 1994; 843: 1–129.

3   Camacho PM, Petak SM, Binkley N et al. American Association of Clinical Endocrinologists/ American College of Endocrinology clinical practice guidelines for the diagnosis and treatment of postmenopausal osteoporosis-2020 update. *Endocrine Practice* 2020 May; 26 (Suppl 1): 1–46.
4   American College of Sports Medicine. American College of Sports Medicine position stand. Progression models in resistance training for healthy adults. *Medicine & Science in Sports & Exercise* 2009 Mar; 41 (3): 687–708.
5   Watson SL, Weeks BK, Weis LJ et al. High-intensity resistance and impact training improves bone mineral density and physical function in postmenopausal women with osteopenia and osteoporosis: The LIFTMOR randomized controlled trial. *Journal of Bone and Mineral Research* 2018 Feb; 33 (2): 211–220.
6   Kistler-Fischbacher M, Yong JS, Weeks BK et al. A comparison of bone-targeted exercise with and without antiresorptive bone medication to reduce indices of fracture risk in postmenopausal women with low bone mass: The MEDEX-OP randomized controlled trial. *Journal of Bone and Mineral Research* 2021 Sep; 36 (9): 1680–1693.

Scene 5 Menopause mix: metabolic and mental health

Dr Anne Latz

On metabolism and mind

Our body and our mind are inseparable. They constantly talk to each other, flooding our bodies with micro signals of neurotransmitters, hormones and other messengers in an unstoppable process of communication and feedback. This can lead to a complicated mix of signals we try to interpret day in, day out. This system needs to recalibrate in various phases of our lives, perimenopause being one of them. Sometimes the language of the body gets louder, when we do not listen or cannot make sense of it. Our body shows symptoms especially in those phases in which the mind struggles to find words for our feelings, sorrows, unconscious conflicts and if it encounters imbalances. Symptoms can be various pains, uncontrollable body functions or more subtle our daily struggles to manage weight and a stable mood. What we experience can be aggravated in challenging life phases of hormonal alterations such as the perimenopausal transition. While hormones sometimes are the loudest voice in the crowd, they are not the only one. The term "psychometabolic health" underscores the bidirectional relationship between mental well-being and metabolic function. Psychological stressors can trigger the release of stress hormones, affecting metabolism and potentially contributing to conditions such as insulin resistance or metabolic syndrome. Conversely, metabolic imbalances, such as intense fluctuations in blood sugar levels, can immediately impact mood and cognitive function. Once we understand the delicate mix of metabolism and mindset, we can master it – in perimenopause and beyond.

Metabolic health – our body's energy crisis

The dialogue between mental and metabolic health starts in the womb – a stressed mother flooding her baby with stress hormones, puts it at greater risk for obesity[1] and continues along the whole life cycle. Truth is: For women the only constant is change. Change in hormones, moods, how our bodies feel or how we feel in our bodies. This is no hokum but based on measurable and complicated hormonal dances. We never stop being detectives reading clues of our bodies. As women enter perimenopause, hormonal fluctuations become more pronounced. The decline in oestrogen levels can impact metabolism and how the body handles blood glucose. Oestrogen is crucial in maintaining metabolic health, and its reduction can lead to changes in fat distribution (increase in fat mass and reduction of lean, fat-free mass), associated weight gain especially around the abdominal area and changes in insulin sensitivity as well as an increased risk of metabolic conditions such as type 2 diabetes[2]. Truth is: We do see significant changes in metabolic and body composition indices in the menopause transition. Especially for women who are already overweight or obese this adds a significant burden[3]. This change in body composition and hormones also makes it harder to manage your blood glucose via exercise or nutrition routines which might have worked so well for you over the last decades. Your energy management is in crisis mode. Blood sugar peaks and dips might occur, leading to hunger urges and cravings, contributing to even more body weight issues. This crisis can be addressed via psychometabolic interventions and strategies based on all five pillars of lifestyle medicine (mind-body-practices, nutrition, exercise, sleep, connectedness). Therefore, it is important to understand the psychological changes associated with this metabolically challenging phase.

Mood changes in menopause

When it comes to women, their emotions and their mood, we are quick to "blame the hormones". Is this justified? What happens with mood and mental health when entering perimenopause? Truth is: The aforementioned hormonal changes of our dynamic duo oestrogen and progesterone can influence mood, and the psychological response to body composition changes can, in turn, affect metabolic health. The hormonal fluctuations can disrupt the delicate balance of neurotransmitters in our brain, which regulate your mood. The phase of perimenopause is not merely a physical transition; it has profound psychological implications with feelings of anxiety, depression and lability in affects and mood being common symptoms.

Why so anxious?

The connection between anxiety and menopause is multifaceted, involving hormone changes, psychological factors and the overall life transition that menopause represents. During this transition, various hormonal shifts can contribute to the emergence or exacerbation of anxiety symptoms. Oestrogen plays a role in regulating neurotransmitters like serotonin and norepinephrine, which are associated with mood. The decrease in oestrogen levels may contribute to imbalances in these neurotransmitters, potentially leading to increased anxiety. Additionally, common symptoms of menopause like hot flushes or night sweats can be physically uncomfortable and disruptive to sleep, contributing to increased stress and anxiety. Sleep disturbances, in particular, can have a significant impact on mental well-being. As already mentioned, menopause often coincides with changes in body composition and the natural ageing process. Some women may experience feelings of loss or changes in self-esteem, contributing to psychological distress and anxiety. In a bigger picture menopause represents a significant life transition, often accompanied by reflections on life achievements and losses, future goals and changes in roles, families and relationships. These midlife changes can trigger existential and identity-related anxieties. All these factors might be especially severe in women with a history of anxiety and mood disorders, making them more susceptible to experiencing anxiety symptoms during menopause. Additionally, environmental stressors or life events can contribute to anxiety during this phase.

It's crucial to recognise that experiences of menopause vary widely among women. While some may navigate this phase with minimal or no anxiety, others may find it more challenging, some getting into a severe crisis. Open communication with trusted people, self-awareness and seeking support when needed are essential steps in managing anxiety during menopause. Healthcare professionals can provide personalised interventions tailored to your individual needs. The options span from self-care practices and new hobbies to psychotherapy which can be beneficial in addressing anxiety symptoms and providing coping strategies. Seeking guidance from a healthcare professional is essential when the symptoms severely impact your quality of life.

Why so sad?

The association of menopause and feelings of low mood and depression is similar to the rise of anxiety symptoms. Psychosocial factors, such as life changes, societal expectations and the ageing process, also contribute to the association between menopause and depression. The challenges associated with transitioning to a postreproductive stage of life, coupled with societal attitudes towards ageing, can contribute to psychological distress. It is important to stress that not all menopausal women will suffer from clinical depression. A history of mental health struggles is a risk factor. Feeling under water and overwhelmed during this phase of life is normal to some extent and can be addressed by lifestyle changes.

What is mostly unknown is the psychometabolic aspect of mental well-being, particularly the effect on risk and severity of depression. Metabolic health conditions like obesity and insulin resistance, causing chronic low-grade inflammation may contribute to depressive symptoms by affecting neurotransmitter function. Hormonal dysregulation, including diurnal cortisol variation, seen in both metabolic disorders and depression, further connect these issues. Poor metabolic health, with disruptions in neurotransmitter balance and mitochondrial dysfunction (hello, energy crisis), can contribute to mood disturbances. Lifestyle factors, such as a sedentary lifestyle and poor diet, play a dual role in both metabolic disorders and depression, emphasising the importance of adopting healthier habits to promote overall well-being. Addressing these interconnected factors means a holistic approach to mental health and metabolic well-being. A tangible example is blood glucose management as a potential way to directly impact cognitive function and stability in mood[4]. Maintaining stable blood glucose levels is essential for providing a consistent energy supply to the brain, which is vital for optimal cognitive performance and emotional well-being. Poor blood glucose control, often seen in conditions like diabetes but also due to lifestyles based on unbalanced diets, may contribute to mood swings, irritability and difficulty concentrating, underscoring the importance of effective blood glucose management for overall mental health[5,6,7]. Lifestyle interventions can improve mental well-being by addressing metabolic imbalances. But how exactly can this work?

A delicate mix: psychometabolic changes

The intricate relationship between mood and metabolic health is evident and easiest to understand in the impact of stress on the glucose metabolism. Feeling stressed or anxious about changes in body composition can trigger the release of cortisol, a stress hormone. Cortisol is a steroid hormone produced by the adrenal glands, and its secretion is regulated by the hypothalamus-pituitary-adrenal (HPA) axis. Oestrogen plays a role in modulating the activity of the HPA axis, which, in turn, affects cortisol secretion. The decrease in oestrogen can impact the regulation of cortisol, potentially leading to alterations in cortisol levels. Furthermore, menopausal symptoms itself can be a source of physiological stress. Symptoms like sleep disturbances can disrupt the natural circadian rhythm. Cortisol follows a diurnal pattern, typically peaking in the early morning and declining throughout the day. Sleep disruptions can alter this pattern, affecting cortisol levels. Same for vasomotor symptoms like hot flushes. These can activate the body's stress response and trigger the release of stress hormones, including cortisol, as a reaction to the perceived stressor. While being high on cortisol can cause uncomfortable feelings like being jittery, on edge and anxious, it also continuously affects the metabolism.

Elevated, unvarying, cortisol inhibits the release of insulin and stimulates the release of glucose – two mechanisms contributing to a high level of blood glucose. Interestingly, cortisol levels may exhibit less diurnal variation in menopausal women, potentially exacerbating the challenges of managing blood glucose levels. As a result, increased blood sugar levels may lead to increased fat storage, particularly around the abdominal area. This not only contributes to more weight gain – one origin of the stress and rise in cortisol – but also heightens the risk of metabolic disorders, themselves being a risk factor for depression. The entry point into a potential vicious cycle. Chronic elevation or disruption of cortisol levels can have implications for overall health, including metabolic health and immune function. Breaking this cycle requires a holistic approach that addresses both the physical and psychological aspects of menopause-related changes. Lifestyle modifications, stress management techniques and psychological support can play crucial roles in promoting overall well-being during this transitional phase.

What you can do to the mix?

Understanding the complex interplay between hormonal changes, daily stressors and metabolic as well as psychological symptoms during menopause is crucial. We learnt that physiological and psychological changes are common in menopause – and closely connected. We can only master a dance if we know the steps. Here's where it gets interesting: managing your blood sugar levels can give a short-term solution to address symptoms of those hard-to-control hormonal changes. Good news: The blood glucose dance is easy to learn. And will impact mental and metabolic well-being. It is known that hot flushes are associated with higher insulin resistance[8] and insomnia is aggravated by diets with high glycaemic load[4]. Understanding hormonal influences on metabolism and blood glucose handling is essential for developing strategies to manage weight and promote overall health and mental well-being during and after menopause.

In other words, taking care of yourself by implementing changes along your lifestyle pillars will help you ride the wave of perimenopausal change more easily and benefit your well-being. Best news: Perimenopause may be the most opportune window for lifestyle intervention, with the onset of unfavourable body composition and metabolic characteristics being a key motivator for lifestyle changes.[9] Empowering yourself with knowledge about the intricate connections between hormones, metabolism and psychological well-being is crucial for navigating the challenges of menopause. Being active and having a healthy weight might be protective for your mental health[10]. And if you are feeling less anxious or blue, you will be able to more easily embrace lifestyle changes. By adopting a comprehensive and proactive approach, you can embrace this life stage with resilience, prioritise your health and well-being and choose positive changes for a vibrant and fulfilling postmenopausal life.

There are five pillars to promote psychometabolic health

- **Mind-Body Practices:** Stress reduction techniques are key to smoothing out those mood swings. When stress is high, it's like driving a car with a lead foot on the gas pedal – things can get a bit out of control. Find activities that help you unwind and relax, like deep breathing exercises, meditation or engaging in hobbies you enjoy. Prioritising self-care and setting aside time for yourself can work wonders in managing stress and promoting emotional well-being. Incorporate mind-body practices such as meditation, deep breathing exercises or mindfulness meditation into daily routines to manage stress and enhance emotional well-being.
- **Nutrient-Dense Diet:** Prioritise a nutrient-dense, balanced, blood-sugar-friendly diet that supports metabolic health and provides essential nutrients for optimal brain function. Focus on a well-balanced diet rich in whole foods, lean proteins, fruits, vegetables (leafy greens!) and whole grains. Avoid excessive consumption of processed foods and added sugars. Include all food groups on your plate (cover your carbs with proteins and fats, e.g. from nuts, fatty fish) and make sure to include fibre (veggies, seeds) in every meal as a starter. Start your day with a savoury meal and sufficient protein. Movement like a 10-minute walk can help to balance your blood glucose after a meal. For snacking: Dark chocolate with high cocoa content contains flavonoids, caffeine and antioxidants. Those can enhance mood.

- **Regular Exercise:** One powerful weapon for mental and metabolic health is regular exercise! Exercise releases endorphins, those fabulous feel-good hormones that can boost your mood and reduce stress. Aim for at least 30 minutes of moderate-intensity exercise most days of the week. It could be a brisk walk, a dance class or even some yoga – whatever gets you moving and brings you joy. Move regularly as it not only supports metabolic health but also has positive effects on mood and cognitive function. Engage in a mix of aerobic and strength-training exercises to boost metabolism, maintain muscle mass and support overall metabolic health.
- **Adequate Sleep:** Just like your car needs a regular service, you need high-quality sleep to rest and perform optimally. Aim for 7 to 8 hours of sleep per night and establish a consistent bedtime routine. Create a calm and comfortable sleep environment, limit caffeine and electronics before bed and practise relaxation techniques to help you unwind. Establish healthy sleep habits to ensure sufficient, restorative sleep, promoting hormonal balance and cognitive function. If you are sleepless in bed, get up, do some reading or housework and then go back to bed when feeling tired.
- **Social Connections:** Foster positive social connections and seek support from friends, family or support groups and health professionals to enhance emotional resilience and well-being and provide a sense of connection during this transitional period. A mental health professional might be helpful to address the psychological aspects of body image and self-esteem during menopause.

Remember, everyone's journey through perimenopause is unique, so finding what works best for you is essential. In essence, psychometabolic health is about recognising and nurturing the intricate relationship between mental and metabolic well-being. By adopting a comprehensive approach that addresses both sides of the conversation, you can optimise your overall health and lead a fulfilling life that integrate the strengths of both mind and body – also in times that feel challenging right now.

The only constant is change.

Judith's Perimenopausal Journey

Background

Judith, a 55-year-old woman, working as an accountant for the last 30 years, began experiencing significant changes in her physical and emotional well-being as she entered perimenopause at the end of her 40s. One of the prominent challenges she faced was unexplained weight gain and heightened anxiety.

Symptoms

- *Weight Gain: Judith noticed a gradual increase in her weight, particularly around her abdomen. The number on the scale did not bother her as much as the way her abdomen started to feel soft and shapeless. Despite maintaining her regular exercise routine and being mindful of her diet, shedding those extra pounds became increasingly challenging.*

- *Anxiety:* Alongside the physical changes, Judith began experiencing heightened anxiety levels. She found herself feeling overwhelmed, restless and at times, struggling to manage daily stressors that she had previously handled with ease. At night she often lay awake, worrying about her children who now live far away. Also, she felt more tense before work and felt her heart racing just when her boss called her. This led to emotional eating to release stress and to reward herself after a stressful day, especially when being alone. This left her with a feeling of losing control.

Thoughts and Concerns

Judith felt frustrated and puzzled by the weight gain, as her lifestyle hadn't undergone significant alterations. She was also concerned about the impact of anxiety on her overall well-being. After her binges she felt full of shame, tried to eat secretly and argued with her inner critic every meal. These changes were affecting her confidence and quality of life, leading her to seek guidance and solutions at her GP.

Potential Solutions and Strategies

- *Mind-Body Practices:* Judith joined a yoga group focusing on yin techniques to calm her nervous system.
- *Nutritional Counselling:* Judith sought the advice of a nutritionist to reassess her dietary choices. Together, they explored nutrition strategies that could support her metabolism during this transitional phase. She learnt to include more proteins in her diet.
- *Exercise Adjustments:* Judith modified her exercise routine to better align with her changing metabolism. Incorporating strength training and aerobic exercises tailored for her age and hormonal profile became essential. She found help at her regular gym to build a training schedule.
- *Sleep Hygiene:* By establishing a sleep routine starting one hour before actually planning to sleep, Judith found a way to wind-down without being confronted with blue light and news tools. Also, she decided to get out of the metro one stop earlier to get in some morning daylight which helped to boost her melatonin, plus to get some extra steps.
- *Community Support:* Judith joined online support groups or sought guidance from friends who had gone through similar experiences. Sharing experiences and tips to eat in a "healthy" way with others navigating perimenopause helped alleviate feelings of isolation and provided valuable insights.

Outcome

Through a holistic approach Judith gradually experienced positive changes and self-efficacy. She got back a feeling of control about her actions and thoughts. Over time, she noticed a gradual improvement in her weight as well as her acceptance of her body, and her anxiety levels significantly decreased. Judith's journey highlighted the importance of personalised strategies based on different lifestyle pillars to address the unique challenges of perimenopause.

References

1 Tate EB, Wood W, Liao Y et al. Do stressed mothers have heavier children? A meta-analysis on the relationship between maternal stress and child body mass index. *Obesity Reviews* 2015 May; 16 (5): 351–361. doi: 10.1111/obr.12262. PMID: 25879393; PMCID: PMC4447110.
2 Cornier MA, Dabelea D, Hernandez TL et al. The metabolic syndrome. *Endocrine Reviews* 2008 Dec; 29 (7): 777–822. doi: 10.1210/er.2008-0024. Epub 2008 Oct 29. PMID: 18971485; PMCID: PMC5393149.
3 Fenton A. Weight, shape, and body composition changes at menopause. *Journal of Mid-life Health* 2021 Jul–Sep; 12 (3): 187–192. doi: 10.4103/jmh.jmh_123_21. Epub 2021 Oct 16. PMID: 34759909; PMCID: PMC8569454.
4 Gangwisch JE, Hale L, Garcia L et al. High glycemic index diet as a risk factor for depression: Analyses from the Women's Health Initiative. *American Journal of Clinical Nutrition* 2015 Aug; 102 (2): 454–463. doi: 10.3945/ajcn.114.103846. Epub 2015 Jun 24. PMID: 26109579; PMCID: PMC4515860.
5 Breymeyer KL, Lampe JW, McGregor BA et al. Subjective mood and energy levels of healthy weight and overweight/obese healthy adults on high- and low-glycemic load experimental diets. *Appetite* 2016 Dec 1; 107: 253–259. doi: 10.1016/j.appet.2016.08.008. Epub 2016 Aug 6. PMID: 27507131; PMCID: PMC515860.
6 Cheatham RA, Roberts SB, Das SK et al. Long-term effects of provided low and high glycemic load low energy diets on mood and cognition. *Physiology & Behavior* 2009 Sep 7; 98 (3): 374–379. doi: 10.1016/j.physbeh.2009.06.015. Epub 2009 Jul 2. PMID: 19576915; PMCID: PMC2775046.
7 Penckofer S, Quinn L, Byrn M et al. Does glycemic variability impact mood and quality of life? *Diabetes Technology & TherapeuticsDiabetes Technol Ther* 2012 Apr; 14 (4): 303–310. doi: 10.1089/dia.2011.0191. Epub 2012 Feb 10. PMID: 22324383; PMCID: PMC3317401.
8 Thurston RC, El Khoudary SR, Sutton-Tyrrell K et al. Vasomotor symptoms and insulin resistance in the study of women's health across the nation. *Journal of Clinical Endocrinology and Metabolism* 2012 Oct; 97 (10): 3487–3494. doi: 10.1210/jc.2012-1410. Epub 2012 Jul 31. PMID: 22851488; PMCID: PMC3462945.
9 Gould LM, Gordon AN, Cabre HE et al. Metabolic effects of menopause: A cross-sectional characterization of body composition and exercise metabolism. *Menopause* 2022; 29 (4): 377–389. doi: 10.1097/GME.0000000000001932.
10 Barghandan N, Dolatkhah N, Eslamian F et al. Association of depression, anxiety and menopausal-related symptoms with demographic, anthropometric and body composition indices in healthy postmenopausal women. *BMC Women's Health* 2021; 21: 192. doi: 10.1186/s12905-021-01338-w.

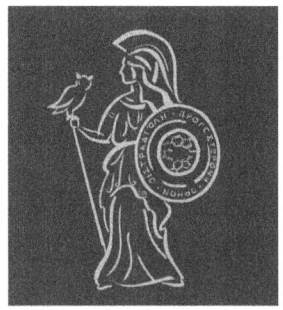

Act 3

Menopause, Sex and Pelvic health

The metamorphosis of Aphrodite

Act 3 Menopause, Sex and Pelvic Health

The metamorphosis of Aphrodite

Dr Nicky Keay

Aphrodite is the Ancient Greek goddess of love, lust, beauty, pleasure, passion and procreation. In the *Iliad*, the Trojan War began after Paris, the prince of Troy, chose Aphrodite as the fairest of three goddesses competing to win the golden apple. After the ensuing turmoil, the Odyssey describes the many challenges a more mature Odysseus overcame on his 10-year journey home, driven by the enduring love he shared with his wife, Penelope.

During her life, every woman experiences a metamorphosis in her personal Aphrodite. Although the element of procreation dwindles during menopause, many aspects remain. Platonic love and physical love endure and transform. The hormonal changes intertwined with this transition can present some physical and psychological challenges. This Act explores the important aspects of menopausal health, focusing on pelvic and sexual health.

Scene 1 No sex after menopause?!

Dr Shema Tariq

Can sex be hot, despite the hot flushes?

Watching TV recently, I found myself almost whooping and punching the air when I saw Jodie Foster (playing a weary, middle-aged cop in Alaska) having joyful, hot sex with someone she wasn't in a relationship with. An old-school booty call. In that moment, I realised how rare it is to see women past the age of 50 portrayed as unashamedly enjoying sex, without any negative connotations.

Is it really true? Do women stop having sex when they turn 50?

Well, no. In 2016, a survey of around 10,000 people in the United Kingdom aged 50 and over found that half of women had been sexually active in the past year. Breaking it down further, two-thirds of women aged 50–59 had had some type of sex in the past year; a very impressive one-in-seven 80+ year olds reported some sexual activity[1].

Ageism and misogyny mean that sex and older women is a taboo subject. Society doesn't view us as sexual, something that's brilliantly parodied by Amy Schumer in the "Last F**kable Day". In this sketch, Schumer comes across Patricia Arquette, Julia Dreyfus and Tina Fey celebrating Dreyfus' official 'last f**kable day' in Hollywood. They tell the younger Schumer how film crews rush them through filming sex scenes before a milestone birthday because *"they think your vagina is going to turn into a hermit crab."* It's both hilarious and painful, even for those of us who aren't Hollywood actresses.

Let's be clear here. Women continue to be sexual beings well into their 50s, 60s, 70s, 80s and 90s. They desire, are desirable and are desired. Using my experience as a sexual health and menopause doctor, I'm going to tackle five myths about sex and menopause.

Myth 1 It's only sex, it's no big deal

> Maya, 52, came to see me in my sexual health clinic. Everything "down there" was itchy and uncomfortable and she wondered if she had an infection. This had been going on for a couple of years now. Sex was painful and she couldn't remember the last time she'd had it, or even the last time she felt like she wanted it.

She hadn't had a period since she was 49. She'd not felt like herself for a few years. We talked. The tears fell. Maya told me how she'd lost her confidence at work. She'd become forgetful and would cry easily, especially when she had hot flushes. She didn't understand what was happening to her and in the end, she'd decided it was better to leave the job she loved. Now she found herself lonely at home, ruminating over the past and avoiding friends. She'd never felt this low before.

Maya deeply grieved the loss of sex and intimacy between her and her husband. He was a kind, supportive and patient partner. She felt guilty that she couldn't be a sexual partner to him anymore and wondered if she should end her marriage or tell him to find a lover. She loved her husband dearly. She missed the sex they had. She missed how sex made her feel about herself.

Maya's story isn't unusual. Over half of women aged 45–60 in the United Kingdom have experienced a sexual problem[2]. We'll get to the reasons for this later. Sexual problems have negative physical and emotional impacts on women, and on their partners and relationships.

In 2018, an international panel of experts got together to develop a vision of sexual and reproductive health rights, demanding that sexual health and well-being be recognised as a central part of people's lives. Their report highlights the importance of bodily autonomy, and the freedom to *"pursue a satisfying, safe, and pleasurable sexual life, free from stigma and discrimination"*[3]. Basically, we *all* have the right to enjoy sex, regardless of who we are (including our age and gender).

We know that sex is good for our physical health. It's good for our heart health, reduces our blood pressure and has even been shown to be good for our immune systems. All of these things become even more important as we get older. Studies have also shown that older adults who stay sexually active are happier than those who don't. For people in relationships, sex increases intimacy and bonding, and improves the quality of relationships. And let's not forget that sex is a form of self-expression and is often a lot of fun.

Peri and postmenopausal women should never feel that issues they are having with sex are no big deal. My job as a sexual health doctor is to support people to have the sex they'd like (happily, safely and healthily), whether they're 16 or 60.

Myth 2 Problems with sex are all in our minds

"Midlife sex slump."

"Health issues and sex in older age."

"Easing painful sex after menopause."

"Sex after menopause is, well, complicated."

If you believe Google (which threw up these pretty depressing headlines), it's all downhill for your sex life when you reach menopause. I definitely don't want to add to this negative view of sex after menopause, but we can't get away from the fact that, for many people, menopause brings physical changes that can impact our sex lives.

Oestrogen plays a really important part in pelvic health. It keeps the tissues and muscles in the pelvis strong, flexible and well-lubricated, and our vaginal walls healthy and moist. When oestrogen levels drop in menopause, it can lead to vaginal dryness, weak pelvic floor muscles and urinary issues. All of these physical changes can make sex uncomfortable and painful and make it more difficult to get aroused. We also experience a drop in testosterone levels, affecting our libido, lubrication, arousal, mood and energy levels.

On top of this, other physical symptoms of menopause (hello hot flushes, difficulty sleeping, muscle aches and tiredness), mean that sex may not feel as easy or as comfortable as it did when we were younger.

The more we understand the physical realities of our bodies as we get older, the more empowered we'll be to find solutions that work for us.

Myth 3 Problems with sex are all in our bodies

OK, so there are physical reasons why sex may not feel as good or not be happening at all. The science of sexual desire helps us understand the role of our brains in all of this. Emily Nagoski, sex educator and author of *Come as You Are*, has helped shine a light on the *"dual control model"* of sexual response[4].

For most women, sexual desire doesn't come out of nowhere. Generally, we don't suddenly feel horny. Instead, there's a delicate balance between our sexual accelerator (the sexual excitation system) and our sexual brakes (the sexual inhibition system) in our brains. Accelerators, or "ons", might include seeing a partner's body, being touched, novelty and trust. Brakes, our "offs", could be things like body image, depression, anxiety, pain, sleep deprivation, relationship conflict, an ever-growing to-do list. Our accelerators and brakes are highly individual, varying both in intensity and what factors trigger them. To complicate things even further, our accelerators and brakes work differently in different contexts. For example, being touched by a partner in bed after a date night is almost certainly going to be received more positively than being touched whilst arguing over whose turn it is to put the laundry away. Same touch, different context, very different response.

Menopause can bring a lot of "offs". Mood changes, changes in our body affecting our confidence, lack of sleep, hot flushes and relationship conflict. Menopause also often coincides with becoming part of the "sandwich generation", where people with children and ageing parents find themselves frankly knackered having to care for everyone. It's not hard to see why this is a time in our lives where the balance is tilted more heavily to offs than ons, and sex goes off the agenda.

Myth 4 This is all way too embarrassing and maybe we just need to live with it

Sexual problems are common during and after menopause. Over 80% of women will experience vaginal symptoms because of menopause, it's just that no one talks about it. It's no good ignoring these symptoms as they don't go away on their own. I have good news though – here are some pretty simple solutions:

1. Find a lube that feels good for you and use it, liberally, during sex.
2. Take time to get properly aroused – use toys, touch yourself, let your partner(s) touch you. And remember that sex does not have to mean penetration – do whatever feels comfortable for you.
3. Use a vaginal moisturiser regularly (special lotions formulated just for vaginas that help restore elasticity and lubrication – think of them as Crème de le Mer for vaginas).
4. Talk to your doctor about vaginal oestrogen. This can be given as a tablet in the vagina or as a cream and have virtually no side effects. They are a much lower dose of hormones than standard hormone replacement therapy (HRT) but relieve symptoms for most women if used regularly.
5. There are some newer medications that your doctor can talk to you about if none of these things work.

Other symptoms of menopause such as hot flushes and mood changes can be managed with changes to lifestyle, which is covered in other chapters, as well as hormone replacement therapy (HRT) for those who would like to take it. Addressing these other symptoms may get rid of some of the sexual brakes we talked about earlier in the chapter.

We also need to understand, accept and lean into our individual sexual desire styles. The majority of women, especially as they get older, have *responsive* rather than *spontaneous* sexual desire. This means we only want to have sex once we've been stimulated or aroused. We need to take time to gear up for sex and allow desire to build. There's nothing weird, wrong or less sexy about this. Both types of desire are normal; it's just that spontaneous sexual desire is what gets all the attention in films and books, leaving us with unrealistic expectations of what sex is. Understanding how desire works, thinking about how we dial up our 'ons' and dial down our 'offs', and communicating all of this with sex partners, are the keys to rediscovering joyful sex.

Finally, once this is all in place, and you're enjoying hot sex again, remember to do it safely. Sexually transmitted infections (STIs) are on the rise in older people, so use condoms, get an STI test and think about contraception if your period was less than 12 months ago because, yes, you can still get pregnant (I say this from personal experience having had a surprise baby in my mid-40s)!

Myth 5 Good sex looks the same for everyone

Sex is whatever floats your boat. One of the many joys of getting older is having the experience and confidence to assert what we want sexually. This might not mean penetration. This might not be heterosexual sex. This might be sex with multiple partners, maybe all at the same time. This might mean long-standing kinks, or the freedom to try new ones. Enjoy and explore your sexuality without shame.

It might also mean the freedom to decide *not* to have sex. I'm reminded here of Kristin Scott Thomas' glorious monologue about menopause in Series 2 of Fleabag, which she ends by turning down Fleabag's advances:

> "Honestly, I can't be arsed darling. I'm going to go back to my room and have one more martini."

Conclusion

> "She wore her sexuality with an older woman's ease, and not . . . like an awkward purse, never knowing how to hold it, where to hang it, or when to just put it down."
>
> Zadie Smith in White Teeth[5]

It's not surprising that sex often becomes tricky as we get older. The physical effects of ageing and changes in hormones, coupled with busy and pressured lives, can have negative impacts on our sex lives. As with so much of menopause, the key to navigating this hormonal and social shift is to be empowered with information. You have a right to healthy and happy sex, and you are deserving of help and support to get there. Maybe honest conversation like this will get us to a point where the sexuality of older women is finally recognised and celebrated in all its forms.

References

1. Lee DM, Nazroo J, O'Connor DB et al. Sexual health and well-being among older men and women in England: Findings from the English longitudinal study of ageing. *Archives of Sexual Behavior* 2016 Jan; 45 (1): 133–144. doi: 10.1007/s10508-014-0465-1. Epub 2015 Jan 27.
2. Toorabally N, Mercer CH, Mitchell KR et al. Association of HIV status with sexual function in women aged 45–60 in England: Results from two national surveys. *AIDS Care* 2020 Mar; 32 (3): 286–295. doi: 10.1080/09540121.2019.1653436. Epub 2019 Aug 14. PMID: 31411046; PMCID: PMC7034538.
3. Starrs AM, Ezeh AC, Barker G et al. Accelerate progress-sexual and reproductive health and rights for all: Report of the Guttmacher-Lancet Commission. *Lancet* 2018 Jun 30; 391 (10140): 2642–2692. doi: 10.1016/S0140-6736(18)30293-9. Epub 2018 May 9. PMID: 29753597.
4. Nagoski E. *Come as You Are*. Simon & Schuster, 2015.
5. Smith Z. *White Teeth*. Penguin Books, 2001.

Scene 2 Goodbye to pelvic health after menopause?!

Dr Gillian Cambell and Christien Bird

The only way is UP!

Background

What is pelvic health and why does it matter?

When we search the internet for a definition of 'pelvic health', the results commonly include symptoms associated with disorders of the pelvic floor muscles such as incontinence (bladder and bowel), pain and pelvic organ prolapse. But pelvic health is so much more, as described by *The Center for Research on Women with Disabilities.*

> *"Pelvic health is the best possible functioning and management of the bladder, bowel, and reproductive organs. It is not merely the absence of disease or weakness in these organs. Pelvic health plays an important role in complete physical, mental, social, and sexual well-being"*[1].

Most pelvic health physiotherapists would go even further and not only include health related to the joints and tissues within and around the pelvis but would say it involves the overall health, emotional and physical well-being of the individual.

Why is pelvic health so important?

Function related to and within the pelvis is integral to everything we do:

 The pelvic organs (bladder, bowel, uterus and ovaries) are integral to reproduction and the elimination of waste, both urine and faeces. The uterus, vagina and vulva are not only essential for reproduction but also for our sexual experience, which, for many women, is an important part of maintaining their relationships.

 The pelvis is central to the control of our movement: the way we stand, walk, run and dance. It connects the lower limbs to the spine and as such is integral to maintaining control in our posture, gait and mobility.

Key anatomy

The pelvic floor is the name for a complex of muscles situated within the bottom of the pelvic cavity (Figure 3.2.1). It is sometimes described as a hammock of muscles and tissues that support the abdominal and pelvic organs when we are upright. They are connected to the pubic bone at the front, the coccyx (tail bone) at the back and the ischial tuberosities (sit bones) to the side. When we contract our pelvic floor, the muscle fibres shorten, which pulls our bowel, vagina and urethra forwards and upwards in a scooping action as seen in Figures 3.2.2 and 3.2.3. It is important that our muscles can not only contract when we need them to but also that they relax when we do not. This movement is an integral part of our ability to maintain continence.

Further the pelvic floor muscles, working in synchrony with the abdominal muscles and the deeper muscles of the spine, provide important support to our spine and the joints of the pelvis as we move and change position.

In summary, the pelvic floor complex supports the pelvic organs, controls voiding and in conjunction with muscles in the back, abdomen and around the hips, controls lumbo-pelvic movement. In a nutshell, it is an essential part of your body, and like the engine in a car, it requires regular maintenance and attention to ensure smooth running. There are key times in women's lives when the maintenance should be optimal and may benefit from a 'full service': puberty, childbearing years and the menopause. This is why we believe that including a chapter regarding pelvic health is a key part of any book about menopause.

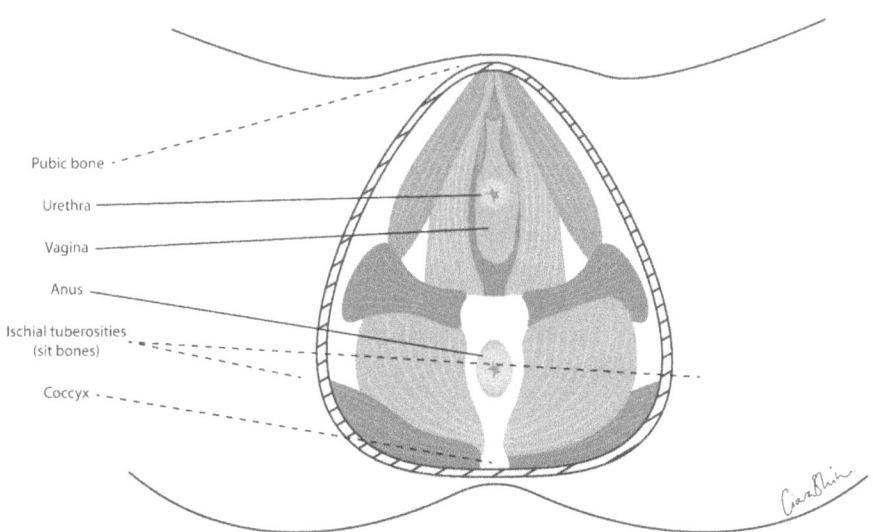

FIGURE 3.2.1 The pelvic floor muscles

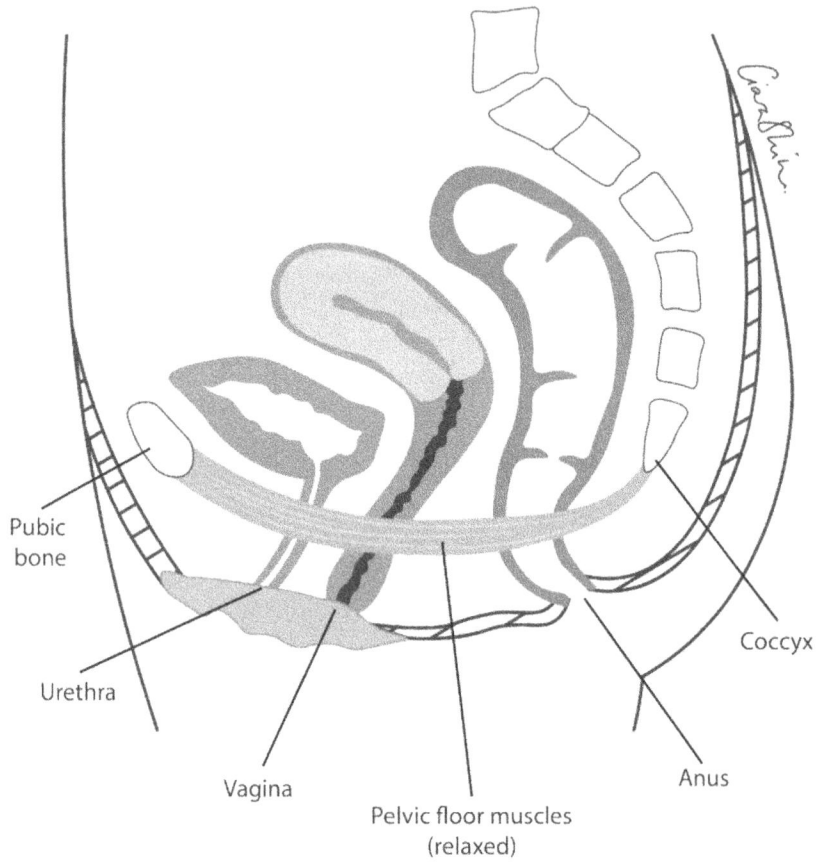

FIGURE 3.2.2 The pelvic floor muscles in a relaxed position

In our clinical experience, many women are very good at 'putting up with symptoms'. Our key message is that there are no medals to be won for putting up with incontinence, pain, recurrent infections or prolapse. Talk to your GP or go and see a specialist pelvic health physiotherapist[2]. Do not give up on your pelvic health, no matter your age. If you have already tried pelvic floor muscle exercises and they didn't work, no matter what, do seek help. There is so much we can do to help manage your symptoms.

Common pelvic health myths

Myth 1

"Since the menopause I can no longer comfortably ride my bike as none of the bike saddles seem to suit me."

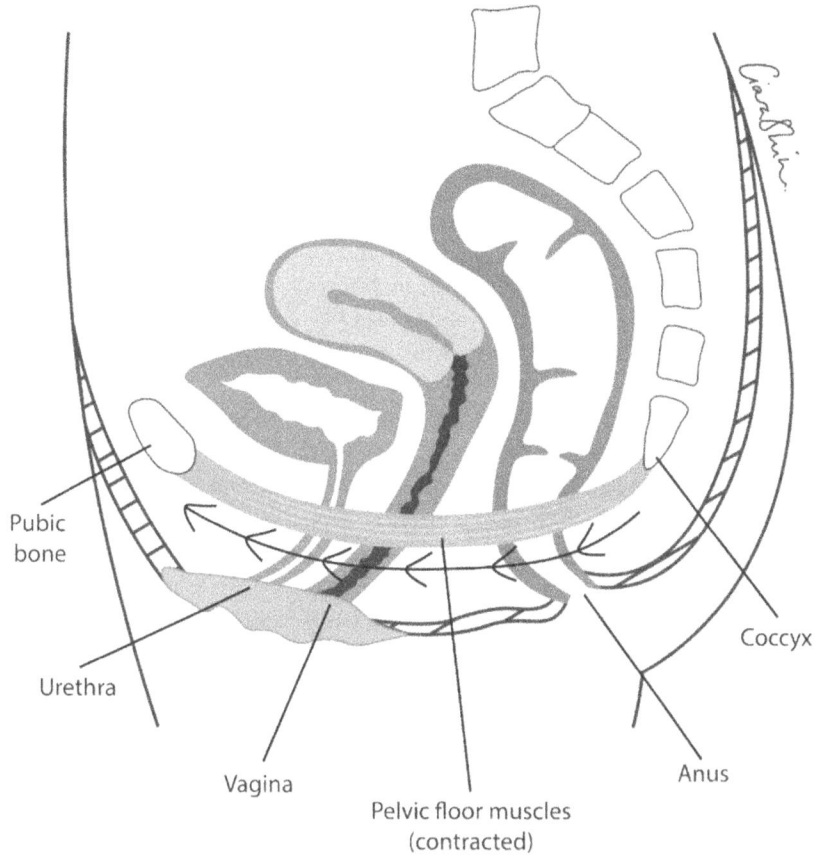

FIGURE 3.2.3 The pelvic floor muscles in a contracted position

Meet Jo:

- A 52-year-old competitive cyclist
- Recent onset saddle pain, despite many years of pain-free cycling prior to menopause.
- Tissue irritation with sex and even with tight jeans!

Jo had been training and racing on her bike for many years and had no saddle issues since her first bike-fit and new saddle at the age of 40. She stopped having regular periods at the age of 47 and initially struggled with common menopausal symptoms such as hot flushes and night sweats. She also experienced weight gain, joint pain and stiffness throughout, as well as some fatigue and brain fog. After being referred to a gynaecologist who specialised in menopause, she was prescribed a low dose of HRT (oestrogen patches and a Mirena® coil) and most of her symptoms had resolved. Five years later, when she attended our clinic, she was still on regular HRT.

Over the previous two years, she had noted increasing issues with saddle pain which occurred after she had ridden her bike for anything over 40 minutes. Initially, she thought that her saddle was probably worn and replaced it with a new version of the same model. She had checked her position, the padding on her shorts and ensured that she used plenty of her usual saddle cream, but was still struggling. Prior to attending the pelvic health physiotherapy clinic, she had paid for another bike fit, this time with a physiotherapist. This fit had included pressure mapping, which enabled the fitter to see how small adjustments to her position and even her shoes and cleat positions, could help to distribute the pressure more evenly. While this had improved her symptoms a little, the saddle pain and tenderness continued.

Presenting problem: Perineal pain associated with cycling after only 40 minutes of riding – lasting for two days. Some irritation from underwear after being on the bike and inability to have sexual intercourse due to the irritation and pain.

No other pelvic health issues, such as bladder or bowel symptoms or heaviness (sometimes associated with a prolapse) were reported.

Assessment: Jo had not ridden her bike for the week before her appointment, and so her vulval tissues were intact, although the skin was noted to be thin. There was some reddening of the skin of the inner and outer labia (just inside the vulva). While able to contract her pelvic floor muscles, she was unable to fully relax them on the left. The pelvic floor muscles on the left side were tense and tender to the touch.

We diagnosed Jo with genito-urinary syndrome of the menopause (GSM), with some associated pelvic floor muscle dysfunction (increased muscle tone on her left side).

What changes and why

GSM, previously known as uro-genital atrophy or vulvo-vaginal atrophy[3] is a common condition of the menopause. Symptoms may start years after the onset of the menopause, so it is common for women not to appreciate that it is associated with menopause at all and to accept it as an unavoidable part of getting older.

Symptoms can be miserable, and so much more than just vaginal and vulval dryness. They may include a watery discharge, pain during sex and general discomfort as well as bladder issues such as urgency, increased frequency and recurrent infections. Women describe general pain, itching, discomfort with walking and some are unable to tolerate wearing a favourite pair of jeans, or, as in Jo's case, a previously comfortable bike setup may just not be bearable anymore.

Reduced oestrogen levels are the primary cause of these symptoms, causing changes in the tissues, the vaginal microbiome and the blood flow to the area as a whole.

Reduced collagen and elastin cause the tissues in the area to become thinner and less elastic, ultimately, in some, causing loss of vaginal length and size. As the top layer becomes thinner, it becomes more vulnerable to damage and the rate of repair is reduced.

When the vagina is healthy, the top layer of cells that line the vagina (superficial mucosa) is shed regularly, releasing large amounts of a sugar called glycogen, which breaks down further into glucose. This process enables the healthy bacteria (lactobacilli) to flourish and convert the glucose into lactic acid, maintaining a healthy vaginal pH of 4.0–4.5. During and after menopause, as oestrogen levels reduce, the amount and regularity of cell turnover diminish, and as a result of this, there is a reduction in glycogen levels and healthy bacteria. Other bacteria, such as *Staphylococcus* and *Streptococcus*, have the opportunity to flourish. Vaginal secretions are reduced and become thinner, resulting in dry, irritated tissues and discomfort[4]. Altered bacterial levels cause the usually acidic pH of the secretions to rise to >5 which can in turn make us more vulnerable to infections, particularly those of the urinary tract infections (UTIs).

An online survey in 2019[5] reported that vaginal dryness was experienced by 35% of all women participating; starting with 26% in the youngest group, from 45 years old, and increasing up to 42% in the 60 to 65-year-old age group. These numbers are reflected in clinical practice.

Despite effective treatment being available, affordable and safe, a large European study reported that urogenital atrophy remains underdiagnosed and undertreated in the United Kingdom[6]. Despite up to 80% of the women presenting with symptoms, they are often not diagnosed as GSM. It is important to reiterate that GSM affects all genital tissues: the clitoris, the labia (outer lips of the vaginal opening), introitus (entrance to the vagina), urethra (tube from the bladder to the outside) and bladder and will not spontaneously resolve unless treated[7].

Many women appear to consider symptoms of GSM a natural age-related process and may consider the symptoms not severe enough to mention to their healthcare professional because they hope that the condition will resolve spontaneously.

The good news is that it can be treated and that the treatment is effective!

Topical vaginal oestrogen is a safe and effective treatment for most women and can quickly improve the health of the tissues and reduce many of the symptoms.

What about the loss of elasticity?

Early studies suggest that pelvic floor muscle training may also have a significant part to play in the management of symptoms of GSM, indicating that regular structured pelvic floor exercises can improve the blood flow to the area and consequently improve vulvo-vaginal elasticity[8]. Further, regular pelvic floor muscle training enables our pelvic floor muscles to contract, relax and respond when we need them.

In a nutshell, improving the tissue with local oestrogen combined with supervised pelvic floor muscle training is what many pelvic health physiotherapists consider to be the gold standard treatment.

Treatment for Jo:

Jo responded well to topical oestrogen prescribed by her GP. This is often in the form of tiny pessaries that are inserted with an applicator. They are designed to stick to the vaginal wall, slowly releasing the oestrogen directly into the environment where it is needed. Topical oestrogen can also be prescribed as a cream or as a gel. In Jo's case, applying the cream directly with her finger proved to be the most effective means for her, allowing her to direct it to the areas that she felt needed it most. She also learnt to contract her pelvic floor muscles effectively and then to fully relax them. The combination of oestrogen and pelvic floor muscle training enabled her to return to her regular training on the bike with minimal discomfort. She felt much more like her old self!

Myth 2

"It is normal to lose bit of wee, 'that oops moment', after we have children and especially as we get older, after all this is what adverts tell us!"

Meet Lesley:

- 53-year-old park-runner.
- Weight gain due to menopause sparked a return to running, 'Couch to 5k', then Parkrun.
- Stress urinary incontinence related to running and coughing or sneezing.

Lesley had previously enjoyed running regularly in her youth, even competing in a few 10 km races. After the birth of her two children when she was 30 and 32, she had stopped due to lack of time. Her periods had stopped at the age of 50 and other than a few hot flushes, she had noticed remarkably few menopausal symptoms other than a little weight gain, particularly around her middle. She decided that, now her children were grown, she would return to running and had hoped that this would help her to lose the extra weight. She started very gently, following the programme in the 'Couch to 5k' App. All had gone well until this year when a friend had encouraged her to come along and join the local Parkrun. She loved the camaraderie and general atmosphere but had noticed that her underwear became damp after the first 2–3 km. She was really keen to continue with Parkrun but was devastated at the thought of wearing a pad for the rest of her life: *"After all this is normal when we get older, just look at all the adverts and this is just the beginning?"*

Presenting problem: SUI is related to running and sometimes with coughs and sneezes. Little or no leaking when running alone or if only running for 10–15 minutes. Otherwise, she was fit and well and felt that the running had started to improve her general health and mental well-being. She even felt better toned, if not any lighter. Despite two vaginal deliveries, Lesley had recovered quickly from both births and had not noted any pelvic floor symptoms at that time. She had done her 'pelvic floor exercises' for the first few months after each delivery as advised by the midwife but had not really thought about it till now.

Assessment: All lumbopelvic movements were full and pain-free. However, when asked to stand on one leg, she struggled to stand up tall and straight on either side. On assessing her pelvic floor muscle function, she was able to contract her muscles from the back to the front as we would hope but struggled to maintain and repeat the contractions. By the fifth contraction the muscle strength had reduced by 50%. When we reassessed her pelvic floor muscle contraction while standing, both the strength and endurance were reduced to around 10%.

We diagnosed SUI due to weakness and poor endurance in the pelvic floor muscles, potentially further compromised by reduced control around the lumbopelvic region and hips. Effectively, while Lesley's muscular control around the pelvis is sufficient for most of her day-to-day functions, such as walking, work and even steady jogging, as soon as she challenged the control by increasing the load (running speed combined with talking and laughing), her muscles failed to respond to the impact from her running.

What changes and why

Our kidneys produce urine all the time and this drains via the ureters to a muscular bag, the bladder. The urine is stored here until it is convenient for us to go to the toilet and pee, via the urethra. The mechanism that keeps us dry is believed to be multi-factorial[9] meaning that it is unlikely in most cases that there is only one direct cause for leaking. For the purpose of simplicity and to guide rehabilitation, however, let's start by thinking about the muscles that control our continence. There are two sets of small muscles that wrap around the urethra, the urethral sphincters. Further, the main part of the pelvic floor muscles (levator ani) is also a huge factor in our control.

It is generally suggested that when the pressure in the bladder becomes greater than what the muscles can withstand, we can leak. This increase in pressure can be associated with anything that raises our intra-abdominal or pelvic pressure overall, such as coughing, sneezing, jumping, running and for some even bending over.

It has been proposed that part of the problem for some may be due to reduced support around the neck of the bladder or the urethra[10] and that improving the overall function of the pelvic floor muscles may help to stabilise these structures. In one study, the runners who leaked were actually shown to have stronger, quicker contracting muscles than the runners who were dry, but at rest, the bladder neck sat lower in those women who leaked[11]. This theory is the rationale for using pessaries to help maintain continence. These are small silicone devices which are placed inside the vagina and are designed to support the bladder neck and push the urethra forward towards the pubic bone. Many women find these really helpful for preventing leaking with exercise, in particular.

Although we are not yet completely sure about the full mechanisms, we do know that pelvic floor muscle training can be very effective in improving urinary incontinence symptoms for many women[12]. (See Figure 3.2.4).

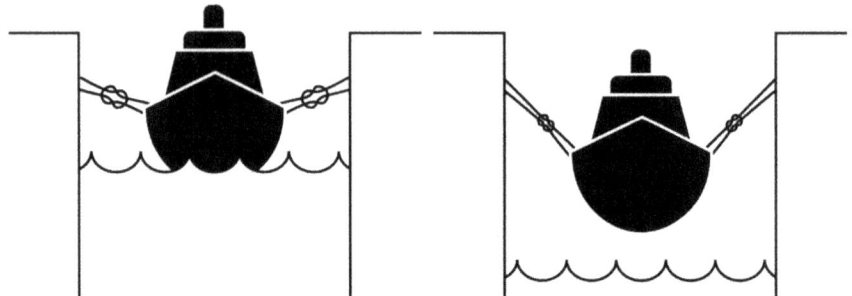

FIGURE 3.2.4 Boat in dock to represent pelvic organs, ligaments, muscles sitting in the pelvic cavity

The reality is that we require all the pelvic supports, for example, both passive (the fascia and ligaments) and active (the pelvic floor muscles), to be functioning well to maintain continence.

It is really important at this point to note that symptoms such as SUI are incredibly common and affect many women of all ages. Studies investigating the rates of SUI in young elite athletes who have never had children reported that the athletes were nearly three times as likely to experience SUI than women who didn't take part in sport[13]. However, in a recent internet survey involving nearly 1,600 women, where 70% of participants reported urinary incontinence, those exercising at a recreational level were no more likely to report leaking than those who didn't exercise at all[14]. Activities involving high impact can cause leaking, but this does not in itself tell us that high impact is a risk to the pelvic floor. Former elite athletes are no more likely to report a problem later in life than women who are not athletic[15]; however, it may be that some women have an increased predisposition to developing symptoms. Given the huge benefits of taking part in exercise in general, it is important to seek help for your symptoms to enable your return to sport and exercise for your overall health and well-being.

Treatment for Lesley: Rehabilitation started with general pelvic floor muscle training to improve both the overall strength and importantly, the endurance of her muscles. As this improved, she also worked on her general lumbopelvic control with exercises to help activate and strengthen the other muscles around her hips and pelvis, making them more effective.

Rehabilitation was progressive, starting with easy non-weight-bearing positions and then progressing to weight bearing and more functional work such as lunges, hopping and even work on wobble cushions to challenge reactivity. As with any musculoskeletal 'injury', return to her main preferred activity was the main goal. As her muscular endurance, strength and control improved, we also factored in gradual increases in her running loads. This was in the form of increased distance, increased speed and more challenging terrain. It is important not to introduce all types of loading at once but rather gradually change and progress one at a time.

She improved well and over time was not only able to increase the distance she could run and maintain continence but also gradually increase her speed. She noted her biggest success was being able to take part in a local fun run, laughing and joking with friends as she ran, staying dry and achieving a 5k personal best!

Myth 3

"It is normal to need to go to the toilet all the time and sometimes leak, as we get older. I am too old to strengthen my pelvic floor anyway."

Meet Rosie:

- 89-year-old, living on her own, independently
- Walking with a Zimmer frame indoors; outdoors uses a mobility scooter.
- Extensive medical history
- Most troublesome symptom: urinary urgency associated with massive leaking.

Rosie booked in for a pelvic health assessment, arriving on her mobility scooter, fiercely independent. Although her medical history was extensive and complex, her main issue was losing her confidence to go out as she was experiencing sudden, strong bladder urges, and if she didn't make it to the loo in time, she experienced urinary incontinence that could wet the floor. This was impacting her independence and freedom more than any of her other medical conditions. She was managing this by not drinking and going to the loo to empty her bladder 'just in case' regularly. She was referred to a continence service but was not getting on with the prescribed pads and had given up using them.

Most of us are familiar with that eye-watering desire to pee, that key-in-the-door moment of pure panic that you might not make it to the toilet in time. This strong desire is called a sensory urge and not making it in time and leaking urine is called a motor urge. Motor urge is when your bladder muscle contracts before you have given it permission to do so, more like the reflex bladder response we see in babies. This is when the bladder starts behaving like an untrained puppy, and sometimes is referred to as overactive bladder. We can often change this, as overactive bladders can respond well to pelvic floor strengthening and bladder retraining.

The relationship between the bladder muscle (the detrusor) and pelvic floor muscles is agonist-antagonist, like your biceps and triceps. When you want to bend your arm, your biceps contract and automatically your triceps relax to allow the movement. When you contract your pelvic floor muscles, there is a similar neural pathway to relax your bladder, which is a helpful strategy when you feel a strong urge. We can facilitate a similar relaxation of the bladder by sitting on a hard chair or crossing our legs to apply pressure to the perineum. It is called the perineo-detrusor inhibitory reflex.

How does this work?

In essence, the empty bladder is a muscular bag sitting within the pelvic cavity and collecting urine, which is produced as the kidneys filter the blood to remove waste. As the bladder fills, it expands and extends above the rim of the pelvis. Stretch receptors in the wall of the bladder are triggered to fire as the pressure rises, and this is what we perceive as the urge or the need to go to the toilet. If it is not appropriate for us to empty our bladder at that time, and we contract our pelvic floor for 8–10 seconds, the reflex causes the wall of the bladder to relax and the bladder to continue filling. We normally go through a series of these episodes before finally going to the toilet to urinate. Once ready and sitting on the toilet, we relax our pelvic floor muscles and the smooth muscle in the bladder wall starts to contract. It will continue contracting until there is no more urine, either in the bladder itself or in the urethra.

The detrusor and pelvic floor muscles working in synchrony are vital to maintain continence. In some cases, the pelvic floor muscles may have a higher level of activity than is ideal and then have difficulty releasing. At other times, they may be weak or not strong enough to control the bladder. There is light at the end of the tunnel; muscles can be retrained at any age.

It is worth mentioning that there is some evidence that women who have urge incontinence sat for significantly longer periods than the women who were dry. So there appears to be a clear link between sitting and experiencing urgency-related urinary incontinence, even for women who are physically active[16]. Don't get comfortable on the couch, at least not too comfortable!

Assessment: Initial observation of the vaginal and vulval tissue in Rosie's case showed signs of GSM. As we discussed before, local vaginal oestrogen is safe and effective for most women[7]. Although her pelvic floor muscles were weaker than ideal, she was still able to contract them and once aware of how these contractions should feel, she felt confident to work on her strength and endurance at home.

Management for Rosie

It took quite a few months before Rosie's tissue started to look healthier. As previously mentioned, pelvic floor muscle training has also been shown to help elasticity[8] of the tissue. Rosie was motivated and committed to do both. Other strategies for Rosie were to increase her fluid intake and stop going 'just in case' so frequently. For 'a good quality pee' you want a reasonably full bladder, giving the detrusor muscle a chance to fully empty and communicate effectively with the pelvic floor.

She started her bladder training at home; when she felt the initial urge, instead of rushing to the loo, she would sit on a hard surface and regain control, then move to the toilet at a normal pace. Another tool in the box can be distraction, for example, counting or mental maths. Depending on how good your mental math is, for most of us, starting from 100 and counting down in 7s is distracting enough for the bladder urgency to lessen.

Although she continued to experience a small amount of urinary leakage, she would no longer wet the floor and felt confident to go out again using only a small pad. In her words, *"the untrained puppy is back on the lead,"* she is back in charge of her bladder.

Myth 4

"I have only given birth by caesarean section so I can't possibly have any issues with my pelvic floor."

Meet Catherine:

- 45-year-old perimenopausal woman for the last two years
- Symptoms of heaviness and dragging, worse by the end of the day and some associated tissue discomfort with tight jeans or leggings.
- Mild symptoms previously associated with just before a period but recently had become worse as her periods became less regular.

Catherine was a mother of two children born, respectively, ten and twelve years previously. Both children had been delivered by caesarean section. The eldest was an emergency operation, but the second caesarean section was planned due to her previous experience. Postnatally, she had not experienced any pelvic floor symptoms, but she had been advised nonetheless to practise her pelvic floor exercises by the midwife. Initially, she had tried to remember, but with everything healing so well and having only had caesarean deliveries, she had not felt it would be important for her to continue. After all: *"If I've only given birth by caesarean section so I can't possibly have any issues with my pelvic floor."*

She had returned to work part-time as a teacher when both children had started school and as a result spent most of her time at work on her feet, carrying heavy piles of books and a laptop from room to room and back home at the end of the day. Over the last few years, she had started CrossFit and loved the feeling of fitness and the toning of her muscles. She was devastated, then, when she started to notice a lump in her vagina by the end of most days. This often coincided with a deep dragging ache which was similar to period pains but was now at any time of the month, not just when menstruating.

She was initially scared and visited her GP, who diagnosed a mild pelvic organ prolapse. She was told to do her pelvic floor exercises and to come back if things did not improve. Catherine could not understand how this could have happened when she had never had a vaginal delivery. Despite trying to do as she was told and following the advice on the leaflet, nothing seemed to be getting better. She was desperately worried that she might need to stop her CrossFit and this was when she was referred for physiotherapy.

Presenting problem: Two-year history of feeling a bulge in her vagina and related dragging and aching increasing as the day progressed. Worse during the week, than on the weekend. Some discomfort with sexual intercourse, including both tissue tenderness and deep aching with penetration.

No other pelvic floor symptoms, such as incontinence, either bladder or bowel.

Assessment: Some very mild irritation of her external tissues was noted. In lying, there was a mild descent of the back wall of her vagina when bearing down. Although able to contract her pelvic floor muscles, there was weakness on the right-hand side, and she could only maintain her contraction for one or two seconds. Palpation revealed some reduction in the bulk of the muscles of the deeper portion of her pelvic floor. When assessed in standing, the back wall of the vagina and the cervix were found to sit lower than optimum within the pelvic cavity..

We diagnosed a grade 1 posterior vaginal and uterine prolapse (this is a mild descent of the uterus and the bowel within the pelvic cavity.). Early symptoms of GSM.

What changes and why

Our pelvic organs are normally supported within the pelvis by two systems:

The ligaments and fascia from which the organs are suspended (passive) and the pelvic floor muscles (active) which support the organs from below.

Some people have described these systems and their support as a boat in a dock where the boat represents the pelvic organs, which are supported by the bulk and the activity of the pelvic floor muscles (the water) and stabilised by the ligaments and fascia (the moorings)[17].

If the muscle bulk reduces and become weaker, then the organs must be supported by the ligaments (the second picture). It has been suggested that during menopause, our collagen (a major component of our connective tissues such as ligaments and fascia) is altered as the ratios of oestrogen and progesterone change and so that the tensile strength is reduced[18]. This has been suggested as one of the reasons why women often only start to notice pelvic floor symptoms such as prolapse as their oestrogen levels reduce during menopause.

While giving birth vaginally and, in particular, assisted vaginal deliveries, for example, forceps, are considered to increase the risk of developing pelvic floor disorders; obesity, chronic constipation and genetic factors can also increase the likelihood of developing problems. Often these risks have a cumulative effect and in the case of many women seen in clinic, these issues have been building up over many years due to jobs where women are on their feet carrying heavy loads all day, every day.

Management for Catherine: In the early stages of her recovery, we discussed 'pacing' during the day so that Catherine incorporated a rest period for her pelvic floor at lunchtime or immediately upon her return from work by sitting with her feet up. Although she believed this would be impossible, she soon discovered that when she got home there was time to sit with a cuppa and chat with her children about their days. This not only ensured her tissues had a short period to rest and recover after a full day of standing, but it allowed her the opportunity to relax and recover generally before starting the evening's tasks. We also discussed the best position to empty her bowel. Advising her to raise her feet on a small stool to lift her knees above her hips alters the mechanics of her bowel and helps to minimise strain when defaecating. Like Lesley, Catherine started a basic routine of pelvic floor muscle training aimed at improving both her strength and her endurance. She noted some improvements quite quickly as the neuro-muscular pathways were activated, but it would take a lot longer to build the muscles in bulk and in strength, just as you would expect when starting a new strengthening routine at the gym. It was important that Catherine understood this to ensure her symptoms would not return if she reduced the level of her pelvic floor muscle training too soon. In the early stages of her recovery, Catherine also benefited from using a self-managing pessary device. These are devices made from plastic or silicone and are inserted into the vagina to support the organs. Pessaries come in different shapes and sizes and a healthcare professional trained in fitting them will discuss the type that might suit you best. It often takes more than one visit to get the right one to address your needs[19]. In Catherine's case, she was fitted with a cube pessary, that filled the space inside the vaginal cavity and prevented the walls from descending. By fitting her cube at the start of the day and then removing it at night, she was able to feel much more comfortable throughout the day.

Catherine's biggest worry before seeking help was that health professionals might tell her to stop going to her CrossFit sessions. We were able to reassure her that, in many cases, taking part in exercise like this can be beneficial for her muscles and tissues. In a large Australian survey of women taking part in CrossFit, there was not found to be any association between lifting heavy weights during their sessions and experiencing symptoms of prolapse[20]. So instead of stopping the CrossFit, which was so beneficial to her mental and physical health, we advised her to listen to her body and work within a symptom-free range. After working hard on her recovery over a period of several months, Catherine became symptom-free and felt like her old self again. She was determined, however, to continue to maintain her pelvic floor strength to prevent any recurrence.

Myth 5

"I haven't had any children and have always done my pelvic floor exercises religiously, so my symptoms cannot be related to the pelvic floor."

Meet Jenny:

- 52-year-old horse rider and runner
- History of painful periods
- Recently started a new relationship.
- Pain during sexual intercourse and urgency-related urinary incontinence.

Jenny was referred to us by her GP, although she couldn't understand what pelvic health physiotherapy could possibly do for her. *"I have always religiously done my pelvic floor exercises even though I have never had children so I can't believe this can be a problem with my pelvic floor!"* She had always experienced heavy and painful periods and when she entered menopause with minimal issues such as hot flushes, it had been a huge relief. No more pain and difficulty controlling the bleeding, which was a particular problem given the fact that tampons had never been comfortable for Jenny. After a difficult divorce in her 30s, Jenny had not had a regular partner for many years, but having decided to get out and meet new people, she had joined the local running club and there met a new partner. When she decided to take the relationship a step further, she had been devastated to find that any type of penetrative sex was prohibitively painful. Her partner was very supportive, but she was desperate to find something that might help. With the new running training, she had also noticed increasing episodes of urinary urgency. These sensations, as noted with Rosie, were on occasion, eye-wateringly uncomfortable, but when she made it to the toilet, she had often found there was little there. This was the incentive to visit the GP. After investigating, they had found that there was no evidence of infection but that her tissues were a little dry and sensitive. She had been prescribed topical oestrogen and referred for pelvic health physiotherapy.

Assessment: Although Jenny described similar desperate urinary urgency to Rosie, she did not report any major leakage and, if anything, was finding it hard to fully empty her bladder. On assessment, as she had been using the topical oestrogen for a little while, her tissues appeared healthy and normal on inspection. When assessing her pelvic floor function, however, it was initially too tender to examine all but the most superficial layer of the muscles. This was how she had described the experience of trying to use tampons when she was younger.

We diagnosed Jenny with increased tone in her pelvic floor muscles, potentially related to her previously painful periods and also her history of anxiety.

Management: Initial work for Jenny involved gentle techniques such as diaphragmatic (or belly) breathing. The benefits of this can be twofold: it has been suggested to promote relaxation and reduce anxiety[21]. Some have further suggested that diaphragmatic breathing can enable us to better relax both the abdominal and pelvic floor muscles and certainly clinically women often find this helpful. Using biofeedback techniques with real-time ultrasound, she was able to see when her pelvic floor muscles were engaged and notice what it felt like when she relaxed them. Working on this over some time started to reduce the increased urinary urgency and frequency she had been experiencing and enabled her to empty her bladder more fully when she went to the toilet.

With respect to the painful intercourse, there is evidence that pelvic floor muscle training that teaches the woman to contract and also to relax can be beneficial[22]. However as many of these cases can be multifactorial, they will often recover best when physiotherapy techniques such as pelvic floor work and, for some, manual therapy is part of a wider treatment plan by a multidisciplinary team. This will often include psychological and medical support in addition to physiotherapy[23]. It was particularly important that she felt confident that there was no pressure from her partner to engage in intercourse before she was ready. To ensure that they were guided to facilitate optimum recovery, they worked with colleagues of ours trained in psychosexual counselling[24]. Through a process that was developed together with the guidance of the counsellor, they learnt ways to enjoy one another without penetration until they both felt that the time was right to do so.

Myth 6

"If I seek help, they will tell me I can no longer do the exercise I love and I will be told off for not doing my pelvic floor exercises sooner."

Meet Rudrani:

- 61-year-old – middle-distance recreational runner
- Vaginal heaviness during runs longer than 5k associated with bowel urgency (does not always make it to the toilet in time).
- shocked and surprised to be diagnosed with osteoporosis despite being a fit person.

Rudrani booked herself in for 'a Menopause Physio MOT', or a general physiotherapy check-up for menopausal women. She was fit and active, running more than 25 km each week. Although she was still running, she found managing her injuries was becoming trickier and reported being generally stiff and sore, especially first thing in the morning and after sitting for any period of time.

She also experienced vaginal heaviness during any runs that were over 5 km. She noted this particularly so if she hadn't opened her bowels before setting off, meaning that on longer runs, the route must be planned to include regular toilets, as at times she reported difficulty controlling bowel urgency and had to rush to the toilet. Sometimes she did not make it in time and noted some faecal leakage, which was incredibly distressing. The strong sense of urge is known as 'sensory urge' and leakage just before you manage to get your pants down is 'motor urge', both are very common and distressing but are treatable.

Finally, Rudrani had also been shocked and surprised to be diagnosed with osteoporosis following a DEXA scan, which revealed low bone density.

Findings: Rudrani, like many of the women we see in clinic did not present with one symptom alone but rather had multiple problems: symptoms of pelvic organ prolapse (heaviness), faecal urgency (difficulty controlling her bowel), joint pain and niggling injuries with any increase in her training programme.

What changes and why

What is the evidence for exercise and joint pain? Does exercise help, or does it increase the pain?

It is a bit of both; of course, exercise can lead to injury, but so can getting comfortable on the couch. It is important to remember the long list of health benefits of keeping active.

In a 2022 review of the latest evidence, 'Moving Medicine' concluded that increased levels of physical activity led to reduced levels of joint pain[25]. In surveys, those who complied with the minimum national physical activity guidelines were less likely to report joint pain symptoms than those who were sedentary. In both peri- and postmenopausal women, physical activity has been shown to reduce many symptoms of menopause, including joint pain[26].

This is such an important message for women, although injury and soft tissue management can be more challenging, and too much training may lead to injury; like Goldilocks, just the right amount of exercise and recovery will help to reduce your joint pain.

For Rudrani's tissue management and injury prevention, we focused on more strength training and adequate recovery. The micro-damage and the consequent repair that occur with exercise, results in tissue adaptation and stronger tissues. Oestrogen, however, is a crucial part of that repair process[27] and when it declines, it becomes even more important to factor adequate recovery into our training programmes.

Recovery is even more important for those women who like to exercise hard, like Rudrani. It is a lovely realisation that you can improve your fitness while you sleep, and for Rudrani, this meant giving herself permission to do so and re-claiming her sleep.

In a further review on sleep by Moving Medicine[28], there was strong evidence that regular physical activity in menopausal and perimenopausal women improves sleep quality. Sleep and exercise seem to partner up well.

So, what exercise is best? The simple answer is: Little is better than nothing, more is better than less, particularly during menopause with the accelerated loss of lean muscle mass.

For Rudrani, we advised her to adjust her exercise to include more resistance and high-intensity interval training (HIIT), as she already does plenty of cardio work, to keep her engine going.

Her strength and HIIT training needed to be multidirectional to improve her bone health so that the muscles pull on the bones in various directions. Running alone is helpful for impact loading, but all the forces are linear. Introducing variety and diversity in her resistance training and impact workouts by applying forces in many directions will better maintain her bone density.

One of the key recommendations within the latest guidelines on bone health published by the *British Journal of Sports Medicine* is that people with osteoporosis should undertake resistance and impact exercise to maximise bone strength[29]; osteoporosis is an indication for progressive muscle strengthening and weight training, not a contraindication. This means that progressive resistance exercises should be prescribed for major muscle groups in order to load those areas of the skeleton most at risk of osteoporotic fracture, such as the spine, proximal femur and forearm. The LIFTMOR study, which recruited 100 postmenopausal women with low to very low bone density to take part in a trial of HIIT exercise over a period of eight months, illustrates this perfectly[30]. Exercises within the intervention included supervised deadlifts, overhead press, back squats and jumping chin ups with drop landings, while the control group followed a home-based program of low-intensity work focusing on balance and mobility. Results showed not only that regular supervised HIIT work improved bone health and general function, but that it was safe, with only one minor soft tissue injury reported in over 2,600 training sessions.

Rudrani was keen to alter some of her training to progressive muscle strengthening. She returned for a follow-up full of excitement. She is loving the lifting!

What about Rudrani's pelvic health issue? (vaginal heaviness, bowel and bladder urgency while running).

Is this due to a hormonal change into the menopause? What is the importance of early risk factors versus hormonal changes into the menopause?

As with most changes in health, ageing and menopause – considering the ecosystems we are – this is multifactorial and complex.

As mentioned with Catherine, there are several risk factors that predispose women to experience pelvic floor symptoms such as urinary incontinence and pelvic organ prolapse. One such risk is vaginal birth, although symptoms may not become apparent until over 20 years after childbirth[31,32]. Other risks include chronic constipation[33], obesity and ageing[34,35]. However, it is often during and after menopause that clinically we find women notice their symptoms become more obvious.

We know that pelvic floor symptoms can be a huge barrier for women taking part in exercise[36] and, as mentioned with Lesley, impact exercise such as running can be a major trigger for women reporting symptoms such as urinary incontinence.[13] Given however, how important regular exercise is in maintaining good health – mental health, cardiovascular health and even reducing the risk of some cancers[37], it is vital that women are enabled to overcome these symptoms and continue with their preferred sport or activities. Research strongly supports pelvic floor muscle training to treat pelvic floor symptoms such as urinary incontinence and prolapse[12] and it is never too late to start this[38].

As pelvic health physiotherapists, we see many women with bowel issues, which range from – difficult defaecation, constipation, slow transit, incomplete emptying to difficulty controlling faecal urgency and continence. Again, pelvic floor muscle training is reported to be effective in managing bowel-related issues such as faecal incontinence and urge[39]. Further, additional advice can ensure that symptoms become minimal.

In Rudrani's case, we discussed diet to help improve her stool formation so that it become soft, formed and sausage shaped, which made it easier for her to empty her bowel completely. We also worked on 'how to have a perfect pooh', as for Catherine, we suggested placing a stool under her feet to improve bowel mechanics and taught her other techniques to protect against straining while emptying her bowels, such as 'splinting' the back wall of her vagina – for optimal voiding. When there is some laxity in the back wall of the vagina, stool can easily 'pocket', these simple techniques can help prevent this. Optimal voiding helped to ensure she was no longer running with stool in her rectum, which had caused the vaginal heaviness and, at times, bowel urgency, for her otherwise asymptomatic back wall prolapse.

The goal we set together was for her to continue with the exercise she loves and to also get stronger and improve her bone health. I bumped into her running in the park, which means the first goal is achieved; she is enjoying her heavy lifting and interested to find out what her DEXA scan will show in terms of bone density in the future. The key message is: there are no medals to be won by suffering in silence, we urge all women to talk to a healthcare professional and keep knocking on doors until you find the right support for you.

References

1. Centre for Research on Women with Disabilities. What is the definition of pelvic health? 2023. https://www.bcm.edu/research/research-centers/center-for-research-on-women-with-disabilities/a-to-z-directory/pelvic-health/what-is-the-definition-of-pelvic-health.
2. Pelvic Obstetric and Gynaecological Physiotherapy. Why choose a POGP registered physiotherapist? 2020. https://thepogp.co.uk/patient_information/why_choose_a_pogp_registered_physiotherapist.aspx.
3. Portman DJ, Gass ML. Genitourinary syndrome of menopause: New terminology for vulvovaginal atrophy from the International Society for the Study of Women's Sexual Health and the North American Menopause Society. *Menopause* 2014; 21 (10): 1063–1068.
4. Lindsay CF. Impact of the menopause on the female urogenital system and sexual function. *Journal of Pelvic, Obstetric and Gynaecological Physiotherapy* 2021; (129): 22–32.
5. Currie H, Moger SJ. Menopause – Understanding the impact on women and their partners. *Post Reproductive Health* 2019; 25 (4): 183–190.
6. Nappi RE, Palacios S, Panay N et al. Vulvar and vaginal atrophy in four European countries: Evidence from the European REVIVE Survey. *Climacteric* 2016; 19 (2): 188–197.
7. Domoney C, Short H, Particco M et al. Symptoms, attitudes and treatment perceptions of vulvo-vaginal atrophy in UK postmenopausal women: Results from the REVIVE-EU study. *Post Reproductive Health* 2020; 26 (2): 101–109.
8. Mercier J, Morin M, Tang A et al. Pelvic floor muscle training: Mechanisms of action for the improvement of genitourinary syndrome of menopause. *Climacteric* 2020; 23 (5): 468–473.
9. Falah-Hassani K, Reeves J, Shiri R et al. The pathophysiology of stress urinary incontinence: A systematic review and meta-analysis. *International Urogynecology Journal* 2021; 32 (3): 501–552.
10. Lovegrove Jones RC, Peng Q, Stokes M et al. Mechanisms of pelvic floor muscle function and the effect on the urethra during a cough. *European Urology* 2010; 57 (6): 1101–1110.
11. Berube M-E, McLean L. Differences in pelvic floor muscle morphology and function between female runners with and without running-induced stress urinary incontinence. *Neurourology and Urodynamics* 2023; 42 (8): 1733–1744.
12. Cacciari L, Dumoulin C, Hay-Smith J. Pelvic floor muscle training versus no treatment or inactive control treatments for urinary incontinence in women: A cochrane review update. Neurourology and urodynamics Conference: 47th annual meeting of the international continence society, ICS 2017 Italy. 2017; 36: S270–S2S1.

13 Carvalhais A, Natal Jorge R, Bø K. Performing high-level sport is strongly associated with urinary incontinence in elite athletes: A comparative study of 372 elite female athletes and 372 controls. *British Journal of Sports Medicine* 2018; 52 (24): 1586–1590.
14 Campbell KG, Batt ME, Drummond A. Prevalence of pelvic floor dysfunction in recreational athletes: A cross-sectional survey. *International Urogynecology Journal* 2023; 34 (10): 2429–2437.
15 Bo K, Sundgot-Borgen J. Are former female elite athletes more likely to experience urinary incontinence later in life than non-athletes? *Scandinavian Journal of Medicine & Science in Sports* 2010; 20 (1): 100–104.
16 Jerez-Roig J, Booth J, Skelton DA et al. Is urinary incontinence associated with sedentary behaviour in older women? Analysis of data from the National Health and Nutrition Examination Survey. *PLoS One* 2020; 15 (2): e0227195.
17 Norton PA. Pelvic floor disorders: The role of fascia and ligaments. *Clinical Obstetrics and Gynecology* 1993; 36 (4): 926–938.
18 Moalli PA, Talarico LC, Sung VW et al. Impact of menopause on collagen subtypes in the arcus tendineous fasciae pelvis. *American Journal of Obstetrics and Gynecology* 2004; 190 (3): 620–627.
19 Pelvic Obstetric and Gynaecological Physiotherapy. Pessaries for prolapse – Patient information 2020. https://thepogp.co.uk/patient_information/womens_health/pessaries_for_prolapse.aspx #selfmanagement.
20 Forner LB, Beckman EM, Smith MD. Symptoms of pelvic organ prolapse in women who lift heavy weights for exercise: A cross-sectional survey. *International Urogynecology Journal* 2020; 31 (8): 1551–1558.
21 Chen Y-F, Huang X-Y, Chien C-H et al. The effectiveness of diaphragmatic breathing relaxation training for reducing anxiety. *Perspectives in Psychiatric Care* 2017; 53 (4): 329–336.
22 Ghaderi F, Bastani P, Hajebrahimi S et al. Pelvic floor rehabilitation in the treatment of women with dyspareunia: A randomized controlled clinical trial. *International Urogynecology Journal* 2019; 30 (11): 1849–1855.
23 Brotto LA, Yong P, Smith KB et al. Impact of a multidisciplinary vulvodynia program on sexual functioning and dyspareunia. *Journal of Sexual Medicine* 2015; 12 (1): 238–247.
24 Medicine IoP. The practice of psychosexual medicine 2024. https://www.ipm.org.uk/about/the _practice_of_psychosexual_medicine.aspx.
25 Faculty of Sport and Exercise Medicine. MSK pain – Reduces pain 2024. https://movingmedicine .ac.uk/evidence/msk-pain-o-reduces-pain/.
26 Javadivala Z, Allahverdipour H, Asghari Jafarabadi M et al. An interventional strategy of physical activity promotion for reduction of menopause symptoms. *Health Promotion Perspectives* 2020; 10 (4): 383–392.
27 Coldron Y. Effects of the menopause on the neuromusculoskeletal system: A narrative review. *Journal of Pelvic, Obstetric and Gynaecological Physiotherapy* 2021; (129): 9–21.
28 Faculty of Sport and Exercise Medicine. Menopause – Improves sleep 2024. https:// movingmedicine.ac.uk/evidence/menopause-improves-sleep/.
29 Brooke-Wavell K, Skelton DA, Barker KL et al. Strong, steady and straight: UK consensus statement on physical activity and exercise for osteoporosis. *British Journal of Sports Medicine* 2022; 56 (15): 837–846.
30 Watson SL, Weeks BK, Weis LJ et al. High-intensity resistance and impact training improves bone mineral density and physical function in postmenopausal women with osteopenia and osteoporosis: The LIFTMOR randomized controlled trial. *Journal of Bone and Mineral Research* 2018; 33 (2): 211–220.
31 Gyhagen M, Bullarbo M, Nielsen TF et al. Prevalence and risk factors for pelvic organ prolapse 20 years after childbirth: A national cohort study in singleton primiparae after vaginal or caesarean delivery. *BJOG* 2013; 120 (2): 152–160.

32 Gyhagen M, Bullarbo M, Nielsen TF et al. The prevalence of urinary incontinence 20 years after childbirth: A national cohort study in singleton primiparae after vaginal or caesarean delivery. *BJOG* 2013; 120 (2): 144–151.

33 Rashidi F, Mirghafourvand M. Pelvic floor disorder and relevant factors in Iranian women of reproductive age: A cross-sectional study. *BMC Women's Health* 2023; 23 (1): 71.

34 Pomian A, Lisik W, Kosieradzki M et al. Obesity and pelvic floor disorders: A review of the literature. *Medical Science Monitor* 2016; 22: 1880–1886.

35 Danforth KN, Townsend MK, Lifford K et al. Risk factors for urinary incontinence among middle-aged women. *American Journal of Obstetrics and Gynecology* 2006; 194 (2): 339–345.

36 Dakic JG, Cook J, Hay-Smith J et al. Pelvic floor symptoms are an overlooked barrier to exercise participation: A cross-sectional online survey of 4556 women who are symptomatic. *Physical Therapy* 2021; 102 (3): pzab284. doi: 10.1093/ptj/pzab284. PMID: 34939122.

37 Warburton DE, Nicol CW, Bredin SS. Health benefits of physical activity: The evidence. *CMAJ* 2006; 174 (6): 801–809.

38 Cacciari LP, Morin M, Mayrand M-H et al. Never too late to train: The effects of pelvic floor muscle training on the shape of the Levator Hiatus in incontinent older women. *International Journal of Environmental Research and Public Health* 2022; 19 (17): 11078.

39 Scott KM. Pelvic floor rehabilitation in the treatment of fecal incontinence. *Clinics in Colon and Rectal Surgery* 2014; 27 (3): 99–105.

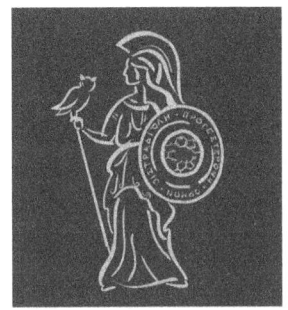

ACT 4

Mastering Menopause

Act 4 Mastering Menopause
How to navigate the female hormone odyssey?

Dr Nicky Keay

Homer's poem of the odyssey demonstrates how perseverance and determination are vital in navigating an epic journey. Fortunately, during the female hormone odyssey we are not at the mercy of capricious gods. Rather, we are in control of our own destiny. This chapter explores the key lifestyle strategies of nutrition, exercise and sleep to master the menopause, dispelling myths that might divert us away from mastering our personal female hormone odyssey.

> *"If we could each individual just the right amount of exercise and nourishment, not too little and not too much, we would have found the surest way to health."*
>
> Hippocrates

Navigating the female hormone odyssey with lifestyle

Over 2,000 years ago, Hippocrates advocated that the surest way to health was by giving each individual *"just the right amount of nourishment and exercise, not too little and not too much."* We now know that hormones explain the link between behaviour and health, as shown in Figure 4.1.1. This approach is as appropriate today as it was for the Ancient Greeks.

As our internal hormone choreography changes on the approach to menopause and beyond, we must review and modify our lifestyle choices regarding nutrition, exercise and sleep.

Bag of the winds

During the Odyssey, Aeolus the Ancient Greek god of the winds gives Odysseus a bag of winds to speed him on his way home back to Ithaca. Odysseus' sailors became envious, thinking that the bag contained gold. Believing that Odysseys intended to keep this wealth all to himself, they opened the bag while Odysseys slept. The winds were released and blew them away from their destination just as the end of their journey was in sight.

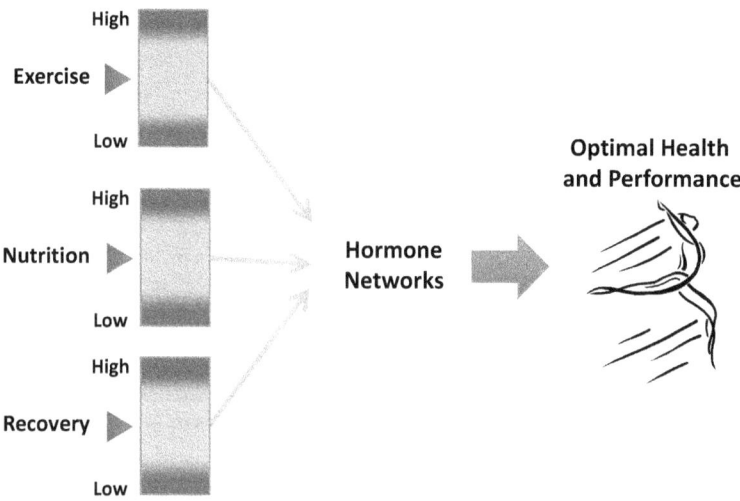

FIGURE 4.1.1 Balancing lifestyle factors to harness hormones. Hormones, Health and Human Potential. Keay 2022. Sequoia books

How is this story relevant to navigating the menopause? It can be tempting to compare yourself to others, who apparently seem to be making plain sailing of this tricky hormone journey. You want to find and use their secret "recipe" for success. It is easy to become envious of others, who appear to take menopause in their stride. What is it that these women are doing that seems to be working? What are the nutrition and exercise regimes that they purport to be following and advocating (generally loudly)? We may be tempted to try to replicate what they are doing. Unfortunately, you might end up exchanging your bag of gold for a bag of wind, leading to disappointment and sailing off course. There is no single approach that works for everyone.

This act is set to dispel the myths and present the facts about the nature of our lifestyle choices. Experts explain how a personalised combination of nutrition, exercise and sleep can support your journey through menopause and beyond.

Menopause diet?

Initially, the myth of a "menopause diet" is examined. It can be tempting to be lured into following highly publicised "menopause diets" that claim to bring quick results. In reality, the key to long-term health and well-being is a review of what you eat and when you are eating it. It is essential to review relative proportions of the food groups required for health (carbohydrate, protein and fats), but never to exclude a food group.

The guiding principle is to adapt to the hormonal changes that accompany ageing and menopause, particularly the declines in the main tissue-building (anabolic) drivers growth hormone (GH) and oestradiol.

There is good evidence to show that increasing the proportion of protein in your diet, can be helpful in resisting the effects of declining anabolic hormones. The timing of protein consumption is important. For example, consuming protein after resistance exercise (anabolic stimulus) promotes muscle and bone formation. The protein casein, found in milk, taken before sleep prevents muscle breakdown overnight and takes advantage of the time when GH release peaks to support muscle formation[1].

What about carbohydrates? Is this food group really the villain of nutrition? Restricting carbohydrates acts as a stressor, resulting in cortisol release, which is a catabolic hormone, breaking down muscle and favouring the deposition of fat: the precise opposite of what you are trying to achieve. Severely restricting calories with a low-carbohydrate diet can cause a slowing of the metabolic rate, with the consequence that weight is regained rapidly as soon as calories are increased[2]. In conclusion, restricting carbohydrates is counterproductive for all aspects of health[3]. The optimal approach is to favour appropriate portion sizes of complex forms of carbohydrate, distributed over the day[4].

Only one type of exercise for menopause?

Ideally, we should already be doing exercise to cover all the elements of fitness: cardiovascular, muscular strength, endurance, flexibility and neuromuscular skills. The approach of menopause offers the opportunity to review the amount and type of exercise you are doing. Just as with nutrition, this does not mean excluding any particular type of exercise, rather consider fine-tuning the ratio of the types of exercise you do. The WHO recommends strength and/or resistance exercise as an element of our exercise choices for all ages[5] and this becomes especially important, on the backdrop of the decline of anabolic hormones, to mitigate sarcopenia (loss of muscle mass and function), adverse body composition (deposition of visceral fat), bone loss and cardio-metabolic issues.

Exactly what type of strength work you do depends on your starting point. If, like me, you are a reluctant gym goer, maybe with medical considerations (like rheumatoid arthritis or double hip replacements), this can be a barrier to doing any strength work. There are alternatives to going to the gym and lifting very heavy weights. Recent research shows that body weight strength work can be effective, if this is the only realistic option for you[6]. Pilates can be a great choice, with resistance bands and apparatus, harnessing all the types of muscle contraction: concentric, isometric and eccentric.

If you are already an enthusiastic gym goer and weightlifter, or this is something you want to develop, then this is clearly the best path for you. Ideally, in addition to intentional exercise, it is best to avoid being sedentary for long periods and to be generally active during the day[7]. Ultimately exercise and nutrition should include some element of enjoyment, in order to sustain consistency in the long term through your menopause journey and beyond.

"Sleep is the chief nourisher in life's great feast"

The words of Shakespeare's Macbeth are apposite for the health of many hormone networks. Regular sleep patterns are important in synchronising hormone choreography and avoiding circadian misalignment, which can have adverse effects on metabolic health. Act 2, Scene 2 explored this relationship and why getting good quality and quantity sleep becomes challenging around menopause and what to do about this. Ultimately you do not want to be in the situation of Penelope, Odysseys' wife who made good progress with her tapestry during the day but undid this good work at night. Although you may be making good nutrition and exercise choices during the day, it is important not to undermine it with poor sleep.

References

1 Trommelen J, van Loon LJ. Pre-sleep protein ingestion to improve the skeletal muscle adaptive response to exercise training. *Nutrients* 2016; 8 (12): 763. doi: 10.3390/nu8120763.
2 Keay N. *Hormones Health and Human Potential.* Act 1 Scene 4 It's all in the Timing. Sequoia Books, 2022.
3 Keay N. *Hormones Health and Human Potential.* Act 1 Scene 3 Harnessing Hormones. Sequoia Books, 2022.
4 Denby N. Menopause: Nutrition and weight gain. *Post Reproductive Health* 2023; 29 (4): 232–234.
5 Bull FC, Al-Ansari SS, Biddle S et al. World Health Organization 2020 guidelines on physical activity and sedentary behaviour. *British Journal of Sports Medicine* 2020; 54 (24): 1451–1462. doi: 10.1136/bjsports-2020-102955. PMID: 33239350; PMCID: PMC7719906.
6 Ogawa M, Hashimoto Y, Mochizuki Y et al. Effects of free weight and body mass-based resistance training on thigh muscle size, strength and intramuscular fat in healthy young and middle-aged individuals. *Experimental Physiology* 2023; 108 (7): 975–985. doi: 10.1113/EP090655. Epub 2023 May 3. PMID: 37133323; PMCID: PMC10988481.
7 van der Ploeg HP, Chey T, Korda RJ et al. Sitting time and all-cause mortality risk in 222 497 Australian adults. *Archives of Internal Medicine* 2012; 172 (6): 494–500. doi: 10.1001/archinternmed.2011.2174. PMID: 22450936.

Scene 1 The menopause diet?

Renee McGregor

Needless to say, there are many myths about diet in general, let alone around this time of life. Nutrition is an endless and controversial topic where, while science exists, it is often overlooked for instant gratification and the latest wellness trend.

While there is some truth in our metabolism slowing as we get older, with a potential further decline in women who become more sedentary, there is no evidence in the benefits of extreme energy deficits and cutting out food groups such as carbohydrates.

For those women who have always been physically active, the aim is always to maintain this, while some modifications may be needed. Research has shown that there are benefits to reducing cardio and endurance training in favour of resistance training. That doesn't mean you need to stop your choice of sport, but it might mean, instead of running 6 days a week, you drop down to 3 or 4 and add 2–3 strength sessions instead. This works on many levels from maintaining muscle mass, which in turn maintains your metabolism, supports bone health, prevents the natural decline and also maintains body composition. For those women who have always been sedentary, this may be the perfect time to start getting active, as research shows that being active can prevent and limit the severity of a number of the common symptoms associated with reducing hormonal levels.

Is there a menopause diet?

So what about diet then? Do we need to change anything major at this stage?

There are a number of myths associated with diet and menopause, but the reality is that, as with most of the population, all evidence points towards a Mediterranean approach[1]. This includes whole grains, plenty of fresh produce, especially fruit and vegetables with an array of colours, nuts, seeds, legumes, fish and then lean meat, poultry and dairy products in moderation. The main focus of this dietary approach is one that supports the gut biome but is also high in antioxidants and anti-inflammatory foods, which support optimal health and reduce the risk of type 2 diabetes, heart disease and osteoporosis[2,3].

The common myths put out about this stage of life include encouraging a keto, that is, a very low carbohydrate approach, or encouraging big calorie deficits, neither of which are suitable nor appropriate.

Carbohydrate: the villain of nutrition?

As we have already mentioned, many women going through perimenopause into menopause, often notice and struggle with changes to their body composition. Cue, current misconceptions and Western societal beliefs and many women at this stage decide that the only way to combat this change is through restrictive diets and removing carbohydrates.

In fact, the latest research shows the complete opposite; declining oestrogen levels mean that the female body is no longer as efficient at fat oxidation, which tends to spare our use of carbohydrate. Thus, carbohydrate intake, especially in those women who remain physically active, is critical not just for performance, but also for counteracting the fatigue often associated with this phase of life.

In addition, we know there is a direct link between carbohydrate availability and thyroid function. When carbohydrate intake is reduced too far in females, this can result in a downregulation of the thyroid gland, and thus metabolism, impacting body composition and energy levels further.

That said, not all carbohydrates are equal and we should encourage the intake of wholegrains, fruit, vegetables and legumes as good sources of complex carbohydrates. Ideally, this should make up one-third of your daily intake.

For those women who are very active, nutrient timing is also critical to ensure appropriate adaptation and progression in their sport.

Protein: why does this become particularly important?

It has been well documented in the literature that muscle mass and strength decline with ageing. In general, muscle mass and strength peak at ages 20–30 years, begin to decline in the 40–50 years, with an acceleration in the decline in the over-70s. And yet, we are seeing remarkable results in both male and female athletes beyond the fourth decade of life.

One key finding from the research across all masters age groups is that any decline in muscle mass is directly linked to physical activity, with inactive and sedentary peers experiencing a more rapid decline. As mentioned earlier in this chapter, resistance training seems to be pivotal in maintaining mass in this population; thus, the addition of 2–3 sessions a week, with a slight reduction in cardio/endurance training, can reap huge benefits.

Staying physically active and incorporating more resistance training is paramount for optimal health during perimenopause and beyond. We have already discussed the importance of carbohydrate in supporting this, but special attention must be placed on the role of protein. Ensuring enough protein in the diet will help prevent the usual decline in muscle mass associated in this population. Studies have shown that those women who are physically active should aim for a minimum of 2.0 g protein/kg body weight (BW) per day, but more likely need up to 2.4 g protein/kg BW per day on very active days.

Those that consume good amounts of protein have been shown to maintain 40% more muscle mass than those that have low intake of protein. Remember, higher muscle mass means you are more metabolically active and thus have improved body composition. In addition to the overall intake of protein, a good distribution throughout the day seems to improve overall retention and encourage adaptive responses. Furthermore, the quality of protein seems to be equally important. Where possible, whole protein sources are recommended. This includes eggs, milk, Greek yoghurt, meat, poultry and fish.

Fats: only deposited as fat?

While many are wary of eating fat, it is important to understand that consuming foods high in essential fatty acids is imperative not just for health but also for brain function.

One key symptom associated with perimenopause is a decline in cognitive function. Many women speak of the "brain fog", and while this is linked once again to declining oestrogen levels, research shows us that the essential fatty acids EPA and DHA play an important role in maintaining brain function. The only real nutritional source of DHA is oily fish, or for those who do not eat fish, you should use a high-dose supplement. In addition, these same essential fatty acids help reduce inflammation and also encourage the absorption of fat-soluble vitamins A, D, E and K.

Details are important: micronutrients and supplementation

Micronutrients are often overlooked. Iron, zinc, magnesium, iodine, calcium, vitamins B12 and D are critical for correct function of muscles, bone, blood and metabolism.

Most of these are needed in small quantities that are easily available if you consume a well-balanced and varied diet.

During perimenopause, bone health becomes a real concern; declining oestrogen levels reduce protection. Ensuring sufficient vitamin D, calcium, resistance training and using HRT can all help to prevent further loss. There are few foods that provide vitamin D, so it tends to be the only micronutrient that routinely needs to be supplemented. Most women will be fine with 1,000 International Units (IU) a day, but in those with darker skin or who have very low levels to start with may need higher doses.

The best sources of calcium come from dairy or soya. During this stage of life, requirements are high at around 1,000–1,200 mg a day.

While there are many supplements available and plenty targeting this population group, there are few that are based on clinical trials and evidence-based research. Vitamin D as we have already mentioned and then B12 and iron may be needed in some individuals due to lifestyle and dietary preferences. The only other supplement that is starting to get quite a lot of traction and has proven to support bone health is collagen. While HRT is important for mitigating bone loss, studies have shown that supplementation with collagen over a 12-month period actually showed an increase in bone density. The optimal dose appears to be 5–10 g a day.

Embrace "good" microbes: the gut microbiome

While still a relatively new area of nutrition, numerous studies have demonstrated that there is no denying a link between the status of our gut microbiome and both our mental and physical health[4].

The gut microbiome includes different types of bacteria that reside in our gut. Collectively, they have a number of functions ranging from synthesising some vitamins, short-chain fatty acids and even neurotransmitters, which are all necessary for optimal health. The more enriched microbial diversity an individual has, the more likely they are to benefit from the positive associations with health. These include a strong immune system, improved mental health and, more recently, there seem to be links with improvements in sports performance.

As women go through perimenopause, hormonal changes can result in gut dysbiosis, a change to the microbial diversity which can then have an impact on digestion and overall health. Our diet is integral to so many aspects of life, from providing us with sufficient energy to allow for all the biological processes that keep us alive, to supporting our adventures and physical activity preferences[5].

When looking at gut health specifically, there are several key nutrients and food types that have been identified which result in the increased microbial diversity that is recommended. A high-fibre diet rich in colourful fruits, vegetables, legumes and whole grain is central to increasing the bacterial diversity in our gut. While our body can't digest a high-fibre diet, there are certain bacteria in our gut that can, and this stimulates their growth, resulting in an improved environment.

Another type of food group that can be beneficial to include are fermented foods. These include yoghurt, sauerkraut, kombucha, kefir and tempeh. It has been found that including more of these foods enhances the function of the microbiome by reducing the abundance of disease-causing bacteria in the intestines.

In addition to food, the inclusion of a probiotic supplement can aid microbial diversity. Probiotics are live microorganisms, usually bacteria, that provide a specific health benefit when consumed. They work on the principle of colonising the gut and benefiting health by changing the overall composition of the microbiome and supporting metabolism. While they can be consumed daily, probiotics have been found to be most effective in restoring the microbiome to a healthy state after it has been compromised.

Care needs to be taken when using probiotic supplements as most are destroyed by stomach acid and so don't make it as far as the gut. That said, one example of a food supplement that does work is the water-soluble probiotic. This live culture is water-based, which means it can pass through the stomach unaffected and be transported into the gut where it can then go on to colonise and benefit its host[5].

A time to review your intake: alcohol

As with most aspects of menopause health, there is very little research on the direct effects of alcohol consumption in this population. That said, recent literature has concluded that in general, there are no health benefits from consuming alcohol for anyone. While we know that every woman's menopause journey is different, there are definitely some symptoms and responses that are common to many.

The main finding around alcohol at this time of life is that for some women, turning to alcohol as a way of coping can become problematic. As we know, perimenopause and beyond is a tricky time of life to navigate. To a certain degree, it feels like puberty in reverse, where once again the unpredictable nature of what our body is doing or not doing and the fluctuating state of our mood and mental health leave us feeling a little off-kilter. Fluctuating hormonal levels cause havoc in our brain, especially in the production of certain neurotransmitters, which can leave us feeling like we can't cope. It is human nature to want to avoid threat; alcohol can be one such avoidance technique. This is definitely something to be aware of. Excessive intake of alcohol is associated with higher rates of depression and suicide[6].

Women generally absorb alcohol a lot quicker than men but also take longer to process it. This is why women often feel the effects of alcohol sooner. As we get older and go through perimenopause, we become more sensitive to alcohol. We do not hold as much water in our bodies and so alcohol is much more concentrated, which is one of the main reasons so many of us experience worse hangovers as we get older[7].

Where we do have some research is that some women find drinking red wine makes their hot flushes and night sweats a lot worse. Similarly, those women who are struggling with menopause-induced sleep disturbances may find this also becomes heightened if they drink alcohol. Additionally, we know in general that alcohol, especially heavy drinking, is not ideal for bone health and can increase our risk of heart disease and depression[8].

While there are no specific guidelines for consuming alcohol at this stage and there are also no recommendations suggesting you need to abstain, what I would recommend is being aware of the potential negative effects it can have on perimenopausal women and being mindful with your consumption.

Fads and trends: too good to be true . . .

As we have already established, perimenopause and menopause are difficult times to navigate, with life feeling very unpredictable, which leaves many women vulnerable and looking for answers and ways to gain control. Enter current trends that promise false gold.

Fasting and intermittent fasting

Intermittent Fasting (IF) was first made popular in the general population as a means of weight loss in 2012 by BBC Broadcast Journalist Michael Mosley when he published his book, *Eat, Fast and Live Longer*. Since then, numerous others have followed in his footsteps, including high-profile individuals.

There are two main versions of IF. The first one involves a prolonged period of fasting and a specific "window" to consume food; the most well-known is 16, 8, where the individual consumes their meals within an 8-hour window but fasts for 16 hours. The timing is up to the individual, but it needs to be maintained. So, if they choose to eat between 12 p.m.–8 p.m., then they would fast from 8 p.m. until 12 p.m. While this is the most popular, new variations have been introduced such as 12, 12 or 14, 10. The second involves 5:2, where you eat "normally" 5 days of the week and then 2 days of the week, your intake is limited to just 500 calories a day. Similarly, to the time-restricted version of IF, different versions of this form of IF have also arisen, including alternate day fasting. This involves eating as normal on alternate days and limiting calorie intake to 500 calories on the other days.

Beyond weight loss, the additional benefits attributed to following an IF model include slowing the ageing process, reduced oxidative stress, improved body composition and improvement in metabolic biomarkers. And it is exactly these potential selling points that entice women going through the perimenopause into thinking this could be "the answer" to all their problems.

While there is a lot of hype, to date there is no credible data to suggest that IF is beneficial to menopausal women; the few studies that have been conducted are based on a very short duration of 1–3 months which doesn't provide us with sufficient evidence to encourage this approach. In fact, what we have seen is that fasting in itself can have more negative consequences for this population group. This includes increased metabolic stress, which often may worsen menopausal symptoms, but also, acceleration of bone loss.

In conclusion, as a weight-loss strategy, while it is not superior to calorie-controlled approaches, it may be easier to follow, especially the time-restricted model where you have a specific window for when food can be consumed. It is this window that restricts the amount of food that can be consumed and thus works similarly to calorie control. With regard to other claims around reduced blood pressure, oxidative stress and body composition, more human studies are required, as presently these are based on animal models.

There is no evidence to support IF and menopause, especially for those that are physically active. However, some individuals whose focus is weight loss rather than performance may find this approach useful and easier than a restrictive eating pattern, especially in the first instance to lose body weight. However, this needs to be caveated by the potential risk to metabolism if continued for long periods of time.

Perimenopause story

"My body was changing and I just felt like I had no control over it. At the same time, I appeared to be a target for all the noise and promotion of intermittent fasting. Every article I read said the same thing, intermittent fasting (IF) was a great way to support weight loss especially if you are physically active. So, I decided to give it a go, and here I am 9 months later, heavier than ever and exhausted."

Montana was 48 years old and a good level runner. She had her sights set on one of the mountain rounds known in the fell running scene. Training had not been going well and she noticed that her body composition had changed; she blamed this for her poor performance. She went to see her GP, who said she was probably in the perimenopause and that she would need to be more mindful of her nutritional intake. The GP also started her on HRT. Two months past and while she wasn't feeling as tired, she still couldn't change her body composition. At this point, she decided to go down the IF route. Nine months later she came to see me.

From Montana's story and her blood tests, it was clear that due to the IF, she was in low energy availability and her body had downregulated, meaning she had actually gained weight even though she was running between 60 and 70 miles a week.

I explained what was happening and although she found it difficult to believe, she decided to trust the process. She stopped doing IF, we increased her energy intake, specifically carbohydrate and she also reduced her running for a few months and swapped two runs for two strength sessions. Within one month, she was running much better and within three months, she was noticing changes to her body composition.

She delayed the Mountain round for a year to ensure she was in the best shape she could be and last summer, she completed it without any difficulties.

A help or hindrance? Continuous glucose monitoring

Continuous glucose monitoring (CGM) has been receiving huge momentum in recent years due to celebrity endorsements, but does it really have a role to play for women at this stage?

The human body is a series of chemical reactions that work on feedback loops. In individuals without diabetes, the body has the ability to regulate blood glucose within normal limits by the hormones such as glucagon and insulin. When we consume carbohydrates, we break them down into glucose, which is then stored in our muscles, liver and brain as glycogen until the body needs it as an energy source. When glucose levels drop, glucagon will release glucose, and when glucose levels rise, insulin will be released by the pancreas to lower glucose levels. This process is part of the homeostasis that occurs in the body. Ironically, it's the body's own CGM.

While the human body likes to keep blood glucose levels within a certain range, this is not an absolute number and hereby becomes the issue with this new craze of CGM. If you believe the hype, you will think that something terrible will happen if your blood glucose is one point off what is deemed "normal". However, if you look at clinical data, it is clear that it's actually normal for blood glucose levels to fluctuate a lot throughout the day. This only becomes problematic if your blood glucose remains chronically elevated, which may be as a result of insulin resistance. But again, despite the noise, this is not something that tends to affect everyone. It is associated with type 2 diabetes and is as a result of a sedentary lifestyle and individuals holding more adipose around their middle. So yes, there is a possibility that during perimenopause you may be at more risk of developing this, but it is a condition that can be reversed by improved lifestyle behaviours.

In contrast, type 1 diabetics have a lifelong condition. Their pancreas doesn't produce insulin as a result of an autoimmune condition, which is usually detectable at a young age and these individuals need to be given insulin extrinsically. In this situation, monitoring glucose is advantageous. However, equally, if you ask any type 1 diabetic, they will tell you that it's often very difficult to predict how their blood sugars are going to respond because **it's not just food that causes glucose fluctuations**. In fact, we know that stress, illness, hormones, dehydration and movement all contribute. Indeed, a number of case studies have shown that even when individuals eat exactly the same food daily for a week, their blood glucose fluctuates significantly. As food is controlled here, it demonstrates how blood glucose is not just as simple as what we eat.

In the perimenopausal population, where we know hormones are fluctuating all the time, it is clear this is going to have some impact on blood sugars, but is this really a problem? Only if, as we said previously, it remains chronically high.

So, what is the problem with CGM in this population, then?

The real issue is the scaremongering around glucose and insulin 'spikes'. In reality, the only real outcome of succumbing to the trend and using a CGM is that it creates anxiety and obsessive behaviours associated with carbohydrate consumption. As stated previously, some individuals may develop insulin resistance, but this is rarely the case for those of us who are active and follow general healthy guidelines around eating[9].

Restrictive eating and eating disorders: do these occur in older age groups?

Brain health is an area that needs more investigation, especially when it comes to perimenopause and menopause. We know that altering hormonal levels leads to many of the symptoms associated with this period of life. Brain fog and changes to our cognition are well documented, but some evidence is emerging that there may also be structural and neurotransmitter production changes that leave us feeling a bit off-kilter.

The menopause transition, as it is often called, is most certainly a time of change. It can also often coincide with big life changes, such as children leaving the family home, ageing parents to care for, as well as elevated risks to personal health. The combination of these factors can often leave a woman feeling out of sorts, perhaps with a sense of falling short or even unworthiness. Humans are hardwired to avoid threats and many of us will look for ways and means to avoid some of these uncomfortable emotions and feelings that are bubbling away under the surface.

An eating disorder is exactly this; it can be a method of coping as it provides distraction, a false sense of security and a method of avoiding feeling. Fixation on how to eat and what to eat can initially feel like an escape, but as with all false refuges, the relief is temporary. The issue with an eating disorder is that it can soon spiral and result in biological consequences that are harmful to health[10].

Women who may have previously suffered from an eating disorder earlier in their life are probably the most susceptible, especially if they didn't fully understand the true purpose of their dysfunctional behaviour[11].

As with all eating disorders, seeking help from a team of qualified practitioners is advised and recommended.

Menopause story

A few years ago, Rosie came to see me. She was in her late 50s and she was struggling as she had noticed that she wasn't seeing any progress in her performance.

She had come to exercise late in her life. She said that she hit menopause and suddenly her body did not feel like hers anymore. She developed a "tummy" and found herself becoming hugely anxious and low in mood.

In an attempt to counteract this, Rosie employed a physical trainer who started her on an intense schedule of weights and high-intensity training. He also prescribed a lower-calorie diet. The weight started to fall off. By the time she came to me, it was clear she had developed a huge exercise dependency, disordered eating and a distorted body image. She was underweight and depressed on presentation.

Over the months we worked together, Rosie started to accept that she had a problem. She realised she was living her life through numerous food rules, which was causing her to miss out on family celebrations and general enjoyment of life. The more we explored, the more it became clear that her relationships with her body and food had changed when she hit menopause, but it was the heightened anxiety that had resulted in developing her exercise dependency, as it acted as a coping mechanism.

It took well over a year to help her achieve her target weight through a combination of modification of training, improved understanding and relationship with food and a combination of behavioural therapy and mindfulness. Prior to menopause, she had never had any issues with food or body.

Conclusions

A "menopause diet" that is effective for all women is a myth. As we are all individuals with different levels of activity and dietary requirements, there is not a universal "menopause diet". This is not the time to adopt exclusion of food groups and extreme eating patterns. Rather, this stage of the female hormone odyssey offers the opportunity to review and revise your eating patterns and make adjustments in step with hormone changes.

References

1 Vetrani C, Barrea L, Rispoli R et al. Mediterranean diet: What are the consequences for menopause? *Frontiers in Endocrinology* 2022; 13: 886824. doi: 10.3389/fendo.2022.886824. PMID: 35546996; PMCID: PMC9084275.
2 Barrea L, Pugliese G, Laudisio D et al. Mediterranean diet as medical prescription in menopausal women with obesity: A practical guide for nutritionists. *Critical Reviews in Food Science and Nutrition* 2021; 61 (7): 1201–1211. doi: 10.1080/10408398.2020.1755220. Epub 2020 Apr 24. PMID: 32329636.
3 University of East Anglia. How a Mediterranean diet could reduce bone loss in osteoporosis. *ScienceDaily* 2018. www.sciencedaily.com/releases/2018/07/180711093133.htm.
4 Peters BA, Santoro N, Kaplan RC et al. Spotlight on the gut microbiome in menopause: Current insights. *International Journal of Women's Health* 2022; 14: 1059–1072. doi: 10.2147/IJWH.S340491. PMID: 35983178; PMCID: PMC9379122.
5 Łaniewski P, Herbst-Kralovetz MM. Connecting microbiome and menopause for healthy ageing. *Nature Microbiology* 2022; 7: 354–358. doi: 10.1038/s41564-022-01071-6.
6 Giannini A, Caretto M, Genazzani AR et al. Neuroendocrine changes during menopausal transition. *Endocrines* 2021; 2 (4): 405–416. doi: 10.3390/endocrines2040036.
7 How to protect your brain health during menopause. https://healthmatters.nyp.org/how-to-protect-your-brain-health-during-menopause/.
8 Why alcohol affects women more in menopause 2020. https://www.healthcentral.com/condition/menopause/menopause-alcohol.
9 Shmerling RH. Is blood sugar monitoring without diabetes worthwhile? Harvard Health Publishing, 2021. https://www.health.harvard.edu/blog/is-blood-sugar-monitoring-without-diabetes-worthwhile-202106112473.
10 Mangweth-Matzek B, Hoek H, Rupp C et al. The menopausal transition—A possible window of vulnerability for eating pathology. *International Journal of Eating Disorders* 2013; 46 (6): 609–619. doi: 10.1002/eat.22157.
11 Baker J, Runfola C. Eating disorders in midlife women: A perimenopausal eating disorder? *Maturitas* 2016; 85: 112–116. ISSN 0378-5122. doi: 10.1016/j.maturitas.2015.12.017.

Scene 2 Where do I start with exercise?

Ally Atkins

Menopause and exercise

There are numerous myths around exercise for women, which can make it highly confusing and even off-putting. The physical and emotional changes that occur can really take their toll, but exercise is one thing that can reap numerous rewards for a stronger and healthier version of yourself. Exercise can be a very powerful ally, offering a multitude of benefits, not only for physical health but for mental health too.

Myth 1 The older you get, the harder you have to exercise to stay in shape

This unfortunately is a very common myth and can cause a lot of stress in women and often pushes women to do less rather than more because it feels like a vicious cycle. The truth is that 'less is more' – less intensity but more frequency. Strength/resistance training is great for building muscle, but what you do during the other hours of the day is just as important as that 30-minute focused workout. You don't have to do anything extreme in your 30 minutes; the most important thing is to feel your muscles working and build those connections. Adding other activities such as walking or cycling to your day is also important. If you're travelling to work or shopping, then try to use stairs instead of lifts. If you're out walking, then increase the pace a little so that you get some good cardio work. It doesn't have to be anything crazy[1].

If you're new to fitness and have started to walk more, then keep going – 20 minutes a day is a good starting point. There are so many health benefits associated with walking, including mental as well as physical health. Walking is brilliant for cardiovascular (heart) health and helps to improve circulation. You can also alter your level depending on your fitness and as you become fitter, you can challenge yourself more by walking uphill or on uneven surfaces to stimulate more muscles and engage your brain to figure out different terrains. I'm a big fan of woodland walking because your brain is constantly communicating with your muscles to maintain balance. It's great for confidence and stimulation. It's especially beneficial if you can combine it with deep breath work. Not only that, but walking can also be a social activity, which gets you out of the house and engaging with people. This in itself is an important part of life and the feel-good factor.

Strength training is hugely beneficial, and great to do as part of a fitness regime that includes walking, because it enables you to focus on specific muscle groups[2]. If you find you're doing a lot of walking but experience low back pain, having balance issues or keep getting cramps in particular muscles, then strength training is well worth your time. Our current lifestyles mean we spend a lot of time sitting, with sporadic walking, running or other forms of exercise.

One muscle group that you really need to pay attention to are the gluteal muscles (glutes), which are located in the posterior hip region. The gluteus maximus is the largest and strongest muscle in the human body, yet your lifestyle (especially the amount of time you spend seated) can hugely impact this muscle and cause instability, pain and poor posture. The simple fact is that when you're sitting, you're not using this large muscle and when you stand, your brain doesn't know to connect. The human body is a linked mechanical system and is designed to compensate during loss of function in any particular area, so if you sit too much and cause dysfunction, then this has knock-on effects. Your brain just wants you to stand but doesn't automatically know what it should be engaging to do so. Over time, this can lead to knee, hip, lower back and hamstring problems while your body tries to find its stability; it can also cause issues with posture because your glutes are important for support. What you may not realise is that you're losing the function of one of the most important muscles in the body[3].

How does this relate to walking versus strength training? If you get up out of your chair and go for a walk, then you may not be engaging properly through your glutes and the rest of your posterior chain. The syndrome of 'flat bottom' is very common among older people and it's not at all surprising. Another very common ailment is tight hamstrings and tight hips while your body tries to find stabilisation from somewhere. If you go out for long walks, using your hamstrings and your hips for stabilisation instead of activating the all-important glutes, then you can make the problems worse and that can put you off walking and instigate the feelings of getting old. You're not old; you're just not functioning as you should. I should say here that the deep abdominal muscles are also important muscles for stability and often go unchecked. The answer to strengthening the core isn't through numerous sit-ups but through targeting the deepest layers of the core through focused engagement. Building the brain-to-muscle connection is key.

This is where strength training alongside cardiovascular activities such as walking is important. Activating the glutes and starting to strengthen those muscles enables you to improve your walking technique and focus. When I'm out walking, I automatically use my glutes because I've strengthened and know how. You can do the same. Once you start using this big muscle group, you'll find you can walk faster and with more stability, which improves confidence and opens up doors for more opportunities with exercise. If you associate exercise with pain, then of course you won't want to do it.

Myth 2 I can't change my exercise habits

The first thing I'll say in response to this myth is that if you believe you won't then you won't. Positivity is never more important than when you get older and start to feel you are a slave to your weaknesses. Is it that your body is letting you down or your mind?

There is a part of your primitive brain called the amygdala and this is associated with the flight or fight response. Its focus is survival; it will do all it can to make it to the next day and if that means conserving energy, then that's what it will do. This is especially true in winter when energy conservation mode is at its highest due to the cold weather, hence why curling up on the sofa is very appealing. Your brain is seeking immediate comfort or pleasure. Once this becomes a habit, then it's harder to break free because your brain feels safe. It's all very instinctive and is part of our hard-wiring[4].

Your brain will never tell you to get out of bed in the morning, look forward to what the day will bring and do some exercise, especially in the early days when you're not seeing rewards for your efforts. This is something you have to train yourself to do and that is where your mental attitude is half the battle. If you've experienced trauma in your life, especially breaking any bones or having a fall, then loss of confidence in your abilities only adds to this caution. Your brain may be telling you to avoid certain exercises because they are dangerous or cause pain. We start to become anxious and do less so that we are safe, when in fact what we need to focus on is our ability to adapt and thrive. You absolutely can turn this around and become stronger and more capable than ever[5].

This is a time when it's important to have goals and plan ahead. We're lucky to have parts of the brain that have adapted – the 'modern brain', which can override these instinctive behaviours. Opting for exercise indoors is a good option so you won't be put off by the weather. There are plenty of ways to motivate yourself and make sure you keep moving whatever the weather, but planning ahead is key. Planning and goal setting are useful tools that help you tune in and get back on track. Don't let negativity hold you back; you need to take control and believe in yourself. First of all, you need to trust yourself and secondly you need to think about strengthening your body rather than weight loss. If you're exercising to lose weight and it's not working, then this in itself is off-putting – change your mental attitude and exercise to be strong. Strength through building muscle is key and it's brilliant for your brain health too. Weight loss will come when your systems are balanced and muscle is a big part of that.

Myth 3 It's too late to improve strength post menopause

As we get older, our muscles gradually decline through a process called sarcopenia and this process begins in our 30s. This natural decline is slow and becomes more apparent as we get older. It also varies between people, which is why our lifestyle is so important. If you are very sedentary, then it will happen faster. Our muscles are like mini factories for energy production – they are home to huge numbers of mitochondria, which are crucial for energy production. Not only this, but muscles are also important for the regulation of blood glucose levels by storing glucose as glycogen. The glycogen can be broken down by the muscle and used as needed. Loss of muscle means protein and energy production is lowered throughout the body, with fewer options for glucose storage[6].

As you lose muscle, you see a decrease in mitochondrial health and that is very important. This alone is reason enough to want to strengthen and build muscle. It's all about looking towards the older version of yourself and what that looks like. With muscle loss can come frailty, falls, loss of independence and loss of function. Weight isn't the focus; the focus should be on what you want for the future you. So why does this decline happen? It's actually a combination of factors, with one of the most important being lifestyle – exercise and nutrition. Not only is it important as well as highly beneficial to exercise, but it's also important to nourish your body with the right foods to help your muscles function and improve[7]. It has been demonstrated that even in the oldest and frailest nursing homes, there has been 'significant functional improvement' through a combination of nutrition and resistance exercises. This is huge! There's no mention of any drug intervention, just changing lifestyle and significantly reducing the onset of sarcopenia or age-related muscle loss. This allows a complete change of mindset, which is that you are in far more control of your future self than you may have realised[8].

Story about getting started with strength work

Emma travelled a lot with work and had started to struggle with putting bags in the overhead locker. She was also beginning to experience knee and hip pain. Emma is in her early 50s and postmenopause, she is very slim and her only exercise regime was running 4 or 5 days a week for around 5 to 7 km at a time. Emma felt like she was very fit but also felt like she was falling apart and needed her arms and shoulders to be much stronger. She couldn't understand why she was losing strength and was worried about frailty at such a young age. It's true that Emma had lost a lot of strength through her upper body, but my main area of concern was her lower body. If you don't have strength through your lower body, then you don't have a good foundation for everything above it. I suggested to Emma that she cut down her running to an amount that kept her mentally happy but didn't push her into stress mode. She settled for 2 days a week and no more than 5 km. The other 2–3 training days became strength training days. Emma went on a programme of body weight strength training, which meant using just her own body weight to strengthen the muscles with good technique. Squats and lunges became a large part of the routine and resistance bands were also useful. We worked on deep core strength (no sit-ups) and gave her hips and knees a rest. We focused on the big muscles of the lower body as these are sites of huge metabolic activity. Emma started to feel better. She felt stronger and her mental attitude also improved. We gradually added some light dumbbell work for the upper body and started forming connections between muscle groups. Emma's knee pain and hip pain gradually improved and she gradually cut down her running to do more strength work along with walking. This is a lady who, postmenopause, managed to strengthen her body, build better connections and reduced her pain. Of course it's possible. You need to believe you can do it.

While this is all highly positive and it's great to know that you have more control over the future version of yourself than you think, it's also important to note that ignoring the importance of strength training can be detrimental[9]. Strength training doesn't have to mean hiring a personal trainer; your daily activities can make a big difference, such as climbing stairs, dancing, cycling, hill walking, carrying shopping home, getting up from a chair without using your hands and many more physical activities.

Myth 4 Loss of balance and confidence are inevitable

Falls are the most common cause of injuries in adults aged 65 and over and are the most common cause of hip fractures and brain injuries. Falls are a common reason why older adults are placed in a nursing home, but the fall risk there is nearly three times higher. Why? It all comes down to being sedentary[8]. If you don't use it, then you lose it. This is an important concept to take on board. A sedentary lifestyle can increase your risk of many chronic problems as you get older. Now is the time to make changes. Ageing leads to a natural loss of muscle strength and flexibility, which makes it more difficult to maintain balance. Most people think ageing starts in their mid-60s but the decline actually starts much younger, as young as your 30s. Can you turn things around? Of course you can!

The majority of ladies I see in my studio, all of whom are over 40, are experiencing a loss of balance to various extents and this in turn affects their confidence. One of the main reasons that I'm contacted is to help with instability and feelings of a 'loss of strength and connection'. It can be unnerving, especially as it may not be at all obvious what's causing it. The good news, of course, is that you can do something about it and having a better understanding of why these things occur is very useful because if you understand it then you can work towards improvement.

Your skeletal muscle holds your bones in place and flexibility within the muscle allows you to move through ranges of motion. One of the biggest contributors to loss of muscle is a sedentary lifestyle[10]. Sitting for extended periods of time not only leads to muscle weakness and loss, but it also causes changes in your structure and posture.

The constant interaction that occurs between your brain, joints, tendons and muscles is hugely important and is called proprioception – the body's ability to sense the position, movement and orientation of its body parts without relying on sight. The inner ear is an important feedback mechanism too – hence why balance can be affected if your sinuses are inflamed. These mechanisms provide us with a subconscious awareness of where our body is in space and how it is moving. A sedentary lifestyle can have a negative impact on all these structures and awareness of our body parts[11]. When the body becomes stiff, weak and immobile due to inactivity, the sensory input from these areas will be diminished or altered, impacting accuracy and efficiency. When tendons and ligaments become too loose, muscles too weak and joints too limited in their range of motion, the sensory receptors become less sensitive and responsive, which in turn can affect balance, potentially leading to falls. Inflammation is another important factor. The older we get, without any interaction, the more out of touch we become with our systems[12].

Muscle motor neurons also play an important role here, causing our muscles to contract or relax following signals from the brain. Generally, each muscle has a supply of multiple motor neurons, which regulate muscle tone and tension. This arrangement allows for precise control of muscle contractions and coordination of movement. When motor neurons stimulate muscle contraction, they generate tension within the muscle fibres, which is detected by proprioceptive receptors. This feedback informs the brain about the current state of muscle tension and position, allowing for precise control of movement and posture[13].

An important point to note here is the impact of stress on movement, stability and balance. If we're stressed, we're likely to be in the fight or flight response, which means tense, tight muscles and rigidity. This is why it's important to be mindful and take time-out. Our body needs to calm down and relax, enabling our rest and digestive functions to take over and help us recover. If you're feeling highly stressed and walking on uneven terrain, then your brain will find it harder to communicate with your muscles and you're more likely to stumble.

The great thing about strength training, even just using your own body weight, means that you can improve your function and coordination as well as your muscle tone. This is where exercise technique is important, as well as listening to your body and incorporating breath work. It's possible to improve your function and your balance; just be patient with it.

Myth 5 You need a gym to strength train

This is a myth and unfortunately the fear of the gym is what can be most off-putting to women when it comes to strength training. Walking into a gym can feel intimidating and is often the last thing a woman wants to do when she is already feeling anxious and off-kilter. They're often not the most supportive and inclusive environments, which is a shame. The great news is you can strengthen your muscles at home with minimal equipment. Your body doesn't know whether you are in a gym, carrying your shopping or cleaning your kitchen at home. Exercises that make you breathe harder are great for cardio – a brisk walk is a brilliant start. Lifting, carrying and moving heavy loads is strength training. What is important is that you are regularly active. Your body and your brain will love you for it.

If you'd like to start a strength training routine at home, then the equipment you'll need totally depends on your fitness level. However, if you're new to it, then no equipment at all is the best starting point. Your own body weight is sufficient for strength building without impacting your joint range; in fact it's preferable to get those joints moving and bring some strength through mobility back.

There are exercises you can do at home that target some of your big muscle groups and really set you on your way to building muscle. Examples and their advantages are listed below:

The tripod foot

Understanding your foot mechanics and how this can feed up the chain to your hips is important and can be quite a game changer for a lot of people. Small daily changes can make the biggest difference. The tripod foot position, also known as the three-point foot position, involves distributing weight evenly across three points of contact on the foot: the base of the big toe, the base of the little toe and the centre of the heel. If you think about this foot position when standing for any period of time, you will relieve stress on your knees and your hips. The number of people I see who lean into one hip when standing still is staggering. Just making this small change of realigning your body weight distribution can really help your mechanics. It's especially important during exercise, such as squats and lunges, where your foot position plays a crucial role.

By evenly distributing weight across the foot, the tripod position provides a stable foundation for performing exercises and helps activate the muscles of the lower body more effectively through efficient transfer of force into the ground. This helps prevent side-to-side or front-to-back shifting of the weight during the movement, enhancing balance and stability. The position helps prevent excessive pronation (inward rolling) or supination (outward rolling) of the foot and reduces the risk of collapsed arches, promoting proper alignment of the ankle, knee and hip joints during squats, as shown in the images below.

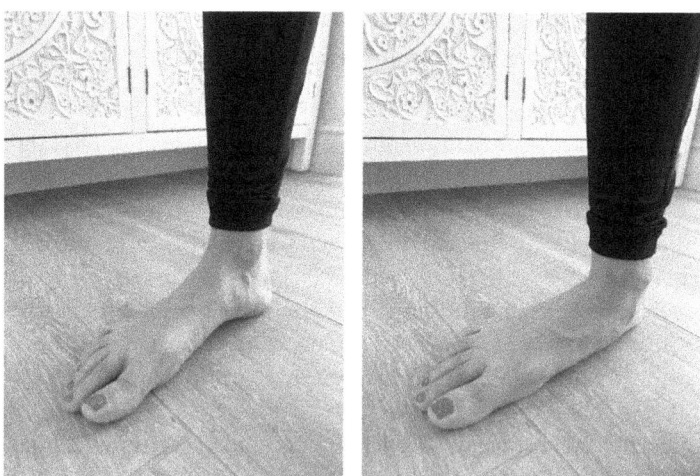

The above photos show a good tripod foot versus a pronated foot and the photos below show a good tripod foot on the left versus a pronated foot in the centre and a supinated foot to the right and how this can affect the alignment through the knees.

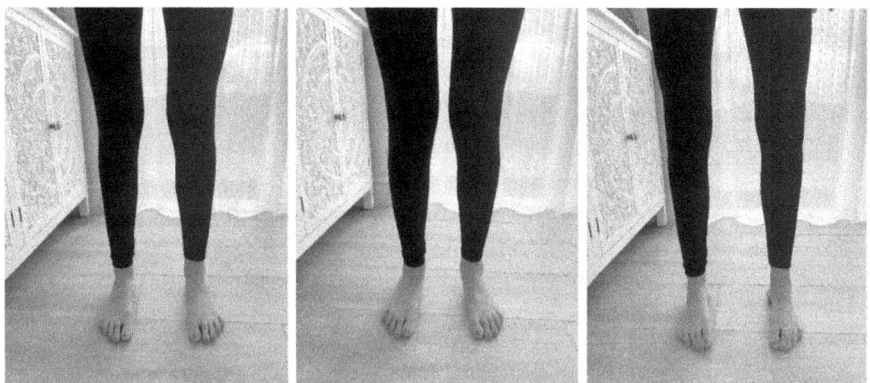

This alignment is essential for efficient force transmission and reduces the risk of injury by minimising stress on the joints. This includes the muscles of the feet, ankles, calves, quadriceps, hamstrings and glutes, optimising muscle recruitment and maximising power output and performance while minimising energy loss.

Focusing on your tripod foot is also important for your brain-to-muscle connection. Proprioception refers to the body's ability to sense its position in space. By consciously focusing on maintaining a tripod foot position during squats, you can develop better proprioceptive awareness, improving your ability to control and coordinate movement.

Static lunges

Static lunges are low-impact exercises that target several major muscle groups, including the quadriceps, hamstrings, glutes and calves, while placing minimal stress on the joints. By strengthening these muscles, you can improve muscle tone and functional strength, as well as boost metabolism by increasing muscle mass. Weight-bearing exercises like these can also help promote bone density and reduce the risk of fractures by placing stress on the bones, stimulating them to become stronger. Additionally, static lunges require balance and stability, which are important for reducing the risk of falls, as well as enhancing mobility and confidence in daily activities. I always recommend starting with just body weight and then you can add weights as you feel stronger, so long as you keep in mind that technique is important. A resistance band can be very useful if you struggle with alignment through your knees.

The images below show good alignment (top images) and poor alignment (bottom images). You can see the impact that poor hip and knee alignment has, but you also need to pay attention to your big toe joint mobility because lack of mobility in the big toe joint can have a knock-on effect and not only impact lunges but also your gait when you walk.

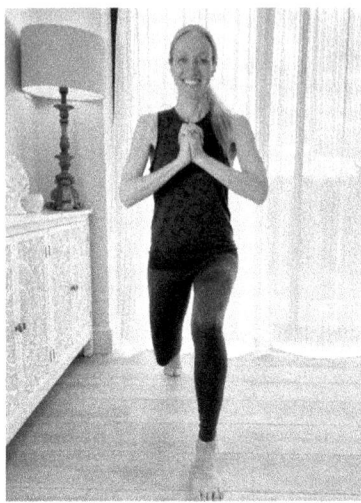 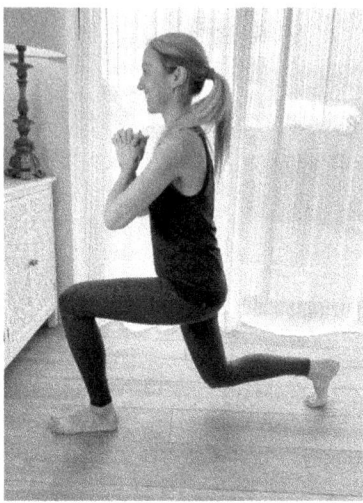

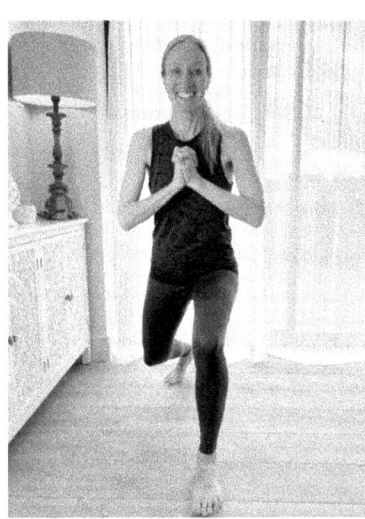 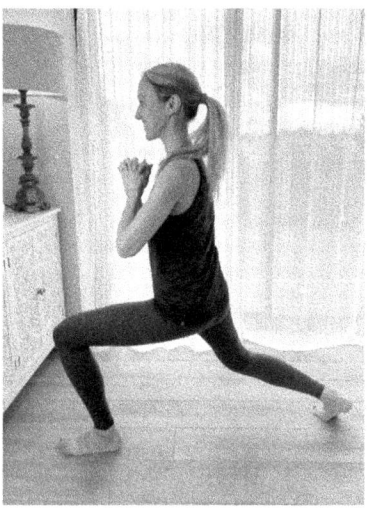

Narrow and wide squats

Squats can be particularly beneficial because they mimic natural movements like sitting down and standing up, making them highly functional for daily activities. By improving strength and mobility in the lower body, squats can enhance overall functional fitness and independence, helping to maintain an active lifestyle.

Squats are another compound exercise that target major muscle groups in the lower body, including the quadriceps, hamstrings, glutes and calves. By engaging these muscles, squats help improve strength, endurance and muscle mass. This is especially important during menopause, as women may experience a decline in muscle mass, exacerbated by hormonal changes, which can increase the risk of functional decline. Squats also help promote bone health by applying stress to the bones, which stimulates bone remodelling and increases bone density[14].

There are different variations and as you gain strength you can add a weight if you feel comfortable with it. They require flexibility, mobility and stability in the hips, knees and ankles and all these can be improved if you start with the basics and gradually strengthen using good technique. It's important to check your knee alignment, as shown in the images below, making sure you don't go so low that your knees buckle inwards. A resistance band can help with this. Performing squats regularly can help improve joint mobility and stability, reducing the risk of injuries and enhancing overall functional movement. Squats are also brilliant for metabolic health because they engage large muscle groups, leading to increased energy expenditure and metabolic rate.

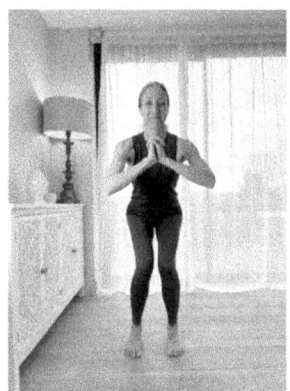
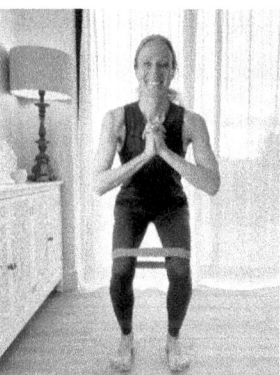
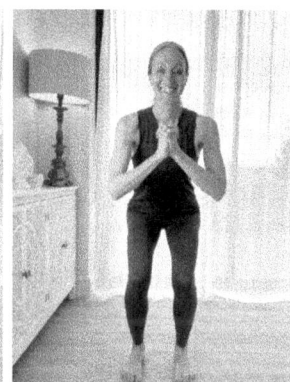

Heel/calf raises

Heel raises, also known as calf raises, can be beneficial for promoting blood flow and lymphatic circulation. Incorporating heel raises into a regular exercise routine, along with other cardiovascular and strength-training exercises, as mentioned above, can help support overall circulatory health and promote optimal function.

Performing heel raises involves contracting the calf muscles. These contractions help stimulate blood flow by compressing blood vessels and promoting the circulation of blood throughout the lower legs. This is why walking is so beneficial, because it naturally forces you to move from heel to toe and stimulate blood flow. A sedentary lifestyle can hugely impact your circulation. If you find yourself sitting for long periods, then heel raises can help.

Your heart does a brilliant job of pumping oxygenated blood around your body, but venous return, the process by which deoxygenated blood returns to the heart from the lower body, doesn't have the same pump action. The calf muscles act as a "muscle pump" that helps propel blood upwards against gravity, assisting in the return of blood to the heart and preventing blood pooling in the lower extremities.

Heel raises are also great for stimulating lymphatic circulation – the lymphatic system is responsible for removing waste products, toxins and excess fluid from the tissues. Muscle contractions facilitate the movement of lymph fluid through the lymphatic vessels and promote detoxification and waste removal. Another great reason why muscles are so important to health.

Heel raises can be a great warm-up and cool-down exercise if you're doing a routine at home. By increasing blood flow to the muscles, heel raises help prepare the lower extremities for exercise, reducing the risk of injury and improving performance. Performing heel raises as part of a cool-down routine after exercise can help promote recovery by aiding in the removal of metabolic waste products, such as lactic acid, from the muscles. This can help reduce muscle soreness and stiffness following physical activity.

To maximise the benefits of heel raises for circulation, it's important to perform the exercise with proper form and technique as shown below. The tripod foot position is an important starting point.

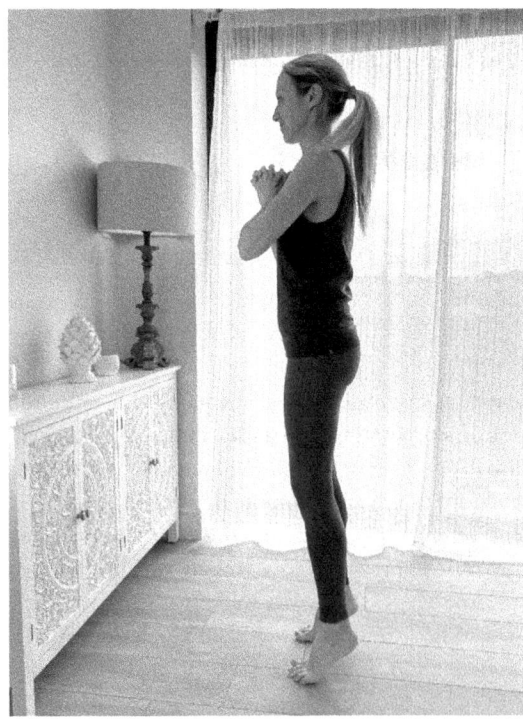

Push-ups

Push-ups are often seen as a man's exercise, but they are beneficial for women too, supporting both bone health and muscle strength. Push-ups are a compound exercise primarily targeting the muscles of the chest, shoulders, triceps and core. The muscles aren't as big as those of the lower body, but using them helps increase energy expenditure and metabolic rate. By regularly performing push-ups, you can improve upper body strength and muscle tone. This is important for maintaining functional strength and independence in daily activities.

Improving bone density is crucial during menopause, as hormonal changes can lead to decreased bone mass and increased risk of osteoporosis. By incorporating push-ups into your fitness routine, you can help preserve bone density, potentially reducing the risk of fractures. Push-ups also engage the muscles around the shoulder and elbow joints, promoting joint stability and mobility.

Push-ups mimic functional movements like pushing or lifting objects, making them highly practical for daily activities. By improving upper body strength and stability, push-ups can enhance overall functional fitness and quality of life. It's important to start gradually and focus on proper form to prevent injury and accommodate individual fitness levels. Modifications, such as performing push-ups on an elevated surface or from the knees, can be used to make the exercise more accessible if you're a beginner or have limited upper body strength. If you use a chair, just make sure it is secure.

The one issue I see most often with push-ups is people leading with their head, thinking they're getting lower, but this can create pain and dysfunction. Lead with your chest and don't worry if you can't get very low; strength building takes time as your muscles need to adapt.

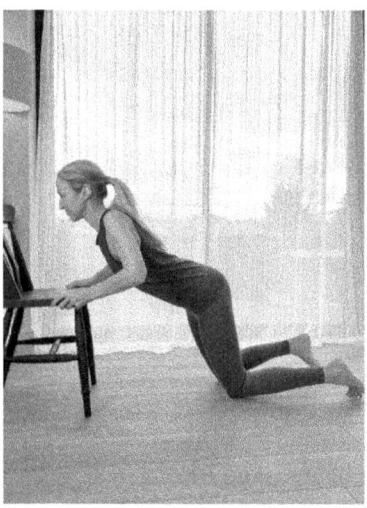 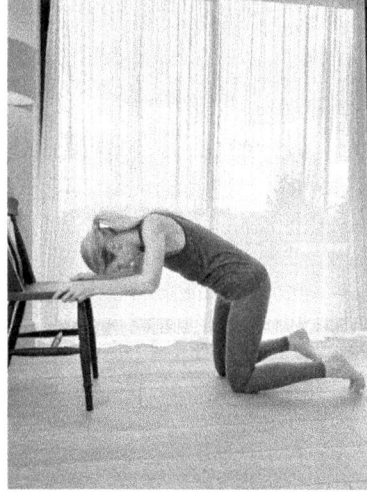

Myth 6 If I build muscle, I'll look bulky

This is a very popular myth that can be off-putting for women who want to get strong but don't want to look like a bodybuilder. The idea that strength training will automatically lead to a bulky physique is a common misconception. In reality, the extent to which an individual develops muscle size is influenced by various factors as shown below.

Women tend to have a higher percentage of slow-twitch muscle fibres, which are more resistant to hypertrophy (muscle building) compared to fast-twitch muscle fibres. This means that women may not experience the same level of muscle growth as men, even with strength training. The type of strength training programme is also important, including the intensity, volume and frequency of workouts, which can influence muscle development. Women who focus on moderate-to-high repetitions with lighter weights, along with proper form and technique, are less likely to experience significant muscle hypertrophy compared to those training with heavy weights and low repetitions.

One very important factor is that you are what you eat and muscle growth requires a calorie surplus and adequate protein intake. Women who strength train without consuming excess calories or following a specific muscle-building diet are less likely to experience significant muscle growth. With proper programming and nutrition, women can achieve a lean, toned appearance through strength training.

Overall, strength training is highly beneficial for women, offering improvements in strength, bone density, metabolism, body composition and overall health without necessarily leading to a bulky physique. It's essential to tailor your strength training programme to individual goals and preferences, whether they aim for muscle hypertrophy, strength gains or simply improved fitness and well-being.

So, how much exercise should you be doing?

If your doctor gives you the go-ahead, there's no reason not to start straight away and begin building connections and gaining strength. The exercises shown in this section are a good starting point, along with cardiovascular exercise such as walking. Starting anywhere is better than not starting at all. Public Health England recommends 150 minutes of moderate-intensity exercise per week, including a mix of cardiovascular exercise and at least two strength-building sessions. If this is off-putting, then start adding 10 minutes a day and go from there. All kinds of exercise can be an effective way to manage stress and stay mentally healthy. You could combine your exercise routine with other evidence-based practices, like mindfulness meditation – or, reap the benefits of some good, old-fashioned fresh air and sunshine by taking a walk outdoors. The important thing is that you find activities you enjoy and stick with them. Start with what you can manage and build from there. Your future self will thank you for it.

References

1. Church TS, Earnest CP, Skinner JS et al. Effects of different doses of physical activity on cardiorespiratory fitness among sedentary, overweight or obese postmenopausal women with elevated blood pressure: A randomized controlled trial. *JAMA* 2007; 297 (19): 2081–2091.

2   Distefano G, Goodpaster BH. Effects of exercise and aging on skeletal muscle. *Cold Spring Harbor Perspectives in Medicine* 2018; 8 (3): a029785. doi: 10.1101/cshperspect.a029785. PMID: 28432116; PMCID: PMC5830901.

3   Buckthorpe M, Stride M, Villa FD. Assessing and treating Gluteus Maximus Weakness – A clinical commentary. *International Journal of Sports Physical Therapy* 2019 Jul; 14 (4): 655–669. PMID: 31440415; PMCID: PMC6670060.

4   Amygdala hijack: When emotion takes over. *Healthline* online 2023. https://www.healthline.com/health/stress/amygdala-hijack. Accessed February 2024.

5   Burnett D. Your brain is hard-wired to avoid exercise. BBC Science Focus. https://www.sciencefocus.com/comment/exercise-brain. Acessed March 2024.

6   Argilés JM, Campos N, Lopez-Pedrosa JM et al. Skeletal muscle regulates metabolism via interorgan crosstalk: Roles in health and disease. *Journal of the American Medical Directors Association* 2016; 17 (9): 789–796. doi: 10.1016/j.jamda.2016.04.019. Epub 2016 Jun 17. PMID: 27324808.

7   Walston JD. Sarcopenia in older adults. *Current Opinion in Rheumatology* 2012; 24 (6): 623–627. doi: 10.1097/BOR.0b013e328358d59b. PMID: 22955023; PMCID: PMC4066461.

8   Lorenz RA, Gooneratne N, Cole CS et al. Exercise and social activity improve everyday function in long-term care residents. *American Journal of Geriatric Psychiatry* 2012; 20 (6): 468–476. doi: 10.1097/JGP.0b013e318246b807. PMID: 22617163; PMCID: PMC4367449.

9   Arce-Esquirel AA, Ballard JE. Effects of resistance training on bone and muscle mass in older women. *Sports Exercise Medicine Open* 2015; 1 (3): 89–96. doi: 10.17140/SEMOJ-1-114.

10 Volpi E, Nazemi R, Fujita S. Muscle tissue changes with aging. *Current Opinion in Clinical Nutrition & Metabolic Care* 2004; 7 (4): 405–410. doi: 10.1097/01.mco.0000134362.76653.b2. PMID: 15192443; PMCID: PMC2804956.

11 Working out boosts brain health. *American Psychological Association* March 2020. https://www.apa.org/topics/exercise-fitness/stress.

12 Suetterlin K, Sayer AA. Proprioception: Where are we now? A commentary on clinical assessment, changes across the life course, functional implications and future interventions. *Age and Ageing* 2014; 43 (3). doi: 10.1093/ageing/aft174.

13 The human balance system. Veda Vestibular Article. https://vestibular.org/article/what-is-vestibular/the-human-balance-system/the-human-balance-system-how-do-we-maintain-our-balance/. Accessed March 2024.

14 Nguyen VH. Exercises aimed to maximize lean mass and bone mineral density at the hip and lumbar spine. *Osteoporosis Sarcopenia* 2021; 7 (1): 42–43. doi: 10.1016/j.afos.2021.03.001. Epub 2021 Mar 18. PMID: 33869805; PMCID: PMC8044589.

Scene 3 Demystifying the myths of exercise

Dr Alyssa Olenick

Menopause: Body and fitness changes

There's a growing awareness about menopause and how it affects women, especially in the fitness industry. Menopause causes hormonal changes that can be confusing and frustrating, particularly when it comes to figuring out the best workouts to manage them. This confusion often leads women to ask, "*What exercises should I be doing?*". It can be challenging for those who haven't had a specific fitness routine before and are now trying to adjust to new workouts while also dealing with changing hormones.

If you're going through menopause and wondering how to stay fit, you're in the right place. But before we talk about what you can do, let's first understand how menopause affects our bodies, why it's essential to stay healthy during this time and how to tackle it.

Before we begin, let me start by saying this: "*I don't want to scare you or add to your worries about the changes that come with menopause. No matter where you are in your journey, you have the power to take control of your health and behaviour.*"

Understanding how menopause impacts muscle, bone and fat

One of the main symptoms of ageing is a loss of muscle mass, known as sarcopenia. The other is bone loss, known as low bone density and osteoporosis. The loss of female sex hormones during menopause, specifically oestradiol (E2), exacerbates this loss of muscle and bone in women. However, this decline may also be partially related to decreases in progesterone and testosterone[3]. Oestradiol is commonly known for being an important hormone that regulates the menstrual cycle and helps maintain female sex characteristics. However, it also plays a vital role in building and repairing muscle tissue and maintaining bone density. Our muscles and bones have receptors that interact with oestrogen, help in muscle growth and recovery, promote muscle health[4] and regulate bone metabolism[5,6].

Sarcopenia occurs with ageing and is the gradual loss of our muscle mass size, strength and how well it works. Sarcopenia is made worse by menopause, which is associated with an increased risk of health outcomes like falling, loss of independence or poorer metabolic health[1,7]. Furthermore, we have two types of muscle fibres. Type I are our slow-twitch, more 'endurance' fibres that help with long-term cardio workouts or daily life. Our type II fibres are our more powerful and thicker fibres, associated with strength and all-out short but hard bouts of exercise. Ageing and menopause are associated with a loss of the total number of our muscle fibres and more specifically with the loss of size of more powerful muscle fibres (Type II fibres) and an increase in the total ratio of our slower and less powerful muscle fibres (Type I fibres)[4]. Menopause may further increase this muscle loss due to an increased inflammatory state, resulting in more muscle loss over time due to an impaired ability of muscles to recover and repair muscle tissue[1,2,8]. These changes are also associated with muscles storing more fat, which may worsen our muscle's metabolism and hurt our metabolic health[1,4,9]. Additionally, our muscle cells can start to die off, and our mitochondria (which help produce energy in our cells) may not work as well as they used to[1,4,9]. This is important because mitochondrial function is essential for endurance performance, weight gain and metabolic health[4,10].

Perimenopause and menopause are also phases of life associated with a rapid decline in bone mineral density, leading to weaker bones[11]. Osteoporosis, a condition that affects 19.6% of women worldwide, is characterised by significant bone density loss[12]. Additionally, 51.5% of women have low bone mass, which increases the risk of developing osteoporosis[12]. The combination of increased fall risk from muscle loss and fragile bones can result in fractures.

Menopause also causes a shifting of fat storage to the belly area instead of the hips and lower body, with a reported average gain of 2–3 kg (5–7 lbs.) during menopause[13,14]. Menopause also increases a specific type of fat tissue called visceral adipose tissue that is stored around the organs and is associated with greater inflammation and poorer metabolic health[15]. Gains in fat mass and muscle loss may result in a condition known as 'sarcopenic obesity'[16], a state of low muscle relative to total body weight. The increased inflammatory state associated with this fat tissue may further result in muscle loss, and loss of muscle mass may contribute to increased fat gain through reductions in total daily energy expenditure, impaired muscle fatty acid metabolism and insulin resistance, creating a feedback loop between muscle loss and fat gain[17-21]. All these changes outlined here and above lead to an increased risk of cardiovascular and metabolic disease in postmenopausal women[22-25].

During menopause, the way we store fat in the body also shifts, causing it to be stored more in the belly than in the hips and lower body[13,14]. Menopause also results in an average reported weight gain of 2–3 kg (5–7 lbs.)[13,14]. However, it is hard to say if this increase in fat mass is due to menopause alone or a combination of lifestyle factors and the challenges of the menopause transition. Additionally, menopause leads to an increase in a specific type of fat tissue called visceral adipose tissue. This fat is stored around the organs and is associated with greater inflammation and poor metabolic health[15]. Together with muscle loss, these changes in body fat can lead to a condition known as 'sarcopenic obesity', which is a state of low muscle relative to total body weight[16]. The increased inflammation caused by increased visceral adipose tissue can further result in muscle loss, which may keep us in a cycle of muscle loss and fat gain[17-21]. Together, these muscle, bone and fat changes can increase the risk of cardiovascular and metabolic diseases in postmenopausal women[22-25].

Muscle, bone, metabolism and health changes can feel stressful when outlined. However, it is crucial to understand what is changing in our bodies so we can separate physiology from shame and avoid beating ourselves up for what is 'normal' even if we don't love the outcome. However, the good news is that exercise (along with good nutrition and sleep) is powerful in maintaining or improving bone, muscle, body fat and metabolic health.

Myth 1 Menopausal women need a unique exercise programme?

It can seem like hormone changes and ageing are the only things impacting our health and fitness. It turns out that less daily physical activity significantly contributes to the loss of muscle, bone mass and strength as we age[26]. As women age, activity levels also tend to decrease. The good news? Physical activity *is* a modifiable factor.

Regarding exercise training and menopause, we need to think less about a 'special menopause exercise protocol' and more about which parts of a good fitness routine become even more critical here. While peri- and postmenopausal women can benefit from any activity, and all activity is good (no shame here around your favourite way to move!), what we want to really start to think about are what I like to call the three main pillars of menopausal fitness: strength, power and intensity. As we have outlined already, muscle, fat and bone changes are some of the biggest risks that come with menopause. The good news? Exercise training is a powerful way to help slow or reduce bone loss, even *build* muscle and decrease things like visceral adipose tissue or central fat changes (alongside good nutrition, of course!). So, let's dive in on what we need and, most importantly, how to do it.

Myth 2 Menopause tanks our metabolism, and it is all our hormone's fault!

Many people associate exercise with the most energy we use or "burn" daily, but this is not entirely accurate. Our daily energy (calorie) expenditure is primarily influenced by our basal metabolic rate (calories needed to keep us alive), the calories we burn while digesting food and our non-exercise daily activities[27]. Menopause can lead to decreased spontaneous movement and physical activity despite women not feeling any different. Research studies are starting to suggest that lower oestrogen levels in humans and rodents result in less daily physical activity, which can reduce daily movement and energy expenditure without being consciously aware of it[28–33].

As mentioned earlier, menopause can have a significant impact on a woman's health and body composition. Muscle mass plays a crucial role in our metabolism[34]. As we age, metabolism doesn't appear to slow significantly until we are 60. However, menopause may still result in a slight decrease in metabolism (<100 kcal/day)[28,29,33,35]. This decrease may be due to lower activity levels, reduced brown adipose tissue activity, muscle loss or a combination of these factors. When coupled with less daily movement, poor sleep and muscle loss, it may lead to a feeling of a significantly slower metabolism in menopausal women.

The good news is you can increase your daily movement by being more intentional if your body isn't doing it without you thinking about it! This can be achieved by taking more daily walk breaks, hitting a total daily step count of 7,000–8,000 steps a day[36] or using small exercise breaks across the day to break up sitting[37]. Gardening, walking with friends or even household chores are ways to achieve this. These things don't have to be extreme, but more mindful practices of moving easily but more often during our days. We can also help maintain or gain muscle through resistance training, which we will talk about further on.

Myth 3 Cardio increases cortisol and cortisol makes us fat, so we shouldn't do it

There is a current trend in menopause to avoid exercises that increase cortisol, such as long-duration cardio or high-intensity exercise. While it is true that menopause is associated with elevated cortisol levels and increased abdominal fat, these are often associated with increases in visceral adipose tissue, or the fat around our organs[38]. It is also true that the cortisol response appears to be higher in individuals with higher body fat and abdominal fat storage[38-40]. However, it is unclear if individuals with a higher cortisol-reactive response gain weight due to this response, or if increased central fat mass elevates this response[40].

Additionally, increased stress levels (associated with elevated cortisol) are possibly related to increased body weight, and an increased cortisol response increases the consumption of fatty and sugary foods[40-43]. However, this response is individual, with some women showing a heightened response to increased food intake in response to this and others showing a decrease[38,42]. The data is not clear-cut on whether cortisol is directly related to body size or if it indirectly causes fat gain due to a relationship between an increased stress response, which results in increased consumption of sugary and fatty foods, leading to increased caloric intake, and this increases weight gain. So, while it may play a role, we can still focus on healthy movement and diet choices!

When it comes to exercise, aerobic and intense exercise do increase our nervous system response, and cortisol is released[44,45]. The amount of cortisol and other hormones made by the adrenal glands (small glands on our kidneys that make hormones), like adrenaline and noradrenaline, increases as exercise intensity increases. This is not a bad thing, though! The release of adrenal hormones during exercise is used as a signal to our bodies to break down carbs or fats in storage to be used during exercise for energy metabolism[44,45]. The cortisol response to exercise is intensity-dependent, appearing to increase at intensities greater than ~60% $\dot{V}O_2$ max (maximal cardio output) and only appears to increase during long-term lower-intensity exercise when we haven't eaten enough carbs and our blood sugar is low

Individuals who habitually exercise will need higher intensities of exercise to reach the same level of cortisol response or have lower exercise cortisol levels at low or similar intensities[44]. While exercise is a stressor, which isn't always a bad thing, adapting to this over time leads to positive adaptations and health outcomes. While there are potential sex, age and training differences in the cortisol and adrenal response to exercise training[46], it is hypothesised that being exposed to this stress response to exercise training in menopausal women may help potentially reduce vasomotor symptoms[47]. However, the data on this is currently very messy and inconclusive.

While cardio gets a bad rap, it (and resistance training) is associated with reductions in visceral adipose tissue[48,49], not increases! In fact, cardio exercise training is one of the best ways to reduce visceral adipose tissue even without total body fat loss changes[50]! Cardio is also related to reduced overall body fat. Therefore, cardio should not be feared or avoided in menopause. Additionally, as we will outline in the section on high-intensity interval training (HIIT), intensity may be something we want to help preserve our muscle tissue and power output during menopause.

Our day-to-day lives bring on many and possibly frequent spikes in our stress or cortisol. The key is not to avoid exercise altogether or fear intensity or cardio. Things we can do instead support our stress management or response to stressors to decrease this within our days. That way, the stress from exercise doesn't 'overdo' what our body can handle. Other approaches that may help are to take breaks from high volume or intense training, like breaks between race training, periods of lower to moderate intensity if we are feeling extra stressed or embracing more rest days as we age to emphasise recovery. While keeping in mind that recovery may be slower as we age, and we may need to take more rest days or do less overall training to get the same results without overdoing it.

Myth 4 We should avoid all high-intensity training

Another approach to cardio training is to balance our intensity or be more specific about intensity in our workouts. This approach often looks like having 1–2 of our weekly cardio workouts spent doing intentional hard-effort training like HIIT, sprint interval training (SIT), high-intensity functional training (HIFT), speed or power work in zones 4–5 or RPE 7–10 (Figures 4.3.1 and 4.3.2) If you are an endurance athlete or someone doing a lot of cardio each week (>3–4 hours), then the rest should be ~70–90% easier effort days like zone 1 or 2 or RPE 2–5 aerobic work (Figures 4.3.1 and 4.3.2). When looking at peri- and postmenopausal women specifically, we may shift this even more so that more of your overall cardio has that high-intensity component to support your muscle and power output, which declines as we age. This would look like 2–3 high-quality hard or intense effort HIIT/SIT/HIFT workouts each week, and the rest being balanced with easier or lower intensity days, lifting days or other activities we love.

One way to add intensity to our exercise is through HIIT, SIT and repeated sprint training, which are types of exercise that involve short bursts of intense activity at near-maximal effort, maximal or beyond maximal effort, followed by periods of rest or low-

ZONE	RPE	BREATH & TALK	% MAX HEART RATE
1	2-3	Very Easy Breathing & Easy To Talk	50-60%
2	4-5	Relatively Easy Breathing & Conversation	60-70%
3	6	Slightly Heavy Breathing & Short Talking	70-80%
4	7-8	Heavy Breathing & Difficult Talking	80-90%
5	9-10	Very Heavy Breathing & No Talking	90-100%

Figure ownership: DR ALYSSA OLENICK LLC

FIGURE 4.3.1 Cardio zones

intensity exercise to recover between (Figure 4.3.3). This type of exercise has been shown to improve aerobic endurance and cardio performance, fat oxidation and mitochondrial oxidation[51,52]. HIIT also has metabolic health benefits like improved mood, lower cardiovascular disease risk, decreased body fat, improved insulin sensitivity and decreased risk of metabolic syndrome, all things impacted by menopause[51].

HIIT decreases total body fat and visceral adipose tissue, improves body composition and increases muscle mass in peri- and/or postmenopausal women[53-58]. While results are mixed on whether this is better than regular moderate-intensity continuous cardio exercise[56,57], HIIT improves body composition like traditional cardio or more! Furthermore, HIIT in postmenopausal women has been shown to improve $\dot{V}O_2$ max (a measure of maximal oxygen uptake and cardio fitness), the ability to use anaerobic energy metabolism and increase power output with training

Therefore, HIIT or SIT training may be advantageous for peri- and postmenopausal women to help maintain muscle performance and health. It's important to note that

RATINGS OF PERCEIVED EXERTION (RPE) SCALE FOR CARDIO ACTIVITIES

1 - 2	Rest or Minimal Exertion
3 - 4	Light Activity, Comfortable & Maintainable
5 - 6	Moderately Hard, Slightly Uncomfortable, but Maintainable
7 - 8	Vigorous Exercise, Hard Breathing, Uncomfortable
9 - 10	Extremely Hard, Maximal Intensity

Source: American College of Sports Medicine.
Figure ownership: DR ALYSSA OLENICK LLC

FIGURE 4.3.2 Ratings of Perceived Exertion (RPE) for cardio activities

HIIT/SIT EXAMPLES

Running, biking, rowing, air bike, or similar:
- 4-6 rounds of 4 minutes all out with 2-3 min recovery
- 4-8 rounds of 2 minutes all out with 2 minutes recovery
- 4-6 rounds of 20-30 second all-out sprints, 1.5-2 minutes recovery

THINK: RPE 9/10 during the intervals, Recovery = full rest.

FIGURE 4.3.3 HIIT and SIT examples

HIIT benefits on muscle power or mass need to be combined with traditional strength training for the best combination of health and performance[55,56].

Myth 5 Lifting and jumping are unsafe for ageing individuals, and they make you bulky!

As women age, they face more risks associated with muscle loss and a decline in their ability to function independently in their daily lives. This makes it crucial for them to maintain their strength as they go through menopause. One of the most effective ways to improve muscle strength, size and functionality is through resistance training

RATINGS OF PERCEIVED EXERTION (RPE) SCALE FOR LIFTING ACTIVITIES

Rating	Description of Perceived Exertion
10	Maximum Effort
9	1 Rep Remaining
8	2 Reps Remaining
7	3 Reps Remaining
5-6	4-6 Reps Remaining
3-4	Light Effort
1-2	Little to No Effort

FIGURE 4.3.4 Ratings of Perceived Exertion (RPE) scale for lifting activities

or lifting weights. This can be done using equipment such as dumbbells, barbells, kettlebells, lifting machines, banded exercises or just your own body weight[61]. These training sessions usually involve sets, reps and effort levels. However, not all individuals know their maximum weight limit. Therefore, a rating of perceived exertion (RPE) can be used as an alternative. The RPE scale measures the level of effort on a scale of 1 to 10, with 10 being the maximum effort or the inability to do any more reps (Figure 4.3.4).

A study conducted in 2021 examined the effects of resistance training on peri/postmenopausal women. Most of the studies used workouts consisting of 8–12 exercises of 2–3 sets of 8–13 reps, lasting up to 50 minutes for 2 or 3 days per week[61]. The results showed that there was an increase in upper, lower or total body strength, including muscle activation, handgrip and knee strength. Furthermore, the studies that looked at functional fitness found that all participants improved daily activities such as standing up, sitting down and walking. This may not seem significant for younger women in the early stages of menopause, but as people age, these activities become more important for maintaining independence and improving muscle function.

One of the most significant risk factors in ageing women is the loss of bone density, alongside muscle power and strength. However, heavy lifting and power or jump training can help reduce this risk[62,63]. To maintain, gain or slow down the loss of bone density, the focus should be on heavy lifting exercises that target the hips and spine such as squats, deadlifts, lunges, step-ups and leg presses, as these areas are at the highest risk of fracture[62,63]. Another effective way to create stronger bones is through jumping, power or plyometric training. A review paper examining bone density in menopausal women found that training at 70–90% of maximum effort for 2–3 sets of 8–12 reps for a year significantly increased bone density[62,63].

In 2019, a review paper analysed the safety and effectiveness of lower body plyometric training for older adults (aged 58–91 years)[64]. Out of 289 subjects, 176 were women. The study found that plyometric training was safe, with no reported injuries. Furthermore, it was observed that plyometric training possibly increased bone density in the femur, spine and hip, and improved muscular power in the lower body. Another review in 2022 found that power training may be more effective than strength training alone, but it is still recommended to combine them[65].

The studies that observed an improvement in bone density were year-long and included up to 50 'hops' a day during the training. The jumping programmes used in these studies ranged from starting with 3 days a week and working up to 7 days a week, with 3-5 sets of 4–10 jumps at a time. If you're just starting out, you should begin with fewer overall jumps (1–2x/week, 2–3 sets of 10 easy jumps) and slowly work up to more frequent jumps (3–5x/week, 4–5 sets of easy jumps) or increase the difficulty of the jumps as you get better at them (Figures 4.3.5 and 4.3.6). There are many ways to do plyometrics, and if you're hesitant, you can start with easy jumps or work with a personal trainer or coach to help you progress safely. When planning your workouts, it's recommended to do your plyometric training after your warm-up and before your lifting.

Starting with too much workout or doing too many exercises may feel overwhelming. To make it easier, a good rule of thumb for those in menopause is to do 2–3 sets of 5–12 reps at a 6–9/10 RPE or effort for each major movement (Figure 4.3.4). These movements should include quads, hamstrings, butt, core, chest, shoulders and back muscles each week (Figure 4.3.7). You can break these down into different types of movements such as hinge patterns for glutes and hamstrings, squat patterns for quads and glutes,

LOWER BODY JUMPS/PLYOMETRICS

Low impact/beginner: Two foot hops, jump squats, two leg vertical jumps, skipping, double leg box jump, jumping rope, standing long jump

Medium impact/intermediate: Single leg hops, tuck jumps, split squat jump, jump over an object, side skip, side to side jumps, lateral box jump

High impact/advanced: Jumping lunges, single leg vertical jump, zig zag hops, single leg box jump, depth jump, depth jump to box jumps.

Source: Davies et al. 2015; Figure ownership: DR ALYSSA OLENICK LLC

FIGURE 4.3.5 Examples of lower body jumps or plyometrics

PLYOMETRICS / JUMPS:

- **Intensity**: Start with low impact and work toward medium or high impact over time
- **Frequency**: 1-3 sessions/week, start with 1.
- **Rest**: 2-3 days between jumping sessions. Take 2-3 minutest of rest between sets.
- **Amount**:
  - **Sedentary adults**: 20-50 jumps per session
  - **Beginner**: 80-100 jumps per session
  - **Intermediate**: 100-120 jumps per session
  - **Advanced**: 120-140 jumps/impact per session

Source: Davies et al. 2015 Figure ownership: DR ALYSSA OLENICK LLC

FIGURE 4.3.6 Examples of programming lower body jumps or plyometrics

pushing patterns for shoulders and chest, pulling patterns for back and upper body, and core for abs, hips and overall stability (Figure 4.3.7).

You should aim to include 2–4 of these lifts each week and organise them by full body, upper body or lower body days (Figure 4.3.9). For most people, 2–3 full body days per week are the best way to incorporate lifting into their training routine. As you progress, you can make your workouts harder or adapt to your fitness level by gradually increasing weight or reps. This process is called progressive overload (Figure 4.3.8). However, it can also be achieved by gaining more confidence in your movements, making lifting feel easier, or trying a more challenging variation.

LIFTING MOVEMENT CATEGORIES & EXAMPLES

Movement	Type	General Example Exercises
Upper Pressing	Shoulder Press	Barbell shoulder press, dumbbell shoulder press, shoulder press machine
	Chest Press	Barbell chest press, dumbbell chest press, chest press machine, push-ups (can modify)
Upper Pulling	Pulling Down	Lat pull down machine, cable pull downs, pull up or chin ups, upward rows
	Rowing	Barbell rows, dumbbell rows, row machine, cable rows, bodyweight inverted rows
Lower Body	Hip Hinging	Barbell or trap-bar deadlift, Romanian deadlifts, dumbbell deadlifts, hip thrusts
	Squat Patterns	Barbell squats, leg press machine, step ups, lunges, single leg squats
	Core/Other	Farmers carries, sled pushes, dead-bugs, planks, hollow holds, etc.

Figure ownership: DR ALYSSA OLENICK LLC

FIGURE 4.3.7 Examples of lifting movement categories and example exercises

WAYS TO PROGRESSIVELY OVERLOAD:

- Increase weight used for rep range
- Improve form used with weight/reps
- Increase reps done AT same weight
- Increase sets done or total training volume (weight used x reps x sets)
- Increase number of days you lift or train
- Maintain lower effort at same intensity / RPE
- Lower RPE at same weight or work demand/Intensity
- Increasing the difficulty of a movement (going from air to goblet to back squat)
- Increase mileage or pace at set mileage

People often over complicate progressive overload and think it means more and more weight each week. Sometimes it's as simple as doing an extra rep at the same weight, or moving up in weight, a lower exertion at the same weight/intensity, or IT simply feeling easier or moving to a more advanced movement pattern!

FIGURE 4.3.8 Ways to progressively overload

Example weekly workout splits:

EXAMPLE:	MON	TUES	WED	THURS	FRI	SAT	SUN
5 DAYS: 2 LIFT 2 CARDIO	FULL BODY LIFT	HIIT/SIT		FULL BODY LIFT		HIIT/SIT OR ZONE 2 20-60 MIN	
5 DAYS: 3 LIFT 2 CARDIO	FULL BODY LIFT	HIIT/SIT		FULL BODY LIFT	FULL BODY LIFT	HIIT/SIT OR ZONE 2 20-60 MIN	
4 DAYS: 3 LIFT 2 CARDIO	FULL BODY LIFT + HIIT/SIT	FULL BODY LIFT		FULL BODY LIFT		HIIT/SIT OR ZONE 2 20-60 MIN	
4 DAYS: 2 LIFT 2 CARDIO	FULL BODY LIFT	HIIT/SIT		FULL BODY LIFT	HIIT/SIT OR ZONE 2 20-60 MIN		
3 DAYS: 2 LIFT 2 CARDIO		FULL BODY LIFT + HIIT/SIT		FULL BODY LIFT	HIIT/SIT OR ZONE 2 20-60 MIN		
3 DAYS: 3 LIFT 2 CARDIO		FULL BODY LIFT + SIT/HIIT		FULL BODY LIFT		HIIT/SIT OR ZONE 2 20-60 MIN	

Please note: these are just examples, and can be rearranged in any order based on your schedule or time you have or what works best for you! There are many ways to set up a week of training.
Figure ownership: DR ALYSSA OLENICK LLC

FIGURE 4.3.9 Examples of how to set up a weekly workout split

Myth 6 Getting started is hard!

For many of you, this may be new information, which can be confusing and overwhelming. However, it does not have to be this way. Here are some tips that can help you get started on your fitness journey:

(1) **Start with small steps:** Begin with 2 to 3 days of training per week and gradually increase from there. You do not have to do everything all at once. Start with what feels easiest for you to fit into your schedule and then gradually build up your workout routine. For example, two lifts and one to three cardio workouts, combined with activities that you enjoy, such as walking, can be an excellent place to start. You do not have to do them on different days, and you can fit them into just 2 to 3 days per week.

(2) **Don't overdo it:** It is not necessary to jump into the most intense or challenging exercise immediately. If you have never lifted a barbell, you can start with machines, free weights or bands to get comfortable. Start with less weight than you think you can handle because you can always add more. Remember, form is a spectrum, and there is no such thing as 'good' or 'bad' form. With time and practice, you will become better at lifting, and your movements will become more comfortable and natural. If you lack confidence in your form or lifting heavier weights or with barbells, consider setting up a few sessions with a personal trainer.

(3) **Use the Rating of Perceived Exertion (RPE):** RPE is a great way to determine if you are going too hard or not hard enough during your lifting or cardio sessions. Use the 1–10 scale to check in with yourself. During your lifts, ask yourself if it feels like a 7–9/10. If you are not sure, keep going until you cannot do any more reps to get a feel for the right intensity (Figures 4.3.2 and 4.3.4).

For cardio, easy workouts should feel like a 2–4/10, and high-intensity workouts like HIIT, SIT or HIFT should feel like a 7–9/10 effort. Another easy way to see if your cardio is intense enough is to check if you can talk during easy cardio but only say a few words or no words during harder cardio.

(4) **Increase the intensity, difficulty or frequency over time:** Progressive overload works for both lifting and cardio. As your lifts or cardio sessions start feeling more manageable, increase the weight you are lifting, the pace you are going at or the resistance of your cardio machine. You can also increase the reps and sets, duration of your cardio or days per week. However, do it gradually so that you can adapt to the new routine and make sure it fits into your life. The easiest way to do this is to increase weight or intensity within the workouts you are already doing (Figure 4.3.8).

(5) **Take rest days as needed:** Menopause may come with a slightly reduced exercise capacity, which means you may need more time to recover, especially between

hard sessions[66,67]. Therefore, spread your heavy lifts or hard cardio across the week with easier workouts or rest days in between. Do not hesitate to take an extra rest day or change the order of your workouts if needed, especially if you are struggling with fatigue due to perimenopause. Aim for 1 to 3 rest days per week, but adjust your workout routine according to your lifestyle.

Conclusion

The world of exercise can be confusing, especially when it comes to menopause. With so much misinformation out there, it's important to find what works for you. However, if you're willing to put in the time and effort, strength, power and intense training a few days a week can be very beneficial. As we age, our goal should be to maintain our muscles, independence and overall function. It's easy to get caught up in the changes that come with menopause, but these training styles can help support our body composition, health and quality of life. So, train to be strong, powerful and to age well. Remember to take time to recover, support your efforts with a healthy diet and most importantly, don't give up – keep pushing yourself. You've got this!

Menopause exercise stories

Michelle's menopause exercise story

Michelle is a 49-year-old woman. Her kids keep harping on her to start lifting and being more active as she ages. She is in the middle of perimenopause and has been active her whole life, but she is new to lifting and plyometrics and doesn't know where to start. She already walks daily and runs two slow and easy jogs a week.

Michelle decided to start with 2 days of heavy lifting and plyometric training and add one HIIT workout each week. She sets up her schedule to do two full-body lifting days each week using the following split. She starts at a 6/10 effort to ease in during the first few weeks, then works up to a 7/10, and then an 8/10 effort as she gains confidence and strength in the gym. She makes sure to hit 1 plyometric, 1 core and one of the major movements or muscle groups each day. For her HIIT, she decides to start with an easy 1-minute work, 1 minute rest for 5 rounds and work up to 10 rounds over the next 6–8 weeks.

LIFT 1
Plyometrics exercise: *3 sets of 10 pogo hops*

Squat/quad exercise: *Leg press, 3 sets of 5–8 reps.*
Shoulder/Press exercise: *Shoulder press, 3 sets of 5–8 reps.*
Back/pull exercise: *Lat pull-down machine, 2 sets of 10–12 reps.*

Deadlift/hinge exercise: *Romanian deadlift, 2 sets of 8–10 reps.*
Core exercise: *Farmer's carries, 2×30 seconds.*

LIFT 2
Plyometrics: *3 sets 4–6 low height depth jumps*

Deadlift/hinge exercise: *Trap bar deadlift, 3 sets of 5–8 reps*
Back/pull exercise: *Row, 3 sets of 5–8 reps.*
Chest/press exercise: *Chest press, 2 sets of 8–10 reps*
Squat/quad exercise: *Step up, 2 sets of 8–10 reps.*
Core: *Dead bugs 2 sets x 30 seconds*

HIIT workout
5-minute easy warm-up

<u>5–10 rounds:</u>
1 minute hard effort (8–9/10)
1 minute easy

5 minute easy cooldown

Mary's menopause exercise story

Mary is a 63-year-old postmenopausal woman. She has been sedentary outside of some daily walking here and there. Still, she has been really frustrated with the changes to her body and life that menopause has brought on. She's very overwhelmed and has no idea where to even start. She wants to start just 3 days a week since that seems feasible with the rest of her life and doesn't feel overwhelming.

When mapping out her training and working with a coach, Mary decides on 3 smaller full-body lifting sessions each week with cardio at the end of each one. She decides on 1 harder effort SIT day, 1 HIIT day and 1 easy cardio day. Then, if she gets super busy, she can move the cardio on their own days if needed. She starts at a 6/10 effort to ease in during the first few weeks, then works up to a 7/10, then an 8/10 effort as she gains confidence and strength in the gym. She starts with 2 low-difficulty plyometric days each week. She tries to hit core and each major movement or muscle group 2x total in her 3 workouts. For her SIT and HIIT, she decides to start with an easy 20-second on, 90-second off SIT workout and a 2-minute on, 2-minute rest HIIT workout. She will begin with fewer total intervals and increase over time as she gains more fitness and confidence in the gym. Then, for her easy cardio day, she will do 20–30 minutes of incline walking or cycling at the gym after her lift at a 4/10 effort. Because she is new to cardio, she is sticking with incline walking or cycling because it will be easier and won't require the skill of running or rowing.

LIFT & CARDIO 1
Plyometrics exercise: *2–3 sets of 20-second skips*
Squat/quad exercise: *Leg press, 3 sets of 5–8 reps.*
Deadlift/hinge exercise: *Romanian deadlift, 2 sets of 8–10 reps.*
Back/pull exercise: *Lat pull-down machine, 2 sets of 10–12 reps.*

HIIT
3-minute easy warm-up

<u>*3–5 rounds:*</u>
2 minute moderate to harder effort (7–8/10)
2 minute rest

3 minute easy cooldown

LIFT & CARDIO 2
Plyometrics: *2–3 sets of 30-second jump rope*
Deadlift/hinge exercise: *Trap bar deadlift, 3 sets of 5–8 reps*
Back/pull exercise: *Row, 3 sets of 5–8 reps.*
Chest/press exercise: *Chest press, 2 sets of 8–10 reps*
Core: *Dead bugs 2 sets x 30 seconds*

SIT
3-minute easy warm-up

<u>*4–8 rounds:*</u>
30-second harder effort (9–10/10)
1.5 minute rest

3 minute easy cooldown

LIFT & CARDIO 3
Shoulder/Press exercise: *Shoulder press, 3 sets of 5–8 reps*
Back/pull exercise: *Row, 3 sets of 5–8 reps.*
Squat/quad exercise: *Step up, 2 sets of 8–10 reps.*
Core exercise: *Farmer's carries, 2×30 seconds.*

CARDIO: *15–30 min, easy effort cardio at a 4/10 effort.*

References

1. Geraci A, Calvani R, Ferri E et al. Sarcopenia and menopause: The role of estradiol. *Frontiers in Endocrinology* 2021; 12: 682012.
2. Buckinx F, Aubertin-Leheudre M. Sarcopenia in menopausal women: Current perspectives. *International Journal of Women's Health* 2022; 14: 805–819.

3. Kim YJ, Tamadon A, Park HT et al. The role of sex steroid hormones in the pathophysiology and treatment of sarcopenia. *Osteoporos Sarcopenia* 2016; 2 (3): 140–155.
4. La Colla A, Pronsato L, Milanesi L et al. 17β-estradiol and testosterone in sarcopenia: role of satellite cells. *Ageing Research Reviews* 2015; 24 (Pt B): 166–177.
5. Manolagas SC, O'Brien CA, Almeida M. The role of estrogen and androgen receptors in bone health and disease. *Nature Reviews Endocrinology* 2013; 9 (12): 699–712.
6. Khalid AB, Krum SA. Estrogen receptors alpha and beta in bone. *Bone* 2016; 87: 130–135.
7. Landi F, Calvani R, Cesari M et al. Sarcopenia: An overview on current definitions, diagnosis and treatment. *Current Protein & Peptide Science* 2018; 19 (7): 633–638.
8. Cioffi M, Esposito K, Vietri MT et al. Cytokine pattern in postmenopause. *Maturitas* 2002; 41(3): 187–192.
9. Walston JD. Sarcopenia in older adults. *Current Opinion in Rheumatology* 2012; 24 (6): 623–627.
10. López-Lluch G. Mitochondrial activity and dynamics changes regarding metabolism in ageing and obesity. *Mechanisms of Ageing and Development* 2017; 162: 108–121.
11. Sirola J, Kröger H, Honkanen R et al. Factors affecting bone loss around menopause in women without HRT: A prospective study. *Maturitas* 2003; 45 (3): 159–167.
12. Neda Sarafrazi PD, Wambogo EA, Shepherd JA. Osteoporosis or low bone mass in older adults: United States, 2017–2018. *NCHS Data Brief, no 405*. National Centre for Health Statistics, Hyattsville, MD, 2021.
13. Marlatt KL, Pitynski-Miller DR, Gavin KM et al. Body composition and cardiometabolic health across the menopause transition. *Obesity* (Silver Spring) 2022; 30 (1): 14–27.
14. Shifren JL, Gass ML. The North American Menopause Society recommendations for clinical care of midlife women. *Menopause* 2014; 21 (10): 1038–1062.
15. Smith JD, Borel A-L, Nazare J-A et al. Visceral adipose tissue indicates the severity of cardiometabolic risk in patients with and without type 2 diabetes: Results from the INSPIRE ME IAA Study. *Journal of Clinical Endocrinology and Metabolism* 2012; 97 (5): 1517–1525.
16. Donini LM et al. Definition and diagnostic criteria for sarcopenic obesity: ESPEN and EASO consensus statement. *Obesity Facts* 2022; 15 (3): 321–335.
17. Guillet C et al. Impaired protein metabolism: Interlinks between obesity, insulin resistance and inflammation. *Obesity Reviews* 2012; 13 Suppl 2: 51–57.
18. Baumgartner RN. Body composition in healthy aging. *Annals of the New York Academy of Sciences* 2000; 904: 437–448.
19. Zurlo F et al. Skeletal muscle metabolism is a major determinant of resting energy expenditure. *Journal of Clinical Investigation* 1990; 86 (5): 1423–1427.
20. Buford TW et al. Models of accelerated sarcopenia: Critical pieces for solving the puzzle of age-related muscle atrophy. *Ageing Research Reviews* 2010; 9 (4): 369–383.
21. Roth SM et al. Inflammatory factors in age-related muscle wasting. *Current Opinion in Rheumatology* 2006; 18 (6): 625–630.
22. Wooten JS et al. Impact of menopause and body composition status on dyslipidemia in women. *American Journal of Health Behavior* 2021; 45 (1): 71–80.
23. Grundy SM et al. Definition of metabolic syndrome: Report of the National Heart, Lung, and Blood Institute/American Heart Association conference on scientific issues related to definition. *Circulation* 2004; 109 (3): 433–438.
24. Marlatt KL et al. Body composition and cardiometabolic health across the menopause transition. *Obesity* 2022; 30 (1): 14–27.
25. Hill JH, Solt C, Foster MT. Obesity associated disease risk: The role of Iinherent differences and location of adipose depots. *Hormone Molecular Biology and Clinical Investigation* 2018; 33 (2).
26. Chambers MA, Moylan JS, Reid MB. Physical Iinactivity and muscle weakness in the critically Iill. *Critical Care Medicine* 2009; 37 (10 Suppl): S337–S346.

27 von Loeffelholz C, Birkenfeld AL. Non-exercise activity thermogenesis in human energy homeostasis. In Feingold KR et al. (eds), *Endotext*. MDText.com, Inc. Copyright © 2000-2024, MDText.com, Inc., South Dartmouth (MA), 2000.
28 Melanson EL et al. Regulation of energy expenditure by estradiol in premenopausal women. *Journal of Applied Physiology* 1985, 2015; 119 (9): 975–981.
29 Day DS et al. Sex hormone suppression reduces resting energy expenditure and {beta}-adrenergic support of resting energy expenditure. *The Journal of Clinical Endocrinology and Metabolism* 2005; 90 (6): 3312–3317.
30 Rogers NH et al. Reduced energy expenditure and increased inflammation are early events in the development of ovariectomy-induced obesity. *Endocrinology* 2009; 150 (5): 2161–2168.
31 Witte MM et al. Female mice and rats exhibit species-specific metabolic and behavioral responses to ovariectomy. *General and Comparative Endocrinology* 2010; 166 (3): 520–528.
32 Melanson EL et al. Influence of estradiol status on physical activity in premenopausal women. *Medicine & Science in Sports & Exercise* 2018; 50 (8): 1704–1709.
33 Gavin KM et al. Modulation of energy expenditure by estrogens and Eeercise in women. *Exercise and Sport Sciences Reviews* 2018; 46 (4): 232–239.
34 Baskin KK, Winders BR, Olson EN. Muscle as a "mediator" of systemic metabolism. *Cell Metabolism* 2015; 21 (2): 237–248.
35 Gavin KM et al. A randomized controlled trial of ovarian suppression in premenopausal women: No change in free-living energy expenditure. *Obesity (Silver Spring)* 2020; 28 (11): 2125–2133.
36 Saint-Maurice PF et al. Association of daily step count and step intensity with mortality among US adults. *JAMA* 2020; 323 (12): 1151–1160.
37 Islam H, Gibala MJ, Little JP. Exercise snacks: A novel strategy to improve cardiometabolic health. *Exercise and Sport Sciences Reviews* 2022; 50 (1): 31–37.
38 Mårin P et al. Cortisol secretion in relation to body fat distribution in obese premenopausal women. *Metabolism* 1992; 41 (8): 882–886.
39 Rutters F et al. Hypothalamic-pituitary-adrenal (HPA) Axis functioning in relation to body fat distribution. *Clinical Endocrinology* (Oxf), 2010; 72 (6): 738–743.
40 Incollingo Rodriguez AC et al. Hypothalamic-pituitary-adrenal axis dysregulation and cortisol activity in obesity: A aystematic review. *Psychoneuroendocrinology* 2015; 62: 301–318.
41 Chao AM et al. Stress, cortisol, and other appetite-related hormones: Prospective prediction of 6-month changes in food cravings and weight. *Obesity* (Silver Spring) 2017; 25 (4): 713–720.
42 Hewagalamulage SD et al. Stress, cortisol, and obesity: A role for cortisol responsiveness in identifying individuals prone to obesity. *Domestic Animal Endocrinology* 2016; 56 Suppl: S112–S120.
43 Epel E et al. Stress may add bite to appetite in women: A laboratory study of stress-induced cortisol and eating behavior. *Psychoneuroendocrinology* 2001; 26 (1): 37–49.
44 Hackney AC, Walz EA. Hormonal adaptation and the stress of exercise training: The role of glucocorticoids. *Trends in Sport Science* 2013; 20 (4): 165–171.
45 Kjaer M. Regulation of hormonal and metabolic responses during exercise in humans. *Exercise and Sport Sciences Reviews* 1992; 20: 161–184.
46 Zouhal H et al. Catecholamines and the effects of exercise, training and gender. *Sports Medicine* 2008; 38 (5): 401–423.
47 Sternfeld B, Dugan S. Physical activity and health during the menopausal mransition. *Obstetrics and Gynecology Clinics of North America* 2011; 38 (3): 537–566.
48 Recchia F et al. Dose-response effects of exercise and caloric restriction on visceral adiposity in overweight and obese adults: A systematic review and meta-analysis of randomised controlled trials. *British Journal of Sports Medicine* 2023; 57 (16): 1035–1041.

49 Verheggen RJHM et al. A systematic review and meta-analysis on the effects of exercise training versus hypocaloric diet: Distinct effects on body weight and visceral adipose tissue. *Obesity Reviews* 2016; 17 (8): 664–690.
50 Vissers D et al. The effect of exercise on visceral adipose tissue in overweight adults: A systematic review and meta-analysis. *PLoS One* 2013; 8 (2): e56415.
51 Atakan MM et al. Evidence-based effects of high-intensity interval training on exercise capacity and health: A review with historical perspective. *International Journal of Environmental Research and Public Health* 2021; 18 (13).
52 Weston M et al. Effects of low-volume high-intensity interval training (HIT) on fitness in adults: A meta-analysis of controlled and non-controlled trials. *Sports Medicine* 2014; 44 (7): 1005–1017.
53 Dupuit M et al. Effect of high intensity Iinterval training on body composition in women before and after menopause: A meta-analysis. *Experimental Physiology* 2020; 105 (9): 1470–1490.
54 Grossman JA, Arigo D, Bachman JL. Meaningful weight loss in obese postmenopausal women: A pilot study of high-intensity Iinterval training and wearable technology. *Menopause* 2018; 25 (4): 465–470.
55 Nunes PRP et al. Comparative effects of high-intensity Iinterval training with combined training on physical function markers in obese postmenopausal women: A randomized controlled trial. *Menopause* 2019; 26 (11): 1242–1249.
56 Dupuit M et al. Moderate-intensity continuous training or high-intensity interval training with or without resistance training for altering body composition in postmenopausal women. *Medicine & Science in Sports & Exercise* 2020; 52 (3): 736–745.
57 Maillard F et al. High-intensity interval training reduces abdominal fat mass in postmenopausal women with type 2 diabetes. *Diabetes & Metabolism* 2016; 42 (6): 433–441.
58 Jabbour G, Iancu HD. Anaerobic and aerobic contributions to repeated supramaximal cycling exercises and their adaptation to high-intensity Iinterval training in obese perimenopausal and postmenopausal women. *Menopause* 2024; 31 (1): 39–45.
59 Jabbour G, Iancu HD. Comparison of performance and health Iindicators between perimenopausal and postmenopausal obese women: The effect of high-intensity Iinterval training (HIIT). *Menopause* 2020; 28 (1): 50–57.
60 Mohr M et al. Long-term continuous exercise training counteracts the negative impact of the menopause transition on cardiometabolic health in hypertensive women - a 9-year RCT follow-up. *Progress in Cardiovascular Diseases* 2023.
61 Ransdell LB et al. The Impact of resistance training on body composition, muscle strength, and functional fitness in older women (45-80 years): A systematic review (2010–2020). *Women (Basel)*, 2021; 1 (3): 143–168.
62 Zehnacker CH, Bemis-Dougherty A. Effect of weighted exercises on bone mineral density in post menopausal women. A systematic review. *Journal of Geriatric Physical Therapy* 2007; 30 (2): 79–88.
63 Benedetti MG et al. The effectiveness of physical exercise on bone density in osteoporotic patients. *BioMed Research International* 2018; 2018: 4840531.
64 Vetrovsky T et al. The efficacy and safety of lower-limb plyometric training in older adults: A systematic review. *Sports Medicine* 2019; 49 (1): 113–131.
65 Balachandran AT et al. Comparison of power training vs traditional strength training on physical function in older adults: A systematic review and meta-analysis. *JAMA Network Open* 2022; 5 (5): e2211623.
66 Mercuro G et al. Impairment of physical exercise capacity in healthy postmenopausal women. *American Heart Journal* 2006; 151 (4): 923–927.
67 Lurati AR. Menopause and exercise intolerance. *Nursing for Women's Health* 2017; 21 (2): 130–136.

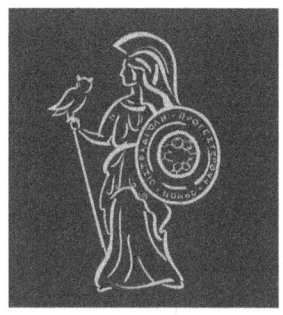

Act 5

Treatment Options
Hormone replacement therapy (HRT)

Act 5 Treatment Options
Hormone replacement therapy
Scylla and Charybdis

Dr Nicky Keay

At a key point in his epic journey, Odysseus had to navigate a passage between the six-headed monster, Scylla, and the perilous whirlpool, Charybdis.

An apparently similar dilemma faces those deciding whether to take hormone replacement therapy (HRT), with proponents expressing strong views, both for and against.

The choice of HRT is a personal decision. The best approach is to gather all the information necessary to make an informed judgement. It is important to dispel myths and lay out the facts about HRT, to help women make the best personal choice, fearing neither Scylla nor Charybdis.

Scylla and Charybdis

Dr Nicky Keay

Setting the scene: What is hormone replacement therapy?

Hormone replacement therapy (HRT) typically contains both oestrogen and a progestogen component. The objective of HRT is to bring internal levels of ovarian hormones up to comparable physiological concentrations seen in women who are having ovulatory menstrual cycles. The purpose of HRT, for women experiencing menopausal symptoms, is to improve quality of life and potentially reduce the risk of long-term health issues. HRT is also the treatment of choice for some groups of premenopausal women with low ovarian hormones to support bone and cardiovascular health. In addressing the myths below, the main reference is the joint position statement by the British Menopause Society, Royal College of Obstetricians and Gynaecologists and Society for Endocrinology on best practice recommendations for the care of women experiencing the menopause.

Myth 1 Menopause is not a medical condition, so is HRT medication necessary?

It is true that "natural" physiological menopause is not a medical condition. Menopause is an expected part of the female hormone odyssey, typically occurring in middle age, characterised by an irreversible drop in ovarian hormone production. Some argue that since menopause is not a medical condition, it does not require medication such as HRT.

Although menopause is not a medical condition, the dramatic changes in ovarian hormone production can make women feel below par, both physically and mentally. HRT is approved by medicine regulatory agencies as a safe and effective treatment that enhances the quality of life of women experiencing menopausal symptoms. Furthermore, at menopause, women lose the health-giving benefits of internally produced ovarian hormones, putting them at increased risk of cardiovascular disease (CVD) and osteoporosis. Although HRT is not given soley for disease prevention, depending on the timing and type of HRT, from the Cochrane review, HRT can extend protection against these risks and reduce all cause mortality by supporting the reduced levels of ovarian hormones. For women experiencing premature ovarian insufficiency (POI) and early menopause, HRT is advised for health reasons, at least up until the average age of menopause.

Physiological menopause is not a hormone deficiency condition, it is argued the word "replacement" in HRT, implies a medical condition of a hormone deficiency that needs correcting. The term, menopause hormone therapy (MHT) is also used. However,

HRT is not exclusively prescribed for menopausal women. Premenopausal women are prescribed HRT for bone and cardiovascular health reasons. These include premenopausal women with premature ovarian insufficiency (POI) and functional hypothalamic amenorrhoea (FHA). Women with POI experience a decline in ovarian function before 40 years of age. It can be a big psychological challenge for a young woman to find out that her fertility is very much reduced, especially for those in their teenage years or early twenties. Although these women with POI may go on to experience early menopause, being offered HRT can be less confronting and arguably technically correct than being offered MHT. Women experiencing FHA, a reversible physiological adaptation, are not menopausal. It is not appropriate to talk about MHT for these women. The term hormone therapy (HT) would cover all scenarios.

HRT differs from non-medical alternatives. As a medical treatment HRT has the advantage of being tightly quality controlled by medicine regulatory agencies for its content, efficacy and safety. In contrast, unregulated treatment options that are not medicines have less certain ingredients, effects and safety profiles.

What about other non-hormonal medications? HRT is licensed specifically to restore ovarian hormones to physiological levels and so manage the underlying cause of symptoms. An alternative might be to treat each menopausal symptom in isolation with non-hormonal medication. However, this approach, known as polypharmacy, results in a burgeoning medical cabinet. Furthermore, antidepressants should be prescribed only for diagnosed clinical depression[1], not as a generic prescription to menopausal women experiencing low mood and/or anxiety.

Some express a view that taking HRT is *"throwing in the towel."* This is not the case. Menopause is a denouement for menstrual periods, but many years of life lie ahead. For many menopausal women, HRT can help navigate the shifts in ovarian hormones, allowing them to continue enjoying life. HRT has a synergistic effect with lifestyle on quality of life and long-term health.

Every woman experiences menopause in a different way. It must be her individual and personal choice whether or not to take HRT after discussion with her GP, who has knowledge of her personal medical history and can weigh up her potential risks and benefits. Women should not be made to feel that taking HRT is a sign of weakness.

It is interesting to reflect that men do not experience the equivalent of menopause, as there is only a slight decline in testosterone by the testes after 50 years of age. Yet there is a trend for men to actively seek out testosterone replacement therapy (TRT).

Myth 2 Does HRT cause breast cancer?

Where does this myth come from? Unfortunately, media headlines were published in the 2000s that HRT "caused breast cancer", referring to a large U.S. study before it had been formally peer-reviewed and published. Understandably this was a major concern for women, many of whom stopped taking HRT as a result. After the dust had settled, three aspects of the study undermined the media panic. Firstly, the study never stated that HRT caused breast cancer, it merely suggested a statistical relationship. A definitive causal link between HRT and breast cancer cannot be demonstrated, as the media headlines stated[2]. Secondly, it transpired that many of the women in the study had an underlying increased risk of breast cancer due to high body weight[3]. Being predisposed to the main risk factor for breast cancer confounds efforts to tease out any possible contributing element from HRT.

The third critique is that in contrast to the methodology of the study conducted over 24 years ago, it would be very unusual in current clinical practice to start a woman on HRT such a long time (10 years) after reaching menopause, using a form of HRT comprising oral synthetic oestrogen and synthetic progestogen. Currently, it is recommended to start HRT as close to menopause as possible to gain maximum benefit. Today, HRT is available containing ovarian hormones with identical molecular structure to those produced by the ovaries, which does not need to be taken orally[4].

Nevertheless, we certainly should be mindful about breast cancer which has an incidence of 23 in 1,000 women in the 50 to 59 years age group. It is also important to highlight that the risk of developing breast cancer (morbidity) does not equate to dying from breast cancer (mortality). Early detection with screening programmes and priority referral pathways means that suspected breast cancer can be promptly assessed and treated appropriately.

The biggest risk factor for developing breast cancer is being overweight illustrated visually in the infographic from Women's Health Concern. In women who are overweight, there are 24 extra cases of breast cancer per 1,000 women in this age group[5]. Modifiable lifestyle factors such as smoking, lack of exercise and drinking alcohol regularly also contribute to the risk of breast cancer. Additional risk factors for developing breast cancer reflect the lifetime exposure to ovarian hormones, namely early menarche and late menopause. Furthermore, the breast tissue is more prone to malignant change in women who have never been pregnant, are older at first pregnancy, had few children and limited time breast feeding[6].

The modest increase of 4 cases per 1,000 women who are taking HRT should be set in the context of extra cases due to controllable lifestyle factors. In fact, the breast cancer risk of taking HRT for menopause is the same as taking the combined oral contraceptive pill or drinking 2 units of alcohol a day[5].

Women who have had a hysterectomy and are taking the oestrogen component of HRT alone have a lower risk of breast cancer than those not taking HRT, 4 fewer cases per 1,000 women. This suggests that for women who have not had a hysterectomy and taking combined HRT, it is the progestogen component of HRT that is important to consider to when it comes to minimising breast cancer risk[5]. Molecularly body identical progesterone is associated with the lowest risk.

Based on all the evidence, The British Menopause Society (BMS) advises that HRT does not cause breast cancer[7]. However, HRT should not be taken by a woman who has been treated for breast cancer, whether this is oestrogen receptor positive or negative. In fact, for many women, a part of the treatment of breast cancer is with anti-oestrogen medication: effectively a "medical" menopause. However, vaginal oestrogen for localised symptoms of vaginal dryness or urinary issues can sometimes be taken with specialist medical discussion.

Having a family member who has had breast cancer may increase the background risk for developing breast cancer. However, the BMS states that this would not be a definite contraindication to taking HRT. This would depend on the exact type of breast cancer a family member had and at what age, and whether the individual woman is a carrier of BRCA1 or 2 mutation which increases the risk of ovarian and breast cancer. A personalised approach is needed to discuss the pros and cons of taking HRT with a medical menopause expert.

The main cause of death in menopausal women is CVD, not breast cancer. HRT reduces all-cause mortality. In other words, HRT has positive health benefits in terms of reducing risk of dying from other disease consequences associated with low levels of female hormones[8].

The main winner when it comes to overall well-being, health and reducing the risk of developing breast cancer is lifestyle. Taking two and a half hours or more of reasonably intense exercise per week reduces the number of cases of breast cancer by 7 per 1,000 women in the 50–59 year age group[5]. This is why lifestyle factors are always a priority, for every woman, for both overall health and reducing the risk of developing breast cancer. When a woman is advised to take HRT before the "natural" age of menopause where ovarian hormones are low due to FHA, POI, or early menopause, then the BMS advise that this does not increase the risk of breast cancer when HRT is taken up to the age of the "natural" menopause.

Myth 3 Women should not take "artificial" hormones

Instinctively taking a hormone that is the "identical" to your body's own production seems best. No HRT can be literally "natural", as the molecules are extracted from natural plant sources not humans. It is important to understand the difference between two superficially similar terms: standardised "body identical" HRT and non-standardised "bioidentical" HRT.

"Body identical" HRT contains hormones with the same molecular structure as hormones produced by the ovaries. The receptors for these hormones throughout the body accept these body identical hormones like old, returning friends. The dose can be personalised to match individual symptoms. The excellent news is that this body identical type of HRT is available in licensed, regulated form in the United Kingdom on the NHS with a prepaid yearly subscription of just £19 at the time of writing. In fact, this prepaid prescription covers all HRT products.

"Bioidentical" HRT is a type of compounded HRT that is unregulated and unlicensed. Some might suggest that the use of similar-sounding terminology is a marketing ploy. The BMS is very clear in its stance on "bioidentical" HRT[9]. Compounding means that ingredients are mixed in varying amounts and so there is uncertainty as to the exact effect.

Regulated and licensed forms of HRT must be compliant in terms of the exact amount and composition of hormones. Licensed HRT has been extensively tested for effectiveness in a specific use, both in the laboratory and in women.

So, what is the lure of the word "bioidentical"? Certainly not the price tag. Maybe for the apparent appeal of exclusivity and personalisation? Yet the licensed and regulated route of body identical HRT can be personalised and is available to all women in a safe and affordable way.

Myth 4 Should all menopausal women take HRT?

Although the only absolute contraindication for taking HRT is a personal history of breast cancer, this does not mean that women should feel pressured into taking HRT.

To reiterate, the main factor in considering HRT is for quality of life[1]. If menopausal symptoms are detracting from your quality of life and overall well-being, HRT could be helpful alongside lifestyle factors such as exercise and nutrition.

What should a menopausal woman do if she is not experiencing troublesome menopausal symptoms. Should she take HRT or not? Sometimes she may be experiencing menopausal symptoms without realising. For example, poor sleep and aching joints are attributed to "just part of getting older". There is a window of opportunity after the final period for getting maximum benefit from HRT, especially in terms of cardiovascular health of up to 10 years. Discussing all the options with your GP is really important. A woman's GP with knowledge of her full medical history is ideally placed to advise on the best approaches, including lifestyle factors as a starting point as discussed in Act 4 Mastering Menopause.

Does HRT help with long-term health? Although this is not the main indication for prescribing HRT, there is evidence that HRT can be helpful. In particular, HRT can be the first line of treatment for poor bone health. HRT can support a significant improvement in bone mineral density, protecting against osteoporosis and osteoporotic-related fractures[10]. Sex steroid hormones, in particular oestradiol, rules supreme when it comes to bone health. This is why menopausal women are at a greatly increased risk of osteoporosis and fractures. The role of oestradiol underpins the temporal use of HRT for premenopausal women with amenorrhoea (lack of periods) associated with low ovarian hormones, including those with FHA and associated poor bone health[11].

Oestradiol has a protective effect on cardiovascular health, by favouring a healthy lipid (cholesterol) profile and supporting endothelial reactivity (lining wall of arteries). Declining oestradiol levels at menopause increase the risk of CVD, making it the main cause of death in menopausal woman (not breast cancer, as many might think). There is evidence that HRT started in women under the age of 60 or within 10 years of the menopause can reduce the risk of heart disease and cardiovascular mortality (death from CVD)[8].

Evidence shows that the most beneficial time to start taking HRT is as close to the menopause as possible. The rational being that cushioning the drop in ovarian hormone levels means that you will be able to ease yourself through menopause and beyond.

For women who experience POI, or early menopause between 40 and 45, for example due to medical reasons (surgical removal of the ovaries, or retirement of the ovaries due to medication), it is very important to start HRT immediately for health reasons and to continue taking HRT at least until the expected age of menopause[12].

Myth 5 HRT is the elixir of youth!

HRT should not be mistaken for the elixir of youth. Alongside lifestyle factors, HRT improves quality of life by helping manage menopausal symptoms. HRT is also helpful in reducing the risk of long-term health issues involving bone and possibly cardiovascular health[13]. However, to reiterate, the primary reason for considering HRT is to improve quality of life. The other consideration is that menopause usually occurs in middle age and ageing involves the decline of other anabolic (tissue-building) hormones such as growth hormone (GH). GH is important in maintaining favourable body composition in terms of muscle mass and resisting increase in visceral fat. Although HRT can potentially bolster well-being and long-term health, this is not a substitute for reviewing and modifying lifestyle. HRT in isolation will not rejuvenate you to a 21-year-old.

HRT story for menopause

Molly was a 51-year-old who had recently experienced menopause. By her own admission she led a very sedentary lifestyle and did not take regular exercise. Furthermore, she was very partial to drinking several glasses of alcohol every evening and knew she was overweight. She was experiencing troublesome menopause symptoms and heard that HRT was wonderful in restoring vitality. Although HRT did help to a certain extent, Molly was disappointed that she did not become slimmer or fitter. HRT by itself does not achieve the optimal outcome. Reviewing and revising lifestyle is always an important starting point and acts in synergy with HRT to improve quality of life and overall health.

Myth 6 When to start HRT?

The main indication for starting HRT is alleviation of menopausal symptoms to improve your quality of life. This is particularly relevant for women not having menstrual periods as the barometer of ovarian hormone production following hysterectomy or as a result of being on hormonal contraception, as discussed in Act 1, Scene 1. For other menopausal women, having menstrual periods, menopause is a retrospective diagnosis based on a year of no menstrual periods. During this time of uncertainty you could be in perimenopause or postmenopause, when menopausal symptoms are typically at their most troublesome. If you begin suffering from symptoms in late perimenopause/early menopause after a full discussion with your doctor, weighing up all the options, including lifestyle, you might decide to start HRT, at the lowest effective dose.

Treatment Options

HRT timing story

Iris was 50 years of age and suspected she was close to menopause as she was getting menopausal symptoms that she had heard about from her circle friends of similar age. Disrupted sleep was not helping "brain fog" and anxiety. Hot flushes were becoming more frequent. Iris was finding it tough to cope and even wondering if she should think about going part-time at work, even though she loved her job as a nurse. Iris had done her research and was following a healthy lifestyle and knew that HRT might help her symptoms, Iris' periods had become very infrequent with her last, light period being about 11 months ago. Iris was relieved to hear that she could potentially start HRT. She was also delighted to hear that body identical HRT was available on the NHS with a prepaid prescription for the year. We explored how to discuss all the options with her GP.

Myth 7 HRT can only be taken for 5 years

The BMS states very clearly that there is no arbitrary limit to how long any woman should take HRT[14]. After a full discussion with your GP, weighing up all the pros and cons, if you wish to stop HRT you should do so gradually to mitigate the abrupt onset/restarting of menopausal symptoms.

How long to take HRT

Mary was 56 years of age. Although she was following a healthy lifestyle, she had struggled to cope with menopausal symptoms and had decided to start HRT age 51. HRT had improved her quality of life, at work, with family and socially. Mary was upset when a friend said she had to stop taking HRT after 5 years. She did not relish a return of her menopausal symptoms. Mary was relieved to discover that it was her choice whether to continue with HRT in discussion with her doctor. The only slight adjustment would be from taking sequential HRT (blocks of micronised progesterone) to continuous evening micronised progesterone alongside continuous daily oestradiol.

Myth 8 There is only one type of HRT

There are many different types of HRT which can be taken in different ways.

Local v Systemic HRT

Local vaginal oestrogen can be really helpful as an additional or a "stand alone" option to help directly with urinogenital issues (urinary issues and vaginal dryness) and also indirectly with libido. Typically, this is in the form of a vaginal pessary or cream containing oestrogen. As vaginal oestrogen is only absorbed locally, it is safe for some women who cannot take systemic HRT and you do not need to take the progestogen component of HRT.

There is the possibility of using the hormone dehydroepiandrosterone (DHEA) locally. In this case DHEA is converted within the cells to oestradiol, through a process of intracrinology[15]. However, DHEA should not be taken for a systemic effect as there is variable conversion to oestradiol and testosterone. Also, for athletes competing under World Anti-Doping Authority (WADA) jurisdiction, DHEA is on the banned list.

Systemic HRT means having effects throughout the body. This is particularly relevant for HRT, as female hormones influence a broad range of systems and cell types.

What are the hormones in systemic HRT? HRT typically includes the two main ovarian hormones: oestrogen and a progestogen component. Progestogen is the generic term that includes progesterone (with body identical molecular structure) and synthetic forms with slightly different molecular structures. Oestrogen and progestogen must be taken in combination, unless a woman has had a hysterectomy (surgical removal of the uterus/womb). The combination of ovarian hormones maintains a healthy endometrial thickness. If a woman has not had a hysterectomy, oestrogen, unopposed by progestogen, can cause the endometrium to become unhealthily thick, increasing the risk of malignancy (cancer). Progestogens, specifically progesterone has other beneficial effects on health and well-being as discussed in Act 1.

How to take systemic HRT? Where possible, taking HRT transdermally (through the skin) and in body identical forms is best for minimising side effects. In tablet form, HRT has to be processed by the liver. The body's hormone receptors are tuned to recognise the specific naturally occurring molecular forms.

What is the "best" form of oestrogen? Oestradiol, the most active form of oestrogen, is well absorbed through the skin, directly into the bloodstream. The transdermal route avoids the first-pass metabolic effect of the liver that occurs when sex steroid hormones are taken orally in tablet form. Oral HRT must first be absorbed from the gut, before passing through the hepatic portal vein to the liver. The liver is a large organ with an important processing role, requiring the induction of liver enzymes. A knock-on effect of inducing liver enzymes is that extra coagulating proteins can be produced, potentially increasing the risk of blood clot formation. Taking oestradiol via the transdermal route has a neutral effect on the way the body breaks down hormones and does not increase the risk of blood clots compared to the risk in those who are not taking HRT.

The oestradiol component of HRT can be taken transdermally in the form of a gel or patch. Typically, gel is applied daily to the inner thigh, whereas a patch is changed twice a week. Arguably oestradiol gel offers a greater flexibility to fine-tune the dose according to the symptoms of the individual. Individual sachets of oestradiol gel are available in the smallest effective amount, allowing a women to adjust the dose with the number of sachets applied, in accordance with guidance from her GP. When travelling, sachets are easier to transport than an oestradiol pump dispenser. It is less complicated and more discrete putting some small sachets in the liquid bag at airport security. The oestradiol in sachets is slightly more concentrated than that from pump dispensers, so minimising a sticky mess scenario. A spray version of oestradiol reportedly dries more quickly. A minor inconvenience of gel is the need to wait for it to dry before dressing. Putting on trousers straight away transfers the oestradiol to your clothes rather than your body. You should also avoid swimming or showering within an hour after applying.

Oestradiol patches offer an alternative to gel, as long as you do not have sensitive skin or do a lot of sweat-inducing exercise. These patches should not come off in the swimming pool, but you may not want to put this to the test, where they may be apparent to others. Although I wasn't bothered by a curious lifeguard asking about the hip replacement scars on my legs (apparently, he had seen a lot of this type of scar on "old" women!), I didn't relish additional questions about patches. I just want to get on with swimming!

What about HRT in tablet form? Although transdermal oestradiol has advantages, the tablet form taken orally can be a good option for women with skin absorption issues. There is new body identical oral formulation of HRT for women where this is the preferred route.

What about progestogen component of HRT?

Progestogen is the generic term describing the family of progestational agents that includes progesterone (with body identical molecular structure) and synthetic progestogens that have slightly different structures. In women with a uterus, a progestogen component of HRT is required to "offset" the effects of oestrogen on the endometrium and prevent thickening of the endometrial lining (endometrial hyperplasia).

The members of the progestogen family are described in terms of the number of carbon atoms and the specific molecular structure. For example, the body naturally makes C21 progesterone. Variants of this molecule, such as C19 forms, have sightly different effects.

Which progestogen is "best"? The body identical form of C21 progesterone is available in HRT that includes micronised progesterone (made from plant sources). This form of progesterone is breast and metabolically "friendly". Micronised progesterone has a neutral effect on the risk of blood clots and a slightly lower risk of breast cancer compared to synthetic progestogens[16]. Body identical micronised progesterone only binds to progesterone receptors and so unlike synthetic progestogens has no side effects of mineralocorticoid (fluid balance) or glucocorticoid (blood glucose control) and fewer androgenic effects. Furthermore, this form of body identical progesterone has effects in the brain on γ-Aminobutyric acid (GABA) receptors to help with mood and sleep. Micronised progesterone has a pleasant soporific effect, which is why it is important to take at night, just before going to bed. Micronised progesterone is taken orally as a soft capsule.

Although progesterone can be taken vaginally, absorption into the blood stream is variable, so this method is not licensed as part of HRT for endometrial protection. Nevertheless, it can occasionally be used on a case-by-case basis for women who experience histamine-related gut issues when taking the oral form. Gel or cream forms of body identical progesterone have variable absorption and so they are similarly not licensed for use as part of HRT for endometrial protection.

Going solo with progesterone? There is emerging evidence from a study in Canada that micronised progesterone, by itself, could be helpful in helping with hot flushes and disrupted sleep[17]. The theory is that progesterone is often the first ovarian hormone to decline, before oestradiol as discussed in Act 1. So, starting with progesterone might be something we will see more of in the future. In a similar way, although women who have had a hysterectomy do not need progesterone for endometrial protection, this hormone's "unsung" benefits may be considered.

Any place for synthetic non body identical progestogens? C19 progestogens, which are more structurally related to testosterone, provide a stronger counterbalance to oestradiol, stabilising the endometrial lining to give better control of menstrual bleeding. Heavy bleeding is common in the earlier stages of perimenopause as internal production of progesterone falls, but oestradiol production maintained. This type of progestogen can be taken as a component of HRT via patch or in tablet form. Potentially, the C19 structural similarity between this progestogen and testosterone might theoretically be helpful as ovarian production of testosterone also declines at menopause. Another option is the intrauterine Mirena® coil which releases continuous progestogen and is licensed to provide endometrial protection as part HRT. This has the additional advantage of being a contraceptive.

Heavy periods in perimenopause

Claire was 49 years old and really struggling with heavy periods. It had got to the point where she was reluctant to go out of the house in case of leakage. Claire was not aware that heavy periods are a sign of perimenopause as progesterone levels fall leaving oestradiol in the driving seat. Claire was experiencing other intrusive menopausal symptoms including hot flushes. Claire wanted to trial HRT and cover contraception. The Mirena® coil provides contraception, stabilises the endometrium to control bleeding and is the progestogen component of HRT licensed to be used for endometrial protection. So, this approach could potentially cover all bases and Claire decided to discuss the next steps and all the options with her GP.

Mix and match?
Figure 5.1.1 shows a suggested decision tree for menopausal women when considering how to take systemic HRT. In the absence of contraindications, all women taking HRT need both oestrogen and progestogen, unless they have had a hysterectomy. The oestrogen component can be transdermal, either with gel/patch or orally in the form of a pill. For the progestogen component, the transdermal route is limited to patch,

HRT Options

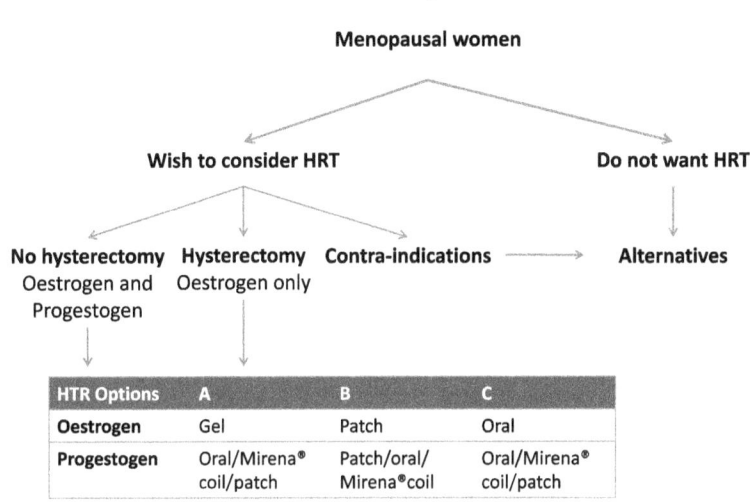

FIGURE 5.1.1 HRT options

as the gel or cream form has variable absorption, which may not provide adequate endometrial protection. There is an oral option including body identical micronised progesterone. The additional option of the Mirena® coil provides continuous release of synthetic progestogen and can be helpful where bleeding is a problem and/or where contraception is sought. This gives women various "mix and match" options according to personal preference which she can discuss with her GP.

To bleed or not to bleed?

HRT can be taken sequentially, typically prompting a withdrawal bleed, or continuously, which does not produce a withdrawal bleed. How to decide what is best for you?

After full discussion with your doctor, then you may choose to take HRT in the sequential way for example daily oestrogen with 12-14 day "blocks" of progestogen. To make it easier to remember when to take micronised progesterone, you can do this on first 12 days of every calendar month. On the other hand, if you have had enough of sanitary wear, you can opt to take continuous HRT as this should not produce any bleeding. For example, a daily dose of oestrogen and daily 100 mg of micronised progesterone. Always check the exact dosing and timing of HRT with your prescribing medical doctor.

For all women starting with sequential HRT, it is advisable to switch to continuous HRT after 5 years for optimal long-term endometrial protection.

Unexpected bleeding on HRT

Bleeding on HRT depends on when you start HRT and the way you are taking HRT. If you are taking the sequential form of HRT, you can expect to experience some bleeding around that time you complete each block of progestogen. If you get any "unscheduled" bleeding outside of this time frame, then you should report this to your prescribing medical doctor.

If you are taking the continuous form of HRT, once established on your personal HRT dose, you should not experience any bleeding. If you do so, this would be "unscheduled" bleeding and you need to report this to your prescribing medical doctor.

The reason that it is important to report any unscheduled bleeding on HRT is that this could be an indication that the endometrial lining has become too thick. Usually, an ultrasound of the uterus and ovaries is performed to check on endometrial thickness and to exclude any other obvious sources of bleeding, such as a polyp. A small sample of the endometrial lining might be taken to check if the cells are healthy.

Myth 9 The dose of HRT cannot be personalised

The dose of HRT can and should be personalised for the individual. Many think that the answer might come by doing a blood test. However, this is not the case as we each have our personal biological response to hormones. Personalisation of HRT dose is based on the alleviation of symptoms, not on blood test results[18]. The situation where a venous blood test might be useful is where poor skin absorption of transdermal oestradiol is suspected. Capillary (finger prick) blood testing can give falsely elevated oestradiol results if gel oestradiol is being used[19].

The most effective way to personalise the dose of HRT, as with many hormone-based medications, is to start at a low dose and gradually increase as necessary within licensed limits. Bearing in mind it can take at least 3 months for HRT to take effect, it is not advisable to increase more rapidly than this. Ultimately, the aim for any medication to use the lowest possible effective dose for the individual to reduce the risk of any potential side effects.

Oestrogen: too much of a good thing?

Oestrogen is a component of HRT and an important hormone in alleviation of menopausal symptoms and long-term health. So, it is tempting to think that the more you take, the more benefit you derive. However, starting on a high initial dose or increasing rapidly can be counterproductive. It becomes difficult to distinguish menopause symptoms from side effects of high oestrogen doses. A phenomenon of tachyphylaxis can arise, where the body effectively protects itself against high doses of a drug. The receptors for oestrogen become less responsive, leading the woman to feel she needs to increase the dose further to have an effect. However, this has an adverse effect on mood[20]. Women taking very high doses of oestrogen may lack adequate endometrial protection with progestogen, unless the uterus has been surgically removed.

Personalisation of HRT dose is important. We are all individuals and our own personal requirements may change as we move through perimenopause to menopause and beyond. This is a gradual, personal, process.

HRT story about dose

Sarah was 51 years of age and struggling with menopausal symptoms. She had heard from a friend who was benefiting from recently starting on HRT. Sarah was eager to try HRT for herself, so she was started on a daily pump of oestradiol and micronised progesterone. However, Sarah was disappointed that after a few days she did not notice any difference. Her friend told her she was taking 4 pumps of oestradiol and testosterone. Sarah saw that she could take more pumps of oestradiol, so immediately increased. However, Sarah reported not feeling any better. She did not realise that rapidly increasing oestradiol dose can be counterproductive. So, Sarah reviewed her lifestyle in terms of exercise and nutrition and went back to one pump of oestradiol as originally advised by her GP. After 3 months, Sarah was feeling much better and felt like the combination of lifestyle and a lower dose of HRT was working well. Sarah understood that modification might be needed moving further beyond menopause, but that rapid changes are not advisable.

Myth 10 I don't need to worry about contraception on HRT?

It is still possible to fall pregnant during perimenopause (unless you have had a hysterectomy). This is because the ovaries may work sporadically. The same applies to women experiencing POI: occasional ovulation is not totally off the cards.

If you are not seeking to become pregnant, it is important to bear in mind that HRT is not contraceptive. The exception is when the Mirena® coil is being used as the progestogen component of HRT. If pregnancy is not desired, you need to continue using contraception for about a year after the final period of menopause has been reached for those over 50 years and 2 years for the under 50s. Barrier methods of contraception, such as condoms or copper coil, could be considered if you are close to menopause, although this will not be helpful for any troublesome bleeding issues that can occur in perimenopause. Or after discussion with your medical prescriber, you might be able to take the progestogen-only contraception pill alongside HRT. However, the progestogen-only pill alone is not licensed for endometrial protection with the oestrogen component of HRT, so this would have to be taken alongside micronised progesterone or patch progestogen[21].

On the other hand, if you prefer to take HRT that also has a contraceptive effect, then at the time of writing, the Mirena® coil (releasing intrauterine synthetic progestogen) is the only licensed progestogen component of HRT providing adequate endometrial protection[21].

Myth 11 Women should not take HRT as this "interferes" with hormones

HRT restores ovarian hormone levels to comparable physiological concentrations found in women having ovulatory menstrual cycles. The underlying network of hormone production remains, unaffected by HRT. To illustrate this point, consider two women, both experiencing amenorrhoea (lack of periods), but for different reasons and with distinct underlying motifs of menstrual cycle hormone choreography. Both take HRT and we will see if the underlying hormonal pattern is altered.

> Susie is 53 years of age and has reached menopause, permanent cessation of menstrual cycles due to reduced ovarian responsiveness indicated by high levels of pituitary control hormones follicle-stimulating hormone (FSH) and luteinising hormone (LH) with low levels of ovarian hormones oestradiol and progesterone. Susie has decided to take HRT to alleviate troublesome menopausal symptoms to improve quality of life. Susie is trying to decide whether to take HRT sequentially or continuously. Sequential HRT is a combination of continuous external oestradiol with cyclical "blocks" of external progestogen, to mimic the fluctuations found in the menstrual cycle. Continuous HRT means a consistent dose of external oestradiol and progestogen. However, Susie wants to know whether the way she takes HRT will alter the underlying reduced responsiveness of her ovaries. Would HRT alter production of her own hormones? Could her own periods return? The answer is no. Although sequential HRT typically produces a withdrawal bleed, this is not a menstrual period as the ovaries remain in retirement, so FSH and LH remain high. This is shown in the upper panel of Figure 5.1.2.

> Suzy is 35 years of age. She is also experiencing amenorrhoea with low levels of ovarian hormones. However, for Suzy this is reversible hypothalamic amenorrhoea with low levels of LH and FSH. Although Suzy is not in menopause, temporary sequential HRT was prescribed for bone health[22], until she can restore her cycles. Suzy wants to know if the withdrawal bleeding from sequential HRT is the same as a period and if taking HRT prevents her own menstrual cycles restoring? I explained to Suzy that the withdrawal bleeding anticipated on sequential HRT is not that same as her own menstrual period, but that HRT does not prevent her own menstrual cycle hormone choreography and associated menstrual periods restoring. In other words, HRT does not interfere with underlying hormone patterns shown in the lower panel of Figure 5.1.2.

Note that in both scenarios, whether HRT is taken in menopause or FHA, the underlying hormone signature is not affected. This is because the doses of hormones in HRT are in line with physiological levels. This is also why it is important to tell premenopausal women like Suzy that HRT is not contraceptive.

Treatment Options

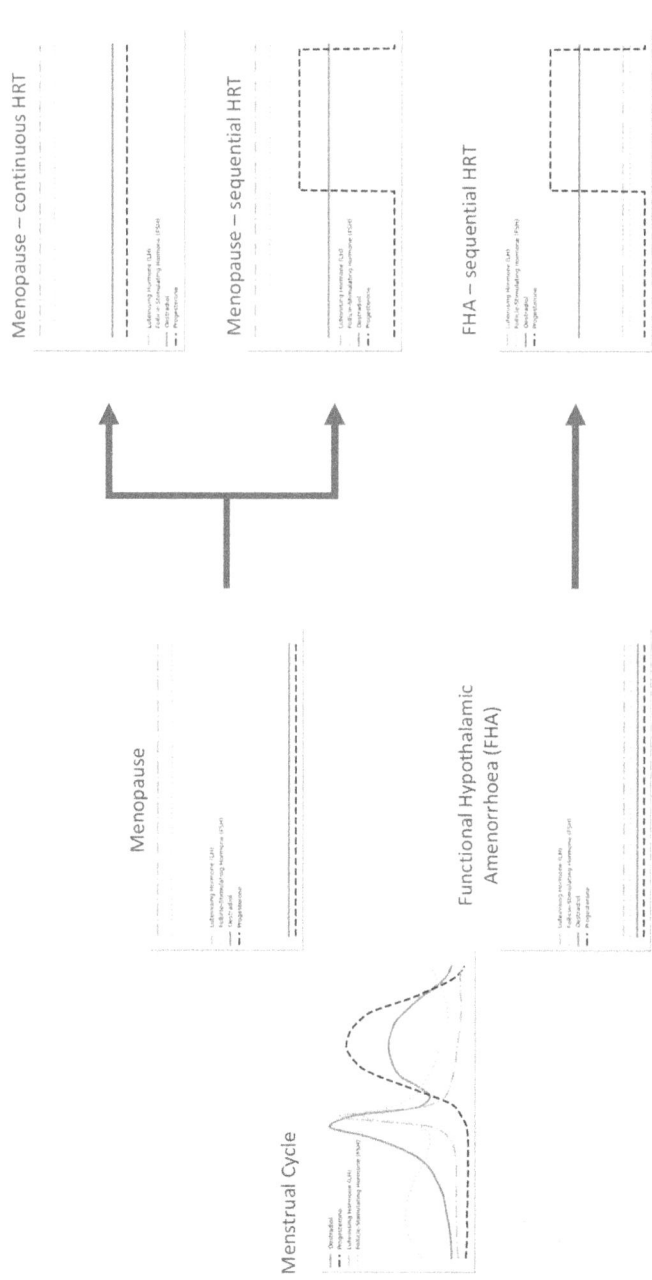

FIGURE 5.1.2 HRT scenarios

In contrast to HRT, many forms of hormonal contraception most definitely do alter internal hormones: suppressing menstrual cycle hormone production. Why the very different outcomes for medications both containing versions of ovarian hormones? Many types of hormonal contraception (like the combined oral contraceptive pill, some progestogen-only pills, injections and implant preparations of progestogen) contain higher-than-natural levels of synthetic versions of ovarian hormones, which suppress the whole of the reproductive axis, resulting in switching off ovarian function, natural hormone cycles and egg production ceases. This is why hormonal contraception is very effective. These hormonal contraceptives ensure that menstrual cycle hormones remain at low levels across the board: FSH, LH, oestradiol, progesterone and testosterone. Some forms of progestogen-only contraception act in a different manner, which may not entirely suppress the natural production of menstrual hormones, though they typically prevent monthly menstrual bleeds.

Hormonal contraception has undoubtedly given women more options. Yet it is strange that, on the one hand, taking external, synthetic hormones to alter and/or suppress female hormone choreography during the menstruating, reproductive years is common practice. Whereas, on the other hand, the choice of more mature women to maintain her physiological levels of these hormones has sometimes been viewed in a negative light. A woman should not feel pressured to make a decision either way about HRT, certainly not based on a myth that HRT "interferes" with hormones. That view is more applicable to hormonal contraception than HRT. Even then, the decision about taking external hormones, must be informed and personal for the individual.

Myth 12 All menopausal women should take testosterone

Just as HRT is not the elixir of youth, neither is testosterone. Despite phases of "testosterone frenzy", no menopausal woman should feel like she is missing out by not seeking out testosterone. The ovaries are the main source of testosterone in women, so when the ovaries retire, levels of this sex steroid hormone decline. Testosterone plays a role in libido. Reduced libido is the only specific clinical indication for considering external testosterone in menopause[23]. The BMS advises that assessing the level of testosterone by a blood test can be helpful to act as a baseline. Generally establishing systemic HRT is the first step, before considering adding in testosterone.

The type of systemic HRT can also affect the amount of circulating testosterone. Oral synthetic oestrogen increases the amount of sex hormone binding globulin (SHBG) by inducing liver enzymes. SHBG binds testosterone, so this type of HRT could indirectly lower active unbound testosterone.

For women competing in sporting events under World Anti-Doping Authority (WADA) jurisdiction, testosterone as an anabolic hormone is banned under any circumstance.

There may be other hormone and non-hormonal factors at play when it comes to libido. For example, low levels of oestrogen can cause vaginal dryness and discomfort with sexual intercourse. This is why it is advised only to consider testosterone, after systemic HRT has been established and/or vaginal oestrogen explored. Non-hormonal lubricants are also worth trying. Other psychological factors involved in libido can be considered.

Myth 13 GPs are not informed about menopause and HRT

Although menopause is not a medical condition, you may have related symptoms and health concerns you wish to discuss with your GP. Furthermore, since HRT is a regulated, licensed medication, it needs prescribing by your GP. As with all professions, some GPs are more expert practising in particular areas.

All medical doctors practising in the United Kingdom must complete medical training and are required to have both annual appraisals and 5-yearly revalidations to keep their licence to practise medicine. All doctors must present evidence of continued professional development (CPD). For doctors with particular interest in menopause, the BMS provides high-quality, extensive CPD opportunities. The updated training course offered by the BMS is aimed to equip medical doctors with the understanding and knowledge to support the vast majority, 95% of all menopausal women[24].

My best advice is to identify a GP at your practice who is empathetic and informed on this particular area of women's health. You can check out the "credentials" of your GPs online and you can always ask the practice manager if there is a GP who has a particular interest and training in menopause.

It also really helps if you can be an informed patient and do your own research from reliable resources (ideally not the Sirens of social media) before you discuss with your GP. I hope this book will help. There is also excellent information on the patient arm of the BMS, called Women's Health Concern[25]. Furthermore, with colleagues at UCL, backed by women's health organisations, we are developing an evidence-based information and support programme for women in the United Kingdom, InTune.

Here is a suggested check list you could take to discuss with your GP. I recommend writing down your points and questions in advance and taking to your appointment:

- Describe any menopausal symptoms, ideally with an outline of intensity, frequency and duration: How long have you been experiencing these symptoms? For example, changed/cessation of periods (where appropriate), hot flushes, disturbed sleep, mood issues, "brain fog", non-injury-related aches and pains, skin dryness, urinary tract symptoms, vaginal dryness?
- Are these symptoms interfering with your quality of life? For example, at work, interactions with family/friends?
- Mention anything you have tried (including exercise, nutrition, etc)
- HRT (systemic and local): even if you have already made a decision about whether you want to take HRT or not, this is your opportunity to discuss HRT options.

- If you do decide on HRT, be sure you are happy with what is being prescribed and you are clear on dose and how to take (e.g. oestradiol gel on inner thigh, micronised progesterone at night)
- Don't forget prepaid NHS prescription for all HRT products at £19 per year at the time of writing!

Myth 14 Alternatives to HRT are equally effective?

Medication: There are some "non-hormonal" medications for the management of menopausal symptoms. The newest of these is a neurokinin 3 receptor antagonist. Neurokinin is a short-range hormone transmitter in the brain that plays a part in modulating the hypothalamus and pituitary gland, the conductor of the endocrine orchestra, in controlling the release of hormones in the reproductive axis. This new medication increases the choice available to women, particularly those who cannot, or do not wish to take HRT. It is likely to offer many women experiencing hot flushes (vasomotor symptoms) improvement in their quality of life[26].

Non-medication alternatives: Care should be taken in considering the range of non-medication alternatives for managing menopausal symptoms. Since these are not medications, they are not subject to the same regulations for effectiveness and reliability of ingredients. This can lead to variable efficacy or none at all. It is advisable to choose good quality options to reduce the risk of this problem. The other aspect to bear in mind that although these types of non-medication options may help symptoms, there will be no effect on long-term bone or cardiovascular health, as with HRT. Nevertheless, some women find these approaches really helpful, especially those with personal history of breast cancer for whom HRT is not an option.

For herbal preparations it is advisable to check that any products have traditional herbal registration mark, to ensure best possible quality. The BMS reports some evidence that black cohosh and *Ginkgo biboba* can be helpful for some women in managing menopausal symptoms. Wild yam cannot be converted to progesterone in the body and currently there is no evidence of effect. There is no convincing evidence that St John's wort is effective and women should be aware that this can interfere with prescription medication, including certain cancer treatments. This is an important consideration for women who cannot take HRT because they are receiving medication for breast cancer[27].

Nevertheless, some women find herbal options helpful. Provided something does not cause harm, it might be worth a try; especially for women for whom HRT is contraindicated from a medical point of view.

Other options include phytoestrogens. These are found in plant food sources rich in isoflavones like soya and legumes, possibly explaining why Japanese women experience less troubling menopause symptoms. Lignans are another plant sources such as oilseeds; they have been reported to be helpful. Cognitive behavioural therapy (CBT) can be effective in managing menopause symptoms[28].

Scylla and Charybdis?

The discussion of HRT in non-medical circles, especially in the context of social media chatter, can give the impression that deciding to take HRT, or deciding not to take HRT are both equally negative decisions. You can feel trapped between Scylla and Charybdis. Whether to take HRT or not, is a very individual and nuanced decision.

Women should be allowed to make informed, personal decisions about taking external hormones, at any age, whether this be for quality of life, health reasons or contraception.

As the former vice president of the Royal College of Obstetrics and Gynaecology, Professor Janice Rymer urges, *"We need to treat women as individuals not statistics."*

References

1. National Institute for Health and Care Excellence. NICE guidelines on menopause. https://www.nice.org.uk/guidance/ng23. Accessed April 2024.
2. HRT: The History. Women's health concern. https://www.womens-health-concern.org/wp-content/uploads/2022/11/10-WHC-FACTSHEET-HRT-The-history-NOV22-A.pdf. Accessed May 2024.
3. Women's Health Concern. HRT: Benefits and risks. https://www.womens-health-concern.org/wp-content/uploads/2022/12/11-WHC-FACTSHEET-HRT-BenefitsRisks-NOV2022-B.pdf. Accessed April 2024.
4. HRT Risks and Benefits Women's Health Concern. https://www.womens-health-concern.org/wp-content/uploads/2022/12/11-WHC-FACTSHEET-HRT-BenefitsRisks-NOV2022-B.pdf. Accessed May 2024.
5. Women's Health Concern. Understanding the risks of breast cancer. https://www.womens-health-concern.org/wp-content/uploads/2019/10/WHC-UnderstandingRisksofBreastCancer-MARCH2017.pdf. Accessed January 2024.
6. Women's Health Concern. Breast cancer. https://www.womens-health-concern.org/wp-content/uploads/2022/12/01-WHC-FACTSHEET-BreastCancer-NOV2022-C.pdf.
7. British Menopause Society. What is the menopause? https://thebms.org.uk/wp-content/uploads/2023/08/17-BMS-TfC-What-is-the-menopause-AUGUST2023-A.pdf. Accessed January 2024.
8. Rymer J, Brian K, Regan L. HRT and breast cancer risk. *BMJ* 2019; 367: l5928. doi: 10.1136/bmj.l5928.
9. British Menopause Consensus Statement. "Bioidentical" HRT. https://thebms.org.uk/wp-content/uploads/2023/10/01-BMS-ConsensusStatement-Bioidentical-HRT-OCT2023-A.pdf. Accessed January 2024.
10. British Menopause Society Consensus Statement. Prevention and treatment of osteoporosis in postmenopausal women. Accessed April 2024.
11. British Association Sport and Exercise Medicine. 'Concerning' lack of awareness of how best to reduce risk of stress fractures in female athletes and dancers, a year after change in NICE Guidelines 2023. https://basem.co.uk/concerning-lack-of-awareness-of-how-best-to-reduce-risk-of-stress-fractures-in-female-athletes-and-dancers-a-year-after-change-in-nice-guidelines/.
12. British Menopause Society Website. Tools for clinicians. https://thebms.org.uk/publications/tools-for-clinicians/. Accessed January 2024.
13. British Menopause Society Consensus Statement. Primary prevention of coronary heart disease in women. Accessed April 2024.

14 British Menopause Society. Ten top tips. https://thebms.org.uk/wp-content/uploads/2022/12/16-BMS-TfC-Menopause-Guidance-Top-Ten-Tips-01-original-NOV2022-A.pdf. Accessed January 2024.
15 Labrie F, Labrie C. DHEA and intracrinology at menopause, a positive choice for evolution of the human species. *Climacteric* 2013; 16 (2): 205–213.
16 British Menopause Society. Progestogens and endometrial protection. https://thebms.org.uk/wp-content/uploads/2023/04/14-BMS-TfC-Progestogens-and-endometrial-protection-APR2023-A.pdf. Accessed January 2024.
17 Prior J, Cameron A, Fung M et al. Oral micronized progesterone for perimenopausal night sweats and hot flushes a Phase III Canada-wide randomized placebo-controlled 4-month trial. *Scientific Reports* 2023. doi: 10.1038/s41598-023-35826-w.
18 Hilard T, Abernathy K, Manoda H et al (eds.). *Management of the Menopause*, Sixth Edition. British Menopause Society.
19 British Menopause Society. Principles and practice of menopause care. Course for healthcare professionals completed 2021.
20 British Menopause Society. Tachyphylaxis with HRT. https://thebms.org.uk/2023/09/tachyphylaxis-with-hrt/. Accessed September 2023.
21 Women's Health Concern. Contraception for the older woman. https://www.womens-health-concern.org/wp-content/uploads/2022/12/04-WHC-FACTSHEET-ContraceptionForTheOlderWoman-NOV22-B.pdf. Accessed April 2024.
22 Keay N. *Hormones Health and Human Potential*. Act 1, Scene 2 In the Red. Sequoia Books, 2022.
23 British Menopause Society. Testosterone replacement in menopause. https://thebms.org.uk/wp-content/uploads/2022/12/08-BMS-TfC-Testosterone-replacement-in-menopause-DEC2022-A.pdf. Accessed January 2024.
24 BMS principles and practice of menopause care. Accessed May 2024.
25 Women's Health Concern. https://www.womens-health-concern.org/. Accessed May 2024.
26 British Menopause Society. https://thebms.org.uk/2023/12/new-treatment-for-vasomotor-symptoms-hot-flushes-and-night-sweats-licensed-by-the-mhra/. Accessed January 2024.
27 Women's Health Concern. Complementary & alternative therapies non hormonal treatments for menopause symptoms. https://www.womens-health-concern.org/wp-content/uploads/2023/11/03-WHC-FACTSHEET-Complementary-And-Alternative-Therapies-NOV2023-C.pdf. Accessed April 2024.
28 Women's Health Concern and British Menopause Society. Cognitive Behavioural Therapy (CBT) for menopausal symptoms. https://www.womens-health-concern.org/wp-content/uploads/2023/02/02-WHC-FACTSHEET-CBT-WOMEN-FEB-2023-A.pdf. Accessed April 2024.

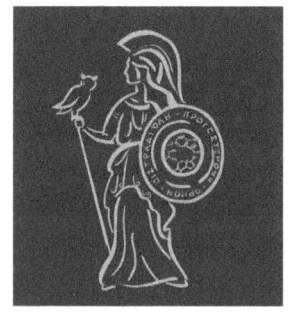

Act 6

Active Women and the Hormone Dance

Terpsichore

Act 6 Active Women and the Hormone Dance

Terpsichore

Ancient Greek muse of dance

Dr Nicky Keay

The hormone dance of life

As you progress through the female hormone odyssey, the hormones that drive adaptation to physical activity change. The internal hormone dance has variations. You can continue to derive the health benefits of exercise by embracing new activities, to remain in synchrony with internal hormone changes. Have you considered tapping into your inner Terpsichore, the Ancient Greek muse of dance? Whether you are a regular dancer or newcomer, all are welcome to the menopause dance.

Dancing is part of my family history. As a child, I clearly remember the pride and awe I experienced watching my mother perform flamenco dancing on stage. Appropriately my grandmother's maiden name was Lightfoot (a source of jocularity at dance auditions!). She lived up to her name as an accomplished ballet dancer, invited by Dame Ninette de Valois to join her company with the likes of Dame Margot Fonteyn. My grandmother took me to my first ballet classes at the age of four. I have never stopped taking ballet classes since.

These photos shown my grandmother and me en pointe at similar ages.

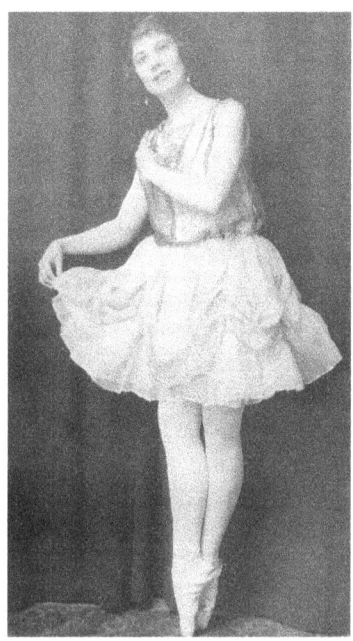

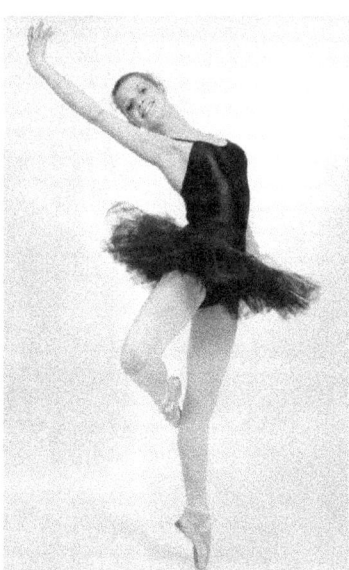

After many years of taking class and performing, ballet remains an important part of my life. Although I have retired from pointe work and my legs don't go as high as they used to, I feel I am a better dancer now than in my youth. Rather than focusing on technique, I relish the joy of movement and expression with music, with my close circle of ballet friends.

As a dancing doctor, I am excited to discuss and present the strong reciprocal relationship between dance and health. You will hear from fellow dancers and dancing healthcare professionals of their experiences of dancing through the female hormone odyssey and the menopause dance and supporting others to do so.

Being medical advisor to Scottish Ballet is my dream job: combining my passions of medicine, health and dance for the professional dancers of the company and the wider community. One of the positive outcomes of this collaboration between health and dance is the initiative in combatting osteoporosis in menopausal women. My first research study, published in the *British Journal of Sport and Exercise Medicine*, investigated bone health in retired female dancers, for which I received the Young Investigator Award (yes, it was many years ago!) from the National Osteoporosis Society (now Royal Osteoporosis Society). This is why I am especially pleased that you will read about the connection between Scottish Ballet and the Royal Osteoporosis Society to support the health of menopausal women through dance.

This Act presents ways to embrace the changes of hormone choreography in a positive, proactive way. Dance is amazing for all aspects of health: physical, mental and social.

Photo: Attitude, Dr Nicky Keay.

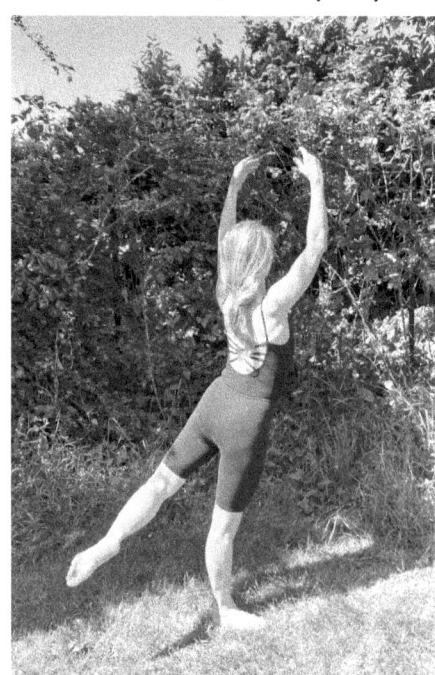

Scene 1 Dancing through menopause

Tiffany Stott

Dance for joy

If you have a heartbeat, you have rhythm. If you have emotion, you can be moved. You breathe in and out every day, so you are never not moving. Bring the three together and you are an expressive, moving being. Denying yourself the joy of movement is like blocking a stream so the water can't flow. We should all let the natural flow of our movement happen without inhibition, fear or judgement. Call it dancing or moving for joy; we cannot deny that humans are innately designed to dance. In addition to joy, dancing can be a way to stay fit for people of all ages, shapes and sizes. There is ongoing research as to the best form of dance to achieve the maximum benefits; but the main thing to consider is what form of dance you enjoy doing?

If you are going to continue with an activity, whatever it is, you have to enjoy it. This is going to be the most important deciding factor as to whether dance will benefit you. Whether it's tango, ballet, African, tap or just dancing around your kitchen, the physical and emotional benefits you experience are real. It is important to also note here as well that you do not have to be "good" at it to experience the benefits of it. So often people get tied up with the notion that they have to be good at something to benefit from doing the activity. Dance does indeed carry with it many misguided preconceptions.

Excuses such as *"I can't dance, I have two left feet"* or *"I have no rhythm"* are banded around suggesting that you need two feet to dance in the first place or that you need to hear to be able to dance. There are many professional and non-professional dancers that all demonstrate the ridiculous nature of these comments marvellously. Dance is not as superficial as this. Dance comes from deeper within us and, as such offers multifaceted benefits that many other physical activities cannot and do not offer.

Dance your troubles away

There are endless physical benefits that dance can offer. Very specific to dance are balance, coordination and agility, as well as motor skills. Dance can develop muscle strength and endurance, as well as improve bone density. Increasing bone density is particularly important as we get older and especially for postmenopausal women to offset the chances of developing osteoporosis[4].

Inherently dance improves posture, balance and stability[5] through the increase in strength but also by creating a physical awareness of one's posture and physical carriage of the body. The nature of the movements, creativity and styles automatically encourage the participants to consider, consciously or not, their deportment.

Increased joint mobility and flexibility throughout the body can be accomplished by working dynamically through wide ranges of movement that explore joint mobility, which an individual may not engage in on a daily basis. If we are to compare the mobility involved in other activities such as walking, swimming or cycling, dance perhaps offers a more varied range of movements on different anatomical planes. Although safely participating in any physical activity can be beneficial, some might perhaps lack the dynamism that dance can offer.

"The ballet staff and musicians create an atmosphere that encourages us to push ourselves. I know my legs are strengthened through the exercise and it just makes me feel amazing after class!"

SB Elevate® dancer

Dance may also help to improve cardiovascular fitness and as such heart and lung health[6]. It may also support healthy weight management. All these physical benefits are important for everyone, especially as we get older, ensuring we stay as strong and mobile for as long as possible and reduce the risk of falls.

Studies show that engaging in creative activities such as dance can positively impact mental health[2]. Dance is a multifaceted activity that provides opportunities for people to be creative as well as physically active, and if done as a group, it also involves social interaction and connection. As with many activities, dance can release the mood-enhancing chemical endorphin, that wonderful natural high. The mechanisms involved in healthy dance practice help reduce anxiety, stress and depression, increase people's confidence and self-image and improve resilience[3]. In addition, dance and movement-based practices have, for a long time now, been used to help support and overcome emotional trauma. There is growing research that suggests that to effectively treat trauma, it is important to treat both the body and mind and, as such implement verbal as well as movement therapy strategies.

"A very motivational session, I felt good while doing the movements and my anxiety levels and tight muscles relaxed immediately."

Health at Hand® dancer

During a dance class, you will be learning new steps, remembering steps or creating your own. Research has once again shown that these elements of a dance class could be neuroprotective and could slow down cognitive decline while increasing cognitive function and memory[7,8].

Dancing is a social activity and can help reduce isolation and loneliness and instead build connections and communities. Evidence shows that society is becoming increasingly isolated, with people reporting feelings of loneliness. This can lead to low mood, low confidence and depression. It is not just older people or people who live alone who are suffering from this. Increasingly, younger people are reporting heightened levels of loneliness and isolation. Increased reliance on social media activities, working from home and the cost of living can all be catalysts. Even those who have busy family and work lives can still feel isolated if they are not truly connecting with people of similar interests and understanding. Once again, the creative and artistic nature of dance can help people connect. Even for those who are socially shy, the non-verbal aspect of dance still evokes connection, communication and a sense of relatedness.

> "It's given me the chance to experience dance again and meet with people who understand my condition."
>
> SB Elevate dancer©

A note on music

We all know the feeling that listening to our favourite song gives us or that toe-tapping beat that just brightens our mood. We don't need any more evidence to support why as humans we love music. We have a heartbeat; therefore, we have internal rhythm and as such our bodies respond to music. Well, as if I need to promote the benefits of dance any more, the icing on the cake is the fact that generally when we dance, we move to music too. What better partnership is there than that? Well, of course, there are Fred and Ginger and Torvill and Dean, but that goes without saying!

It is said that movement is medicine; well, then dancing to music has to be medicine with a "spoon full of sugar". For those who are not entirely sure of the benefit of music, here are just a few. Music has been evidenced to activate multiple brain networks during listening, responding and performing. With one of the most important functions of music being to create feelings of cohesion and connectedness. Listening to music engages and stimulates the brain and can help increase learning capacity. MRI scans show active areas of the brain light up when music is played, and music can also increase memory function and slow down cognitive decline.

Listening to music also triggers the release of a number of neurochemicals that play an important role in brain function, mood and mental well-being. Dopamine, which is associated with the reward centres and pleasure, oxytocin that helps us to feel connected and serotonin to support immunity and reduce the stress response hormone cortisol. Music has also been shown to reduce fatigue as well as motivate and improve physical performance. Music therapy is becoming more common practice these days in the management of pain and trauma.

With all of this in mind, it is hardly surprising that people's commitment to dance is often better than participating in exercise.

> "I decided to take up dancing because I wanted to do something for me. . . . I don't really enjoy traditional exercise and find going to the gym lonely and outfacing. I would find any excuse not to go."

"I love music and although I never danced before I really enjoy watching it. The dance class environment provides me with the opportunity to be with and socialise with other people who enjoy the same thing, so it is less lonely and isolating then going to the gym. . . . My body feels freer, I have more mobility and I am definitely stronger and more coordinated since dancing regularly. In addition, I have the opportunity to be creative and to express myself. When I dance, I don't think about anything else, I am completely absorbed in what I am doing. I might be feeling distracted and anxious when I go in but by the time I come out I am calm, relaxed and yet energised and focused. I certainly find my mental agility as well as my physical agility has benefited since dancing."

Anonymous

Dancing for everyone

There are many examples of dance classes offered to the wider community. These classes cater to those people who do not dance for a living but dance for the joy of it, for well-being, fitness and connecting with people and themselves.

Many of these classes are set up and run by independent dance teachers who will deliver in the style they are trained in. This might be ballet, ballroom, Bollywood or various other forms. Many independent dance schools often offer community classes for adults alongside the children and young people's classes. Many dance companies also offer community classes.

Scottish Ballet is Scotland's national dance company and a National Centre for Dance Health. They offer a range of community programmes and projects for people across the life cycle, including young people's mental health and well-being projects, weekly ballet classes for a range of experiences and abilities, well-being resources for health and social care staff and resources for people living with long COVID.

They also offer three neurological weekly dance programmes: Dance for Parkinson's Scotland, dementia-friendly Time To Dance® and SB Elevate® for people living with multiple sclerosis. Classes are delivered in the studio, online, in hospitals and care homes, in schools and online via free pre-recorded resources.

This wide range of community dance means there are many access points for people to enjoy dancing and movement.

For over 15 years, Scottish Ballet has also been delivering a ballet programme called Regenerate. These classes are specifically designed for people aged 60 and above; they offer an accessible route into ballet for people who may or may not have danced before.

The teachers are experienced and skilled in working with an older group of dancers. Participants can enjoy a safe and enjoyable way into dance, knowing that the teachers understand their specific requirements as a mature dancer.

It is very important in any physical activity to take into account the individual's age and experience in order to avoid injury. An adolescent body versus a highly trained adult body versus a more mature body with less experience all require a different approach to the activity. As our bodies grow, develop and age, it is important to consider how we might need to adapt physical movement to ensure we remain injury-free and are able to continue to move optimally for as long as possible. How we tailor this movement will depend on each individual's unique body and movement history, as well as what other physical activities they are doing.

Some people may be put off or feel uncomfortable attending a class where they might be one of the oldest in the group. It may be less appealing to attend a general dance class if they feel that their needs are not met, and the teacher may not be experienced in working with people their age. Regenerate offers the participants a chance to dance for enjoyment as well as safely offering them the potential physical benefits of improved dynamic balance, stability, strength, posture, mobility, range of movement and stamina.

In addition to the physical benefits that might be experienced, the Regenerate dancers also describe how the classes provide them with an opportunity to socialise and connect with their peers who appreciate dance. Many of the class members have developed long-term friendships over the years and as such have grown their social circle as a result.

> *"I'm convinced the Ballet exercises have been material in keeping me fit into my eighties, Scottish Ballet changed my life (for the better) in old age. I was performing in public, which I never expected to do. I've made wonderful friends and I feel privileged to be associated with and representing Scottish Ballet and in particularly in The Elders Company."*
>
> *Regenerate and Elders company dancer*

A number of the Regenerate dancers were also members of the Scottish Ballet Elders Company (SBEC). SBEC was a performance group run by Scottish Ballet. Members of this group were required to audition to take part. They rehearsed weekly and experienced the chance to work with a variety of professional choreographers. This saw them performing all across Scotland and the United Kingdom at various events and locations, including Sadler's Wells. Some of their work were also intergenerational, which provided both the older and younger dancers a chance to work together to create, collaborate and connect with different generations.

> *"I'd done dance fitness for many years, but it was really about exercise, not dancing; although I loved it. But joining Regenerate and actually performing in public introduced me to a whole new world, which, while I found it terrifying, made me realise that I had probably always been a frustrated dancer. The sense of achievement, particularly in old age, is incredible."*
>
> *Regenerate and Elders company dancer*

Dancing bones

Research has shown that for menopausal women engaging in dance can positively impact a number of physical[9] and psychological factors associated with the menopause.

Menopausal women are at a greater risk of developing osteoporosis. This is due to a reduction in the hormone oestrogen. Oestrogen is important for maintaining healthy bone density. A reduction of bone density leads to a reduction in bone strength and a greater risk of breaking bones. Strength training and weight-bearing impact exercises can help to ensure bone density is maintained. Dancing with the right degree of weight-bearing and impact can be an enjoyable and effective exercise choice to protect against osteoporosis.

To weight bear, your whole-body weight needs to pull down on your skeleton. To add impact to this, you need to add an additional force. This can be anything from jogging to walking or jumping. In addition, a variety of movement is good, particularly moving in different directions and at different speeds. The Royal Osteoporosis Society suggests that dance is particularly good for this.

To generate movement, muscles need to pull on bones. In turn, this pull on the bones causes them to renew themselves and, as such maintain their strength. As muscles get stronger, they pull harder and this leads to an increase in bone strength.

To strengthen muscles, they must move against resistance. To increase their strength, they must reach overload. Lifting weights, working with resistance bands or performing bodyweight movements can all help to ensure muscle strength.

The Royal Osteoporosis Society has recently released a dance resource for people with osteoporosis, Dance for your Bones. The dance resource has been designed to ensure that there are adequate amounts of impact placed on the musculoskeletal frame to aid the improvement in bone density. The dance resource is structured in a way that allows people to follow along and learn the routine in their own time. Although this resource is aimed at people who already have osteoporosis, the same principles would apply as a preventive tool.

Evidence also supports how dance can improve pelvic floor muscles and as such reduce stress urinary incontinence[10], which is another potential symptom of menopause. In addition, other research has shown lowering of cholesterol and improvements in lipid profile. During menopause, due to the reduction in oestrogen levels, there is an associated risk of an increase in cholesterol and other lipids. This is because one of the functions of oestrogen is to regulate these lipids. An increase in cholesterol, in turn may increase the risk of heart disease. Engaging in exercise, including dance, may help to manage this risk[11].

Anxiety and depression are other common symptoms of menopause. To help women manage this, it is often treated with medication, which in turn can have side effects. As we now know, dance can reduce anxiety, depression, improve mood, self-esteem and self-image in the general public. Dance has also been evidenced to reduce feelings of depression and anxiety for menopausal women[12]. Therefore, dance may be a successful non-pharmaceutical intervention for managing some of these symptoms without the side effects.

> "I had recently moved to the area with my family and was struggling to meet new people as I work from home for myself. I moved from a busy city to a rural community, so it was quite a cultural shock. My children are teenagers and so my interaction with other parents is also limited now. I was feeling quite lonely and isolated and to make matters worse also going through the menopause. The combination of re-locating, no friends, prepubescent children and going through the menopause was causing me to really struggling with my mental health, feelings of loneliness, disconnect and lack of identity, confidence, fatigue and depression. . . . I have always loved the arts and dancing in particular. I was lucky enough to hear about an adult ballet class that was going on in my village. I was nervous to attend at first but they were all so welcoming. A large group of people of different ages all from different backgrounds and all attending for different reasons. The class has allowed me the chance to connect with other people and build my confidence as well as physical strength. I have so much more energy now, I am more mobile, I have less pain, I feel stronger and my posture and balance improved. I find I can focus for longer and by having to remember steps and figure at the moves I am sure my mind is sharper and memory better. I am sure my children will disagree though!"
>
> "I love the creativity of the class, the music and opportunity to express myself uninhibited as I am amongst other people who all feel the same way. I have made new friends in this class and spoken to a number of others who, to my surprise, had also joined the class for similar reasons. My friendship group and support network has grown and I have now started attending another dance class in the week as well as making sure I move every single day. I have learnt that for me to be the best version of myself I need to move, dance, express myself and connect with likeminded people. . . . I am just shocked that it has taken me till this age to discover these simple facts!"
>
> *Anonymous dancer*

Révérence

The benefits you might enjoy from engaging in dance may support well-being on many levels and form a part of a healthy lifestyle. More and more in our culture, we are becoming sedentary, with jobs that require us to sit behind computers all day, travelling in cars or public transport. With demanding lives and limited time, it is hard to ensure we are moving our bodies well and enough. Consequently, the physical, psychological and mental impact of not moving is often felt as we get older. By not moving well and regularly, we see a reduction in mobility, strength, balance, coordination and motor skills. Lack of movement can lead to obesity, injury, poor posture, increased risk of falls and, as such fractures.

Building regular movement into your life is vital to ensure we all age well both physically and psychologically. This investment in ourselves is like putting money in a savings account. We are preparing for the future and safeguarding our bodies for whatever life throws at us. A strong healthy mind and body are more likely to weather the storms of life if they are protected, have reserves and take a preventative approach rather than a reactive one.

For women, these principles are vitally important to ensure they mature and age well. It is never too early to start implementing healthy lifestyle choices. The key is that they have to be achievable and enjoyable for you to commit to them. You must feel good doing it or enjoy how it makes you feel afterwards. If dance is your movement choice, there are so many options to choose from. Try different styles, different classes, take a friend, go on your own, join an online class or find one of the thousands of free online tutorials. The research behind the amazing multifaceted benefits makes us realise why humans have always danced. We do not need research to prove this, just give ourselves permission to do it and enjoy it! So, what is stopping you? Put some music on and just dance wherever and whenever you can.

References

1. Fong Yan A, Cobley S, Chan C et al. The effectiveness of dance interventions on physical health outcomes compared to other forms of physical activities: A systematic review and meta-analysis. *Sports Medicine* 2018 Apr; 48 (4): 933–951. doi: 10.1007/s40279-017-0853-5.
2. Amaro Moratelli J, Veras G, Bellani Lyra V et al. Evidence of the effects of dance interventions on adults mental health: A systematic review. *Dance Medicine & Science* 2023 Dec; 27 (4): 183–193. doi: 10.1177/1089313X231178.
3. Burgess GS, Burwitz L. Effects of a 6-week aerobic dance intervention on body image and physical self-perceptions in adolescent girls. *Body Image* 2006 Mar; 3 (1): 57–66. doi: 10.1016/j.bodyim.2005.10.005.
4. McGrath RP, Kraemer WJ, Vincent BM et al. Muscle strength is protective against osteoporosis in an ethnically diverse sample of adults. *Journal of Strength and Conditioning Research* 2017 Sept; 31 (9): 2586–2589. doi: 10.1519/JSC.0000000000002080.
5. Hwang W-NP, Braun KL. The effectiveness of dance interventions to improve older adults' health: A systematic literature review. *Alternative Therapies in Health and Medicine* 2015 Sep–Oct; 21 (5): 64–70.
6. McCrary, Redding E, Altenmüller E. Performing arts as a health resource? An umbrella review of the health impacts of music and dance participation. *PLOS ONE* 2021 June 10. doi: 10.1371/journal.pone.0252956.
7. Hewston P, Kennedy CC, Borhan S et al. Effects of dance on cognitive function in older adults: A systematic review and meta-analysis. *Age and Ageing* 2021; 50 (4): 1084–1092. doi: 10.1093/ageing/afaa270.
8. Muiños M, Ballesteros S. Does dance counteract age-related cognitive and brain declines in middle-aged and older adults? A systematic review. *Neuroscience & Biobehavioral Reviews* 2021; 121: 259–276. doi: 10.1016/j.neubiorev.2020.11.028.

9. Sun J, Yao C, Wang Z et al. The beneficial effects of square dance on musculoskeletal system in early postmenopausal Chinese women: A cross-sectional study. *BMC Womens Health* 2022 Jun 21; 22 (1): 247. doi: 10.1186/s12905-022-01832-9.

10. Tang Y, Guo X, Wang Y. Rumba dance combined with breathing training as an exercise intervention in the management of stress urinary incontinence in postmenopausal women: A randomized controlled trial. *International Journal of Environmental Research and Public Health* 2022 Dec 28; 20 (1): 52. doi: 10.3390/ijerph20010522.

11. Teixeira GR, Cruz Veras AS, Rodrigues Rocha AP. Dance practice modifies functional fitness, lipid profile, and self-image in postmenopausal women. *Menopause* 2021 Oct; 28 (10): 1117–1124. doi: 10.1097/GME.0000000000001818.

12. Gao L, Zhang L, Qi H et al. Middle-aged female depression in perimenopausal period and square dance intervention. *BMC Womens Health* 2022 Jun 21; 22 (1): 247. doi: 10.1186/s12905-022-01832-9.

Scene 2 Gracefully ageing (we hope) forever swans

Astrid Sherman

My hormone history, looking back is definitely a *". . . hmmm"* moment. As I write, I reflect on how much I had no idea of and how little anyone around me knew and, more tragically, how little clear advice was given by the medical field at the time.

My generation was likely the first generation to seek out female gynaecologists. I remember speaking with friends and fellow dancers in my late teens and early twenties about awkward, uncomfortable experiences and hearing from some who had magically found the first lady gynaecologists in the community. These women empathised and listened to us dancers.

As a dancer, I was typical of one who incurred a "late puberty". I was 18 before my body kicked in and was absolutely horrified at the changes as it timed exactly when I arrived at a ballet postgraduate pre-professional training school. Overnight, I went from a "skinny-malinky long legs" (as my mum called me) to curves arriving in places that teachers at the school called "disaster zones".

So, very quickly, I followed my "friend's" advice and saw the friendly doctor who started me on a combined oral contraceptive pill which would regulate my wild hormones. Very quickly, I grew very comfortable with the routine that the "pill" offered me. I could prepare for the bleeding week. I knew when it was coming and could plan.

In my late forties, perimenopause called. The dependable schedule on "the pill" was no longer as dependable. I consulted "Dr Google" and started missing out the week off the combined contraceptive pill to control the break though weird bleeding of perimenopause. Unfortunately, at the time, I was between doctors (and countries) so my medical advice was haphazard. After all, I had been on this pill for over 30 years and thought myself educated.

A couple of years later, in my early fifties and during the pandemic (and still between countries and medical systems), short-term gain for long-term pain was about to come knocking. I had stayed on my combined oral contraceptive pill when I read conventional practitioners simply pick an age (typically 50) and move you directly to HRT. What is the difference, I thought?!

I suffered a Deep Vein Thrombosis (DVT) on an intercontinental flight. I was/am fit, not overweight and have no other health concerns or conditions. I nearly died walking off that plane!!!

In typical dancer fashion, mid-flight when my calf muscle seemed to "cramp", I did my piano toes, calf stretches, ABC ankle rolls and rolled a lacrosse ball, only when my heart started racing and my energy went from hero to zero and I was puffing like I had completed 132 and not 32 changements did I think something might be wrong!

So began my REAL journey into perimenopause . . . the emergency ward! I had to stop my contraceptive pills overnight. Besides the blood thinner heparin being injected directly into my stomach, the experience of coming off the contraceptive pill was hardly pleasant. Even though I was on a low-dose combined oral contraceptive pill, going "cold turkey" after so many decades of use, resulted in some very unpleasant "withdrawal" symptoms. Apparently, our bodies train/adapt over the years to depend on these synthetic hormones and make fewer of their own. And so, I heard (or rather felt) the first whisper about the "muzzle effect" that the contraceptive pill had put on my endocrine system.

Once the haematologist back in Los Angeles had ruled out any genetic causes and pointed to a "perfect storm" of age, long flight and the combined oral contraceptive pill, I was kept on blood thinners for the next 6 months and *no* oral contraceptives. However, I seemed to bleed for weeks on end, relentlessly. So, a decision was made to re-allow progestone to control the bleeding and I was prescribed the progestone-only mini pill. Other options were negligible, as it was discovered I had very large fibroids. Now there was an added debate as to whether these fibroids were induced by my too high synthetic oestrogen levels over too many years.

The progestone-only mini pill did help. For a while, I savoured just *not* bleeding.

At the same time, I was planning an educational series for dancers regarding hormones in dance for International Association of Dance Medicine and Science. What I learnt from Dr Nicky Keay between hosting these sessions was mind-blowing.

What I had not really understood/ taken the time to learn/ been made aware of from medical doctors, in over thirty years, was that synthetic hormones are not the same as natural ones. Nor did I appreciate or have any awareness of the difference between controlling hormonal fluctuations and flatlining your natural hormones.

I'm now on natural progesterone, which works wonders for my menopausal body. I have no weight gain, no moods, no night sweating and wonderful, wonderful sleep. In fact, at 9 p.m. I'm looking at the time asking myself if it's too early to go to bed?! I am in *love* with sleep again. I think I have years of sleep deprivation to catch up on!

It's clear that concrete inroads in the research world of the dos and don'ts of taking a contraceptive pill for athletes and dancers need to be made more public. The differences between natural versus synthetic and whether you should allow yourself a bleed can be life-changing facts. My generation is having such a journey of learning by experience. The next generation will have all the information at hand from great researchers and dance lovers like our Dr Nicky Keay!

Photo: Astrid Sherman, fourth position on the golf course.

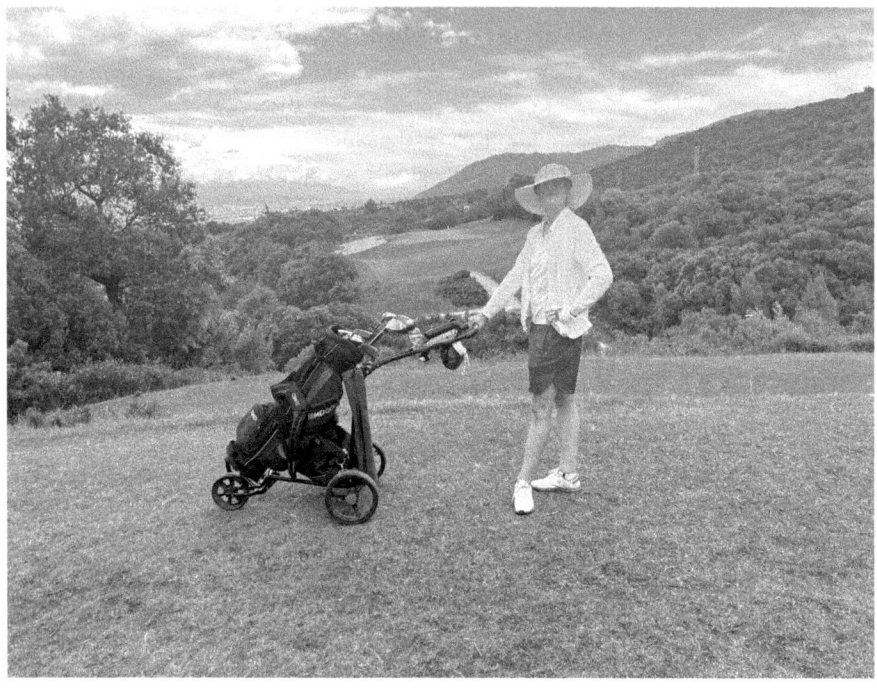

Scene 3 Menopause flamenco!

Nikki Crane

Having worked in the arts and health field for the past 25 years, I am acutely aware of the power of the arts to improve health and well-being and transform lives. As arts and health professionals, we see this transformation at work in our daily encounters with unforgettable workshops and performances and tirelessly make the case for funding through building the evidence base for health outcomes. But there's nothing quite like experiencing this impact firsthand and so it was when I went through my own health challenges during menopause, and my weekly flamenco classes took on a whole new significance in my life.

I've been dancing since I was four and went on to fulfil my dream of training as a dancer when I was accepted into the new dance degree course at the Laban Centre in London back in the 1980s. Ballet and contemporary dance had always been at the core of my training, but it took a move to South Humberside for my first proper job as a community dance worker to find the dance form which would be transformational in my life.

Controversial in its history, it is generally agreed that flamenco is an eclectic mix of the music of the many cultures that have played significant roles throughout the centuries in Andalusia, southern Spain, the most important of these being Muslim, Jewish, Byzantine, Indo-Pakistani and the Romani people, also known as Gypsies. The Romani people, most commonly associated with flamenco, brought their music, dance and folklore from India to Spain. What we are more certain about is that flamenco as we know it today did not begin its development until the sixteenth century when minority groups in Spain were expelled in an effort to promote pureness of race and religion. It is thought that flamenco emerged from the common experience of these persecuted peoples, evolving over centuries into a unique art form developed by an outcast society. Flamenco combines music, dance, singing and *jaleo* (rhythm accentuation and reciting) to express pain, joy, sorrow and longing and over the years has often been used as a form of protest against oppression and social inequality.

With such a seemingly remote and exotic background, it might seem unlikely that I would stumble across a flamenco class in a tiny church hall in a rural village just outside Scunthorpe in South Humberside, but this was my first encounter with this elusive art form. The sound of the live flamenco guitar, castanets, palmas (rhythmic clapping) and stamping feet through the open door was like a call from the wild after so much restrictive ballet training. I took up flamenco there and then and will be forever grateful that it was firmly embedded in my life when the onset of menopause began to turn my life upside down in my late 40s. By my early 50s, I was struggling with anxiety, a paralysing loss of confidence, mood swings, poor sleep and brain fog, all very destabilising while trying to hold down a senior leadership position, in which I felt huge pressure to perform and not let others down. I decided early on not to go down the medical route but to find other ways of dealing with the changes that were coming at me thick and fast. Flamenco, not surprisingly with its history of survival through adversity, seemed like the perfect medium to channel so much turmoil and uncertainty and so my weekly classes became the mainstay of my health and well-being during this time. There is nothing like a flamenco dance class with its combination of highly technical footwork (zapateado) and lithe body movements to provide a full mind and body workout. Absolute focus and presence in the body are required to execute the complex rhythms, interacting minute by minute with the musical accompaniment while expressing the full emotional range of each dance, from the mournful one moment to defiant and explosive the next. Flamenco teachers have a favourite instruction to be more 'sentada', literally meaning "seated", where they are calling for their students to be more grounded, centred and connected to the earth – such a powerful metaphor when your mind is churning and you feel you have lost your anchorage.

Robert Vidal, a famous classical guitar professor, once said: *"I love flamenco because it is an art form, which you don't listen to with your ears but with your intestines. First you have to feel the music before you can think about it."*

Feelings of disembodiment through the menopause were hugely disconcerting, a sense of being disconnected from oneself and also from others; thus, the social connection that classes provided was an ongoing source of sustenance – an encouragement to stay engaged with the world when it was so tempting to withdraw. I was fortunate to be dancing with such a supportive, caring group of people, mainly women of my own age, led by a teacher who was adept at picking up all the different moods and emotions at play in her class. After all, expressing and communicating with raw emotion is what flamenco is all about. Of course, there were times when I didn't feel like being sociable, but there was space to accommodate this too in the sympathetic environment of the class and also within the all-encompassing flamenco-dance repertoire. I was drawn particularly to the soulful *Solearas* (derived from the word "soledad" meaning "loneliness"), one of the *jondo* (profound) dances – often a trigger for some deep emotions but at the same time a sanctuary for stillness and calm. It was also a relief on low-mood days to be lifted up and out of myself through one of the more upbeat (chico) dances – *Tangos or*

Alegrias – an opportunity to bring out the extrovert, delight in being visible again and experience the sheer joy of dancing.

> "Throughout periods of fluctuating depression, flamenco has served as my version of mindfulness, or meditation. It is the concentration on the complex choreography and almost mathematical foot patterns & rhythms that forces me to be completely in the moment, banishing the external world & thus gives me mental respite. So that part is the cerebral challenge. But, once the choreography is finally mastered, you get the 'reward': the pleasure of letting the music flow through your body & making it move; & the emotional release that comes with expressing something, however intangible, through dance; which, when it happens, is the most wonderful therapy!"

Unsurprisingly, I did struggle sometimes to find the motivation to go to class, often feeling exhausted and lacking the confidence to face the immense challenges of flamenco. It is not a dance of half measures. The thought of being exposed when asked to get up and perform one of the terrifyingly complex choreographies in front of so many proficient dancers was enough to make me go into hiding. However, I had a very strong instinct that withdrawing behind closed doors was not the answer, so I pushed myself to attend. Putting on my flamenco gear, the classic polka dot skirt (la falda) and elegant high-heeled shoes (with reinforced nails under the toes and heels!) certainly helped to give me the boost I needed and signalled the transition from home and work into another world.

> "It is all about stress release for me, unwinding and tapping into a different part of yourself when dancing . . . stamping and flouncing was a major release from the stress of my job. I can remember doing 'planta' (pressing into the ball of the foot) and thinking of all the people who had driven me mad that day!"

Post menopause, eight years on, many of the health and well-being challenges still remain, and losing my mother recently taught me that bereavement shares a good deal of common ground with menopause – a sense of loss, grief and irreversible change, but also an opportunity to accept and move on with new insight. Both these experiences brought the gift of self-discovery and new meaning to this next phase of my life. I couldn't have had a better companion than flamenco along the way.

Photo, Nikki Crane, Flamenco

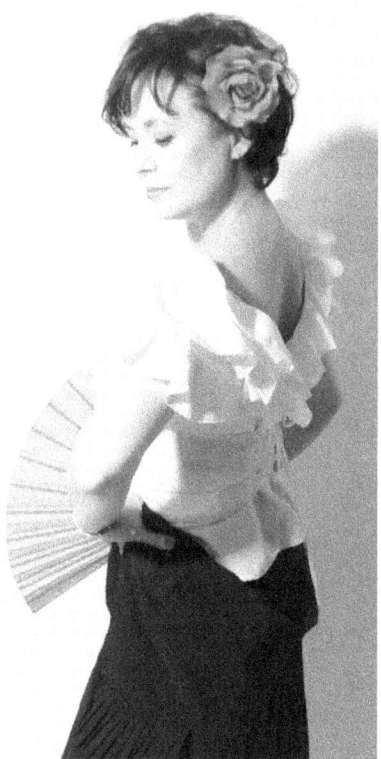

Scene 4 Everybody leaks?!

Dinah Hampson and Dr Brooke Winder

> "I feel like the foundation of my house is crumbling.
> "I have no energy, but I can't sleep."
> "I feel like my body is taking one step forward and two steps backward."
> "I pee a little when I jump."

These are sentiments we've heard from professional dancers moving through their 40s as they continue their careers in dance. If you're thinking right now . . . *"but these are the fit ballet artists who we see moving magically across the stage and through the air! If they are feeling these things, is there any hope for me, a regular human?"*

Yes, there is. We are your pelvic floor physiotherapists, here to chat about your pelvic floor and the role of physical therapy as you journey through menopause. I'm Dinah Hampson, a registered physiotherapist, who works in high performance, leads professional dancers through strength and conditioning classes 10 times a week, works full time and I am mother of two daughters. Did I mention I'm turning 55 this year and I had extensive pelvic surgery due to pregnancy/delivery complications? And I'm Brooke Winder, a licensed physiotherapist and university professor, who clinically researches and treats pelvic floor health in performance athletes, and who leads performing artists through strength, conditioning and injury prevention. I am also a mom in my 40s, navigating changes in my own body.

We wish that people had been talking long ago about the pelvic floor, including how to properly engage the core and the role of exercise well beyond the boring sit-ups and push-ups we were made to do in gym class. What is pelvic health, and why do we need to talk about it as we take this hormonal journey through perimenopause and menopause?

Why do we need to talk about pelvic health?

We need to talk about pelvic health because it is an uncomfortable subject that people don't like talking about. We need to talk about it because any human with a uterus will experience hormonal changes throughout life that will impact their overall physiology.

We need to talk about it because there are effective management strategies available that people simply need the right information about to incorporate properly into their lives.

The increase in life expectancy results in females living over a third of their life post-menopause, or more than 30 years past menopause[1]. Participating in physical activity, including high-performance sport/dance should be normal for this postmenopausal population. It's interesting that at the age when many women find their parents might be passing on and, if they have children, the children are becoming independent adults, this is the exact moment that menopause layers itself into our world. So now what? Well with 50% of women over the age of 50 experiencing urogenital symptoms that require treatment to improve, we need to let women know what those treatment options are[2].

The women have spoken, and the menopausal pelvic void that seemed present in medical texts, clinical practices and cultural expectations is now being filled with wonderful research and powerful evidence supporting women to accept nothing less than their best lives. In a study by Dumoulin et al. that reviewed pelvic floor muscle training in groups versus individually, they found that group pelvic floor strength training is not inferior to individual[3]. Women should be encouraged to participate in group physical endeavours throughout and postmenopause. Furthermore, if there are no options for individual or group pelvic floor therapy close-by, women should be encouraged to look to virtual therapy options. The global COVID pandemic brought virtual treatment options to the forefront of physiotherapy and in a 2021 study by Bernard et al., symptoms of urinary leakage were reduced for 87.5% of study participants using a home exercise program with telephone check-in with the physiotherapist[4]. It is important to us that women everywhere understand that they do have options and access to quality pelvic floor care.

There are some common myths regarding pelvic health and menopause – you may have heard or expressed these yourself

Everybody leaks.

It's normal to pee when you sneeze.

It's normal to pee when you do physical activity.

Leaking is normal over age 50.

Being over 50 means you can't keep up.

Lifting weights will make me bulky.

I can get all my strength training through yoga and Pilates.

I've been training this way since I was a teenager, so I don't need to change course.

"What's going on down there?"

Most women (most people, really) are not taught enough or even correct terminology when it comes to female pelvic anatomy, including the pelvic floor and female genitalia. Therefore, though many women can experience symptoms of dysfunction with the pelvic floor throughout their life phases, including in menopause, it is quite common that women have very limited knowledge of the pelvic floor itself[5-7]. So, when changes arise during perimenopause or menopause, not only can women feel embarrassed or uncomfortable talking about these issues, they might not even feel like they have the right words to describe their concerns about their own body or they may feel that asking the questions might open a pandoras box of issues they aren't sure they're ready to discuss. Therefore, we will next discuss some pelvic anatomy to help women know a little bit more about this area of the body. This will help women better understand changes or symptoms one might experience in the pelvic floor, why this may occur during menopause and have confidence in asking what to do about it.

Introduction to pelvic anatomy: It's not your hoo hoo or vajayjay

The bones of the pelvis form a heart shaped bowl, with the hard pubic bone area at the front and the tailbone (technically known as the coccyx) at the back, shown in Figure 6.4.1.

Internally, the pelvis contains the bladder, uterus, cervix, fallopian tubes, ovaries, vagina and rectum, as well as many blood vessels, nerves and connective tissue (which is body tissue that acts as support to the organs and other structures of the region) shown in Figure 6.4.2.

The vagina is the fibromuscular tube connecting the cervix to the vulva — it is lined with specialised skin called mucosa, arranged in folds or ridges known as rugae, atop a layer of smooth muscle. There are three "openings" in female pelvic anatomy: the urethra (where urine exits), the vaginal opening and the anus[8,9].

The external aspect of female genitalia is known as the vulva; this is the part of a female's anatomy that touches the underwear. The vulva includes the following structures: the mons pubis (a mound of skin and fatty tissue extending from the pubic bone to the clitoral hood), the urethra (the opening where urine is excreted), the vestibule (where the vaginal opening meets the vulva), the labia majora (outer skin folds that enhance sexual pleasure and protect the vaginal opening), the labia minora (the inner folds that circle the clitoris, engorge with sexual stimulation and enhance sexual pleasure) and the clitoris (sex organ analogous to the glans penis in males, for producing sexual pleasure). The clitoris is an inverted Y shape, with two sets of arms that surround

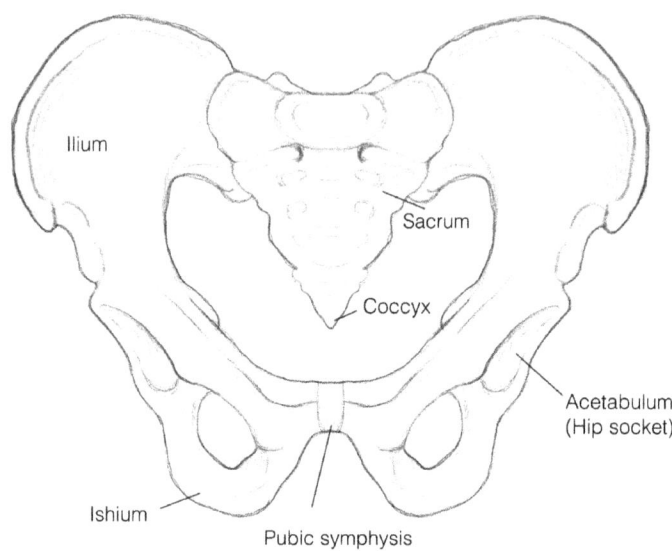

FIGURE 6.4.1 Bones of the pelvis

the urethral opening. The glans clitoris is the only visible portion of the clitoris — it is the folder tip of the Y, partially covered by the clitoral hood. Illustrated in Figure 6.4.3.

There are many responsive nerves and erectile tissue in all parts of the clitoris for sexual stimulation and orgasm[9-11]. Normal, expected hormonal changes that occur in menopause can affect the tissues of the vagina and the vulva, and we will discuss those changes later in the chapter.

Pelvic floor muscles

At the base of the pelvic "bowl", the pelvic floor muscles span from front to back (pubic bone to tailbone) and side to side (between the sitz bones, or the two prominent bony structures one can feel at each buttock when sitting). There are three layers of muscles in this region shown in Figure 6.4.4a Superior and 6.4.4b Inferior view of pelvic floor muscles.

The muscles closest to the surface of the body are mainly focused on "closing the openings", keeping urine and faeces in until we respond to the call to urinate or empty the bowels. The muscles farthest from the vulvar surface of the body, closest to the organs, are also known as the pelvic diaphragm muscles. These muscles serve as support like a hammock just below the organs. When the pelvic floor muscles contract, they pull in towards the centre of the perineum as well as up towards the inside of the body[9,12-15]. Many people know this as a "kegel".

The pelvic floor muscles serve several typical functions[16]:

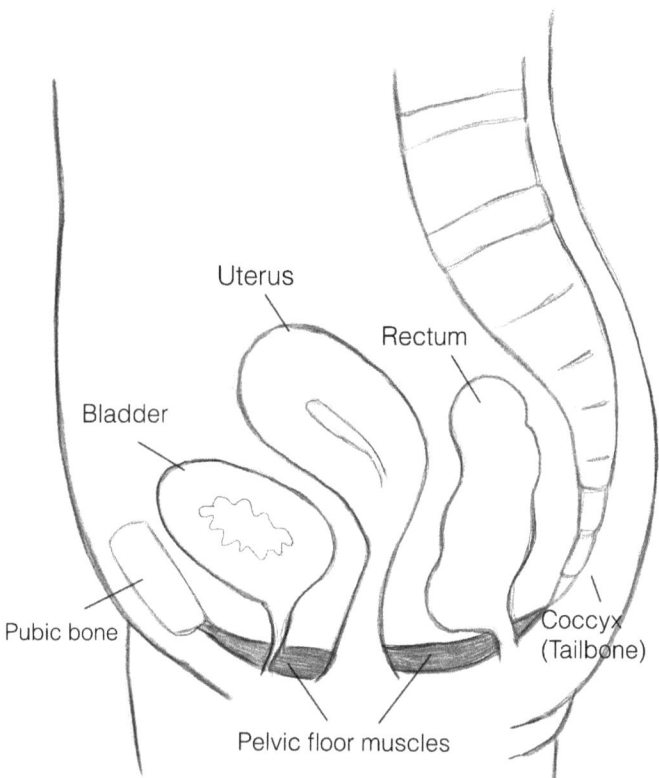

FIGURE 6.4.2 Lateral view of organs in pelvis

Sphincteric: As mentioned earlier, one of the major functions of the pelvic floor is to maintain some resting tension, and to contract further when needed, to keep us continent (make sure we aren't leaking urine or faeces). These sphincter muscles also need to relax to allow for comfortable urination and bowel movements.

Support: Also mentioned earlier, these muscles help to lift and support the pelvic organs, especially against daily forces and changes in pressure from above (pressure changes occur all the time, including during vocalisation, coughing, sneezing, lifting, jumping, running or other exercise activity)

Sexual function: These muscles are important in arousal and producing an orgasm.

Stability: The muscles span across the pelvic bones, helping to contribute to stability across the pelvis.

Breathing: These muscles move automatically during breathing, typically following the movement of the respiratory diaphragm (the umbrella-shaped breathing muscle at the base of your ribs that helps you move air in and out of your

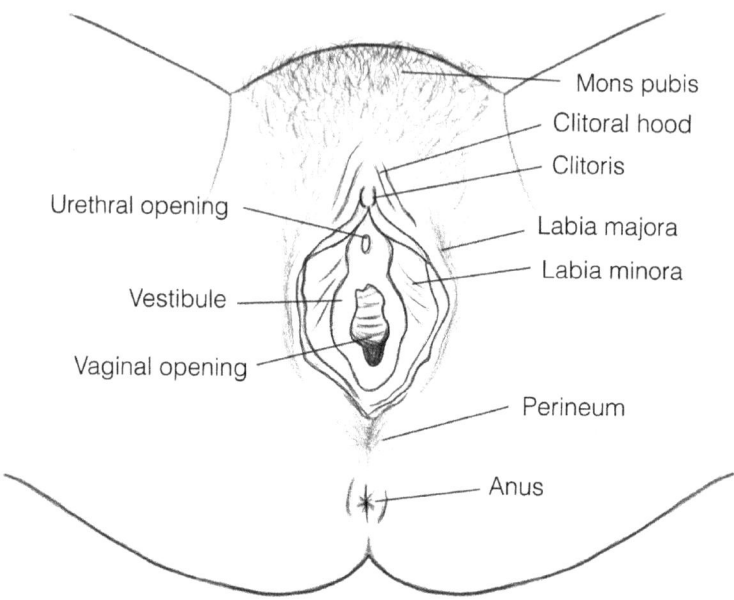

FIGURE 6.4.3 External female genitalia

lungs). In a relaxed breath, when one inhales, the respiratory diaphragm moves downwards to allow air into the lungs, and at the same time, the pelvic floor muscles will slightly lengthen. In an exhale, the diaphragm will move upwards, as will the muscles of the pelvic floor[17]. This coordination certainly has more complexity, but starting with this basic information can be very empowering, because the main thing to remember is that the pelvic floor muscles coordinate with breathing. So, one can help optimise pelvic floor function by practising lots of different breathing techniques.

Intra-abdominal pressure and core control: The pressure maintained within our trunk is known as "intra-abdominal pressure". Increases in pressure occur during daily movements, athletic activity, coughing, vocalising, lifting etc. The pelvic floor muscles regularly respond to these increases in pressure from above to help protect the pelvic organs and maintain continence against this pressure. Research also shows that the pelvic floor muscles work together (or, synergistically) with the abdominal muscles, so they are part of our core[18–22].

What is a Kegel, anyway?

In 1948, Kegel exercises were first described by Arnold Kegel for pelvic floor muscle strengthening. Dr Kegel noted that with pelvic floor strengthening the symptoms of urinary incontinence could be reduced.

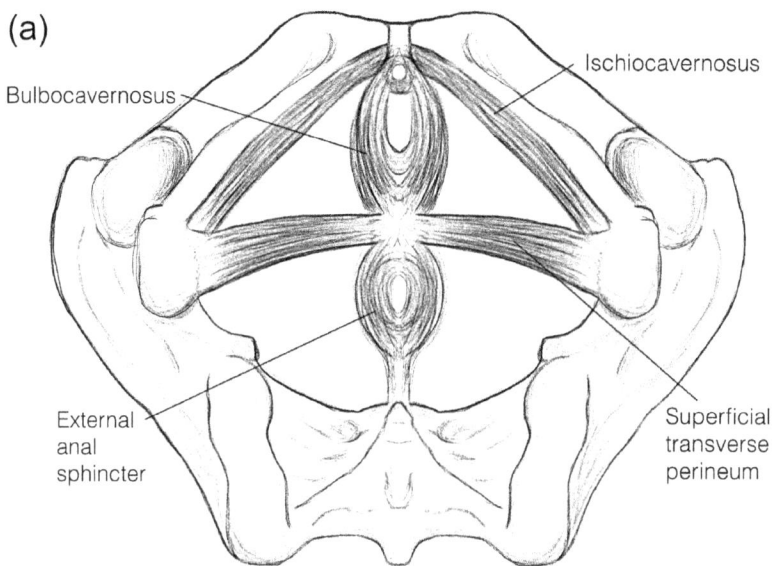

FIGURE 6.4.4A Superior view of pelvic floor muscles

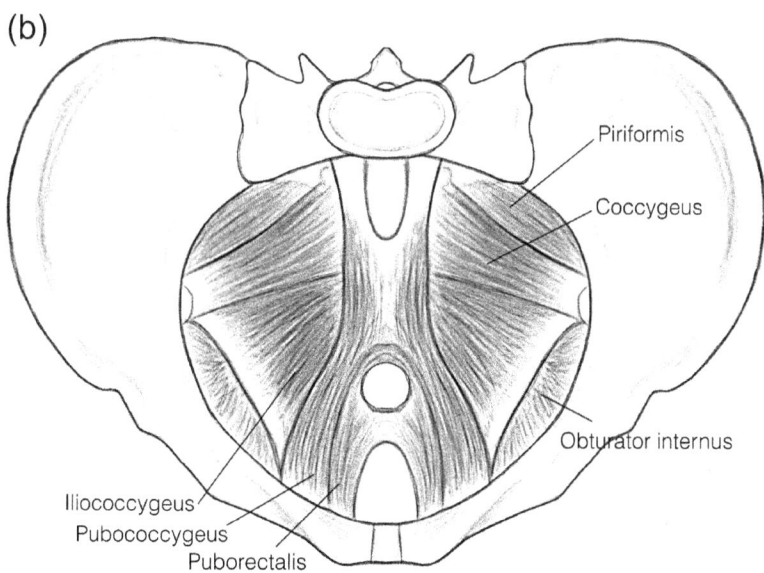

FIGURE 6.4.4B Inferior view of pelvic floor muscles

What does it feel like to "do a Kegel"? We use descriptions like "vacuuming a milkshake off the ground", "lifting a kleenex off the ground, 4 corners upward", or "drawing a blueberry into the vagina and feeling the upward lift of the pelvic floor".

We know these analogies sound ridiculous, but by making them so ridiculous, we hope you can feel the actual closing and lifting of the pelvic floor as you sit in imaginary puddles of spilt milkshake and piles of blueberries. Once you have performed the contraction, make sure to allow yourself to soften and relax the muscles (Figure 6.4.5).

Some information about the bladder, urethra and their regular functions in keeping leakage away

Maintaining "continence" (keeping urine from leaking), involves a combination of the structural support of the body's anatomy and the complex timing of the body's nervous system. Normally, leakage is avoided by keeping the pressure of urethral closure higher than the pressure of the bladder, so that urine stays in the bladder until one is ready to empty[8,9]. The urethral sphincter muscle, a circular structure surrounding the wall of the urethra, is a big factor in maintaining this closure pressure against daily forces, along with the compressor urethrae muscle, the urethrovaginal sphincter, the bulbocavernosus muscle and smooth muscle support. Support for the urethra is also provided by fascial structures like the endopelvic fascia and the fascial structures that attach to the side walls of the pelvis like cables of a suspension bridge. The levator ani muscles also help keep urine from leaking by compressing the vagina, urethra

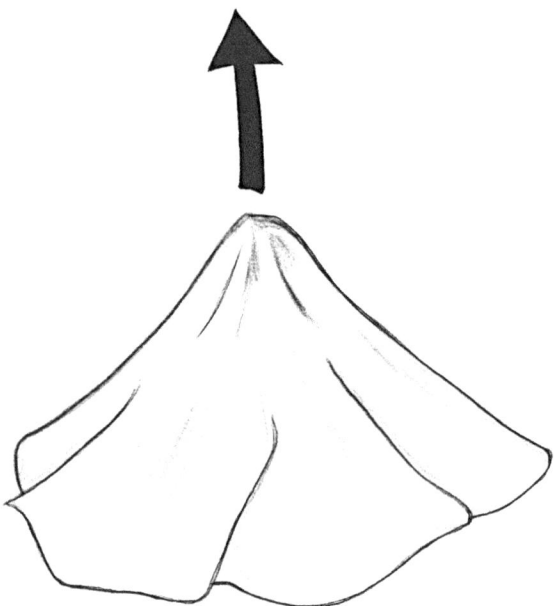

FIGURE 6.4.5 Kleenex image to assist visualisation of a Kegel

and rectum against the pubic bone and creating a lift of the pelvic floor and organs slightly upwards. The levator ani muscles maintain closure of the "urogenital hiatus" at rest, against regular pressure from gravity as well as abdominal pressure. During daily activities the levator ani muscles are recruited more to maintain closure and continence during increased intra-abdominal pressure and loads that naturally cause downward movement of the organs[9,23].

There is also a large (and complex!) neural component to bladder control. The bladder is surrounded by smooth muscle known as the detrusor. As the bladder fills in early stages, the body senses the gradual stretching of the bladder through sensory nerves in the bladder wall, but the body's nervous system automatically suppresses the contraction of the bladder muscle (the detrusor). Typically, about halfway through bladder filling, the body's nervous system sends signals of bladder filling and a desire to void that now becomes consciously noticed in the brain, and the brain can help resist bladder emptying through suppressing the contraction of the detrusor. When the bladder fills more, the desire to void becomes more apparent. The brain can still help inhibit the contraction of the bladder muscle, and there is some pelvic floor muscle activity that increases to keep urethral pressure high until one reaches an appropriate place and time to empty. When one begins to urinate, there is a relaxation of the pelvic floor muscles, an inhibition of the "suppression", and the detrusor muscle of the bladder will contract to help initiate the flow of urine[8,9,24,25].

"Everybody leaks . . . right?"

> *"I've noticed that I pee a little now when I run or jump."*
>
> *"I dribble a little bit after I have finished going to the bathroom."*
>
> *"I feel like I have to pee all the time. Sometimes it's like "I gotta GO and then I am a little wet by the time I get to the bathroom."*
>
> *"I am afraid I will leak if I try that. Maybe I should be doing lower impact exercise now."*

Leaking urine can be distressing. "It seemed so ridiculous; she did not think to ask for pelvic floor advice. When she called to say, 'I was wondering if this might be a pelvic floor problem?' she recounted the daily experience of reaching the staircase beside her home and feeling the sudden urge to pee. Then one day, the pee just happened, and she found herself soaked through on a public staircase, hoping the world might afford her enough privacy to get inside her house and change".

Leaking urine, otherwise known as urinary incontinence, is an experience that affects roughly 25–45% of women worldwide of various ages – though reported percentages differ from study to study, with some studies showing higher percentages[26–29]. Stress urinary incontinence refers to leaking urine with things like coughing, sneezing, laughing or exercise. Urge urinary incontinence refers to a very strong urge to urinate followed by an inability to make it to the bathroom without leaking. Some people can experience both types, which is referred to as "mixed incontinence"[30,31]. Leaking is common, so if this is something you experience, you are certainly *not* alone! Though this can be such a common occurrence, it is often highly stigmatised, and many women don't seek support because it can feel embarrassing or uncomfortable to talk about. In fact, studies show that less than 50% of women with pelvic floor issues seek care[32,33]. On top of this, 1 in 2 women who experience urinary leakage report that this symptom interferes with their participation in exercise (one of the most important things we can do for our health, especially through menopause and ageing)[34]. What many women *don't* know is that urinary incontinence can be treated — so, if you experience leakage, you do *not* just have to live with it! (More on this later.)

Does leaking urine become more common during or after menopause? Well, the short answer is yes – many women experience an initial onset of urinary incontinence after their last period[1]. But this is not the whole story. Menopause *can* be a factor, but it is also important to note that it is not the only factor, because the risk of experiencing leakage also increases with age[29,35,36]. There are also several other factors that increase a woman's risk for developing incontinence in their lifetime, including pregnancy, childbirth (higher risk with vaginal birth), obesity, chronic constipation, smoking tobacco or a history of chronic urinary tract infections (UTIs)[36]. Therefore, your own experiences prior to menopause may or may not contribute to symptoms you may now notice. For example, a woman could experience an onset of urinary incontinence postpartum due to birth injury to the nerves, muscles or connective tissue that supports the bladder or urethra. Perhaps this is something she has been told is "just a normal consequence of having a baby", and has not been informed that treatment options are available. Perhaps she lives with it, and maybe with time and natural muscle recovery it doesn't happen too often. Then, as menopause approaches, there are changes to hormones and muscles, and perhaps even a decline in physical activity – this could be a time that the factors accumulate to their tipping point and the leakage becomes more of an issue.

What is it about menopause itself that might contribute to women experiencing urinary leakage, perhaps even a new onset of leakage? Well, as you learned earlier in this book, there are oestrogen receptors all over the body – including within the urinary system. The drop in oestrogen leads to a multitude of tissue changes in both the urethra and bladder, as well as changes within the signalling system for bladder function[1,37]. Such changes are associated with Genitourinary Syndrome of Menopause (GSM), the changes to the urinary and genital systems that occur due to the drop in oestrogen and other sex hormones that occur in menopause[1,38]. Now, if stress urinary incontinence in menopause were *only* due to a drop in oestrogen, it would likely be resolved with hormone replacement therapy – HRT (menopausal hormone therapy) – but studies show this is not necessarily the case[39,40]. Some studies do show that local vaginal oestrogen may be helpful in reducing incontinence and other urinary issues in women, so this could be a tool to explore[40]. Overall, the exact connection between hormone changes in menopause, pelvic floor muscle strength and the development of pelvic floor issues like incontinence is still not totally clear[40,41].

Really, the good news here is that it seems that it is not menopause *alone* causing leakage; it is likely what we call "multifactorial". People who study injury risk in sports know that this is often the case with other types of muscle/skeletal dysfunction or injury – unless there is one obvious fall or trauma, most injury risk seems to evolve from an accumulation of factors. As mentioned before, one risk factor that does seem consistently linked with pelvic floor dysfunction after menopause is age.

So, what might be going on with our muscles and normal ageing? We do know that in skeletal muscles elsewhere in the body, the loss of muscle mass and force-production ability with age, also known as sarcopenia, leads to decreases in strength over time[42]. Studies are beginning to show that with age, the pelvic floor muscles show a decrease in cross-sectional area (overall size), changes in stiffness and alterations in other mechanical properties that likely impact their capacity for bearing load and producing optimal force, all of which are consistent with degeneration associated with ageing muscles[43–45]. This may seem like bad news (*"Ok, I'm just getting old, so I have to just accept that my pelvic floor muscles will be weaker with every year?"*), but it's not. Why? Well, for one thing, studies show that even in very elderly adults, resistance training increases muscle size and muscle strength, and physical activity and strength training are good for maintaining skeletal muscle health and mitigating these deteriorations in muscle as we age[46,47]. Another thing to consider in muscle health is that with ageing it can be common to simply become less physically active for a multitude of reasons – perhaps some of the muscle degeneration seen with ageing is also related to decreased activity levels. Good news, because activity levels can be changed! In fact, physical activity is a big mitigating factor when it comes to age-related muscle weakness[48]. The challenge is that with urine leakage many women can feel even *more* restricted from participating in physical activity[34]. This can become a cycle — perhaps some developing weakness is contributing to the leaking, and the leaking causes women to start decreasing their activity levels. This is a cycle we want to help women avoid during and after menopause.

So, you're saying I can do something about the leaking?

How might this information about muscle ageing and the positive effect of resistance training and physical activity apply specifically to the pelvic floor and to problems with leaking? Well, here is some good news about training the pelvic floor muscles at any age: pelvic floor muscle training is considered *the* "first-line treatment" for urinary incontinence, and this is supported with a significant body of research. Pelvic floor muscle training reduces leakage, improves quality of life and sexual function and increases self-esteem for women with stress incontinence, urge incontinence and mixed incontinence[49–51], yes, even women in menopause and post menopause[52]. It's also good to know that both individualised and group pelvic floor muscle training seems to be effective for decreasing leakage[3].

Pelvic floor muscle training is a supervised treatment that involves exercises to increase awareness of and strengthen the pelvic floor muscles, with the aim to improve pelvic floor muscle strength, endurance and coordination[53]. For stress incontinence, improving pelvic floor muscle support likely helps with supporting the bladder neck and the urethra more optimally against the increases in pressure from above. For incontinence related to urgency, it is theorised that pelvic floor muscle training helps inhibit the contractions of the bladder muscle, the detrusor, helping to manage the urgency and prevent leakage[53]. According to the National Institute for Health and Care Excellence in the United Kingdom (https://www.nice.org.uk/guidance/ng123), as well as the International Continence Society, a trial of 3 months of pelvic floor muscle training should be the first step in treating urinary incontinence.

Typically, pelvic floor muscle training is guided by a pelvic floor physiotherapist who has undergone specialised training in this area. Supervised pelvic floor physical therapy will involve an assessment of your pelvic floor muscle strength, endurance and control, followed by exercises to help improve these muscle qualities. Pelvic floor specialists can also help guide you in your breathing techniques and how you manage pressure in your trunk with activity, in how to incorporate pelvic floor muscle training with whole body strength, and in how to optimise bladder habits and manage issues like constipation (reducing constipation can also help reduce leakage). Other research-backed recommendations for reducing urinary incontinence include modifying fluid intake (increasing, decreasing or altering timing depending on your individual needs) and reducing the intake of bladder irritants (for example, caffeine).

If you find that you are having trouble locating a pelvic floor physiotherapist in your area, don't forget that research has shown that group training and virtual pelvic floor physical therapy are also great options. There are also many online resources and databases one can search to find qualified pelvic floor physiotherapists, depending on the country you live in.

"I can't be far from the toilets now . . . "

Many women begin to feel frustrated that they can't get through a night of sleep without waking to pee, sometimes much more than 1–2 times per night. And they wonder why this started to slowly become the case as they entered menopause. They may also feel concerned about getting through a long plane or car ride without needing to pee several times.

Some urinary issues, besides leakage, that might surface for women in menopause include more urinary frequency (having to go more often than every 2–4 hours during the day), nocturia (frequent urination disturbing sleep), urinary urgency, painful urination and recurrent UTIs. Many of these symptoms are commonly associated with GSM. Urge incontinence (a strong urge to go followed by leakage, mentioned briefly in the last section) becomes more common with age compared to rises in stress urinary incontinence.

If you are experiencing strong urges to pee, heading to the toilet more than 6–8 times a day and find that the amount you void is less than 2 oz, you should consider keeping a bladder diary for 3–4 days. Recording the fluid that comes in and the fluid that goes out will give you a very objective record of frequency and volume. Often, seeing the voids written down in a daily 24-hour clock is enough to tell the brain if you are voiding in reasonable patterns or if you need to change your habits. Bladder retraining techniques involve breathing exercises, distraction techniques and altered habits. The morning is a good time to empty the bladder and then immediately fill by drinking 32 oz of water. The bladder learns to fill completely and empty completely. Your pelvic floor physiotherapist will walk you through this too.

Please note that if you are experiencing recurrent urinary urgency, frequency and discomfort, you should also check to make sure this is not a symptom of a UTI. UTIs can become more common post menopause because oestrogen deficiency affects the urethra and inhibits the growth of vaginal *Lactobacillus* flora, which normally help maintain vaginal pH and prevent colonisation by pathogens that can cause infections. In fact, 10–15% of women over 60 years old have recurrent UTIs[54-56]. Note that there is research to support the use of low-dose vaginal oestrogen to treat urgency/overactive bladder symptoms and also to prevent recurrent UTIs. There will be a bit more information on low-dose vaginal oestrogen when we discuss painful sex[57,58].

"Exercise will break my vagina"

"Lifting weights makes leaking worse"

"I feel out of place in a gym"

Exercise is important. Research clearly demonstrates the importance of regular physical activity for good cardiovascular health, reduced excessive weight gain, improved cognitive function and reduced risk of dementia[59]. Furthermore, exercise has been shown to mitigate progressive physiological changes like lean muscle loss (sarcopenia), bone density loss (osteopenia), type 2 diabetes, certain cancers and osteoarthritis. Being fearful of exercise can lead women to avoid it and miss the vast positives associated with physical activity. While there is some concern in the literature that high-impact training, particularly at young ages can increase the risk of stress urinary incontinence, the evidence does support women participating in regular low and moderate impact training without negative impact on the pelvic floor muscles and greater overall health benefit from physical activity.

Incorporating weight training in combination with pelvic floor training results in faster improvements in urinary incontinence[60]. Other studies show that combining hip strengthening along with pelvic floor muscle training shows a better decrease in daily frequency of urine loss compared to pelvic floor muscle training alone, indicating that adding strength to areas outside the pelvic floor is beneficial for those who leak[61].

If issues like leakage or urgency interferes with your ability to run, lift weights, dance, swim or jump, pelvic floor specialists who understand your chosen physical activity can be a great help. There are many ways to approach exercise technique while respecting the pelvic floor. Incorporating a pre-lift kegel or "knack" technique is one method used to control leaking. This well-timed, pre-load contraction prepares the pelvic floor for the increased load about to come. For runners, changing stride by increasing cadence/step rate between 5–10%, thinking of keeping the chest over the pelvis or a slight feeling of forward lean or thinking of making your footfalls lighter if they tend to be heavy, could reduce leakage[62]. For those lifting weights during resistance training, changing the timing or pattern of breathing, playing with posture alterations and changing the cues for holding tension through different areas of the body can be helpful to explore to reduce or resolve symptoms of leakage during exercise.

"My organs are going to fall out of me"

> *"I learned what 'queefing' was rather awkwardly on returning to Pilates following the birth of my second child. I was feeling great about getting back to exercise and flipped into a Pilates roll over (basically lying on my back with my legs flipped over my head) and as I contracted my post-partum core muscles to lower my legs, air was pushed out of my vagina, and I thought everything would slide out along with it".*

Queefing, technically termed vaginal flatus, is the release of trapped air from the vagina. It is important for you to know that vaginal flatus can occur with anyone who has a vagina (because it is a space that air can occupy); it is not in and of itself a sign of anything wrong. However, it can feel so embarrassing when this occurs in the middle of Yoga class or during sex. This is also a symptom that many people with pelvic organ prolapse (POP) can experience. So, what is POP?

POP is something that sounds scary, especially if you go scrolling on the internet. But it is important for you to have proper information about POP and the fact that it does become more common as we age. POP is defined as changes to the tissue support of the organs such that there is a descent of the front or the back vaginal wall or of the cervix. Symptoms commonly associated with POP are feeling or seeing a vaginal bulge, a sensation or pressure or a falling-out feeling, a feeling of incomplete bladder emptying, difficulty with bowel movements, a need to "splint" for more complete urination or bowel movements, and/or bladder urgency. Recurrent UTIs can also occur with POP due to difficulty with emptying urine[28,64]. Common risk factors for developing POP include pregnancy, childbirth, obesity, congenital or acquired connective tissue abnormalities, chronic constipation, a family history of POP, denervation or weakness of the pelvic floor, menopause and ageing[63].

Symptoms and severity of POP seem to increase with menopause – but, as we discussed with the onset of urinary incontinence, it is difficult to fully determine how much of this is due to oestrogen dropping in menopause and how much is due to ageing and its associated alterations in connective tissue and muscle support[27,63,64]. Similar to with urinary incontinence, research seems to indicate that vaginal oestrogen does not seem to be too successful in preventing or limiting POP. It is important for women to know that POP is relatively common, and that it is not always symptomatic or bothersome. Also, the symptoms women experience might not always correlate well with the anatomic severity of the prolapse.

The first-line intervention for POP is conservative – pelvic floor muscle training, bowel and bladder habit training, managing constipation and modifying activities that increase symptoms[63]. Several meta-analyses show that women with symptomatic mild POP treated with pelvic floor muscle training undergo significant improvement in prolapse symptoms and POP severity[65–67]. With guidance from experts, women with POP can also elect to use a pessary for support. Vaginal pessaries are passive mechanical devices designed to support the vagina and hold the prolapsed organs back in the anatomically correct position. With proper fitting (guided by a trained healthcare practitioner) and use, pessaries can improve quality of life, reduce vaginal and sexual symptoms and improve mental health for those with POP[68–70]. For women who are not interested in exploring pessary use, they can try an over-the-counter/non-prescription option for support (an example would be Poise® Impressa Bladder Support devices.)

Women with symptomatic prolapse who have not responded well to conservative management are candidates for reconstructive surgery. There are different types of surgical procedures available depending on the individual, and surgical treatment of symptomatic POP has been shown to result in improved quality of life[71,72]. There is no indication for the surgical repair of POP as an isolated procedure if it does not cause any symptoms.

"Sex will hurt"

As oestrogen levels drop along with changes to other sex steroids, there are changes to both vaginal and vulvar tissue in women post menopause related to GSM. Vulvar tissue can become more fragile and lose the ability to stretch, with skin thinning and increased dryness. Oestrogen dropping also affects the glycogen deposition in the vaginal mucosa, reduces cervical mucus, reduces the rugae of the vagina and makes the tissue of the vagina drier, thinner and less tolerant to stretch. Vaginal dryness is the most prevalent genitourinary issue experienced with menopause, with 60% of postmenopausal women reporting this symptom[1]. The increased fragility of the vaginal tissues can cause sex to be painful, with some women also experiencing burning, fissuring, and/or post-coital bleeding[73]. Lack of lubrication is a primary reason for painful sex post menopause. These issues can also decrease the pleasure of sex, and some women post menopause also report difficult reaching orgasm[74].

Though studies estimate that between 32–41% of postmenopausal women experience pain with sex[74], it is difficult to get a fully accurate picture for several reasons. First, a very low number of physicians tend to ask women about sexual activity, especially post menopause. And, many women do not report the pain they experience with sex, that they avoid sex altogether because of pain, because they think this is just an expected part of ageing, they feel embarrassed to discuss it or they might simply be unaware that there are treatment options available.

If GSM is a main contributing factor to vaginal dryness and painful sexual activity, the International Menopause Writing Society specifies that lubricants and moisturisers should be the first line of treatment. Lubricants, which are available in water-, silicone-, mineral- or plant oil-based forms, are applied to the vagina and vulva (and/or the penis or sexual tool) prior to sex to reduce pain by providing a slippery barrier and reducing friction. Vaginal moisturisers are used to rehydrate dry mucosal tissue and restore healthy microbiota. They are absorbed into the skin and adhere to the vaginal lining, thereby mimicking natural vaginal secretions, and can be used several times per week[58,73,75].

Low-dose vaginal oestrogens, in the form of tablets, inserts, creams or a slow-release ring, have been shown in recent systematic reviews to be the second most used treatments for symptoms of GSM. Low-dose vaginal oestrogen helps restore vaginal pH and microflora, relieves dryness, itching, irritation, painful sex and urinary symptoms including recurrent UTIs and overactive bladder[73].

There are circumstances when hormone-based therapies are not appropriate nor medically recommended for women. In these instances, there are some alternatives you can consider. For example, fractional CO_2 laser therapy is something to discuss with your doctor, and although more rigorous and sham-controlled studies are needed, the CO_2 laser may be an option for women who have been advised or prefer not to use ospemifene, vaginal DHEA or local vaginal oestrogens. The CO_2 laser is considered a medical, not a cosmetic device, and should not be used for vaginal "rejuvenation" or "tightening" for the treatment of stress incontinence, sexual satisfaction in the absence of vulvovaginal atrophy, low libido or impaired arousal[73].

It is important to note that regardless of whether it contributed to the development of pain with sex, the pelvic floor muscles can develop dysfunction if pain is present. Pelvic floor physiotherapists can assess whether this is a contributing factor and help postmenopausal women via techniques like myofascial release, pelvic floor muscle training and relaxation strategies, guidance on use of vaginal dilators or the use of a collision bumper to control depth of penetration[58,76,77]. Pelvic floor muscle training has been shown to help women who experience pain with sex by improving blood flow to vulvovaginal tissues and help with the capacity for the pelvic floor muscles to relax[74,78].

Takeaways

"Can you see now why we love helping people know more about their pelvises? After reading this chapter, we hope you feel much more informed and empowered about navigating your pelvic floor experiences through perimenopause, menopause and beyond. There

are so many common experiences in the pelvic floor region during this time of life, even if not enough people are talking about them (yet)! Now, you have the language to better describe what you are feeling and where, and *you* can start talking about it. And last, you now know that there are a lot of research-based solutions available to help you move from being distressed and confused by pelvic floor symptoms to enhancing the joy in your pelvis and in your life.

References

1 Sarmento ACA, Costa APF, Vieira-Baptista P et al. Genitourinary syndrome of menopause: Epidemiology, physiopathology, clinical manifestation and diagnostic. *Frontiers in Reproductive Health* 2021; 3. doi: 10.3389/FRPH.2021.779398/FULL.
2 Barlow DH, Cardozo LD, Francis RM et al. Urogenital ageing and its effect on sexual health in older British women. *BJOG* 1997; 104 (1): 87–91. doi: 10.1111/J.1471-0528.1997.TB10655.X.
3 Dumoulin C, Morin M, Danieli C et al. Group-based vs individual pelvic floor muscle training to treat urinary incontinence in older women: A randomized clinical trial. *JAMA Internal Medicine* 2020; 180 (10): 1284–1293. doi: 10.1001/JAMAINTERNMED.2020.2993.
4 Bernard S, McLean L, Boucher S et al. An in-home rehabilitation program for the treatment of urinary incontinence symptoms in endometrial cancer survivors: A single-case experimental design study. *International Urogynecology Journal* 2021; 32 (11): 2947–2957. doi: 10.1007/S00192-021-04981-X/TABLES/3.
5 El-Hamamsy D, Parmar C, Shoop-Worrall S et al. Public understanding of female genital anatomy and pelvic organ prolapse (POP); a questionnaire-based pilot study. *International Urogynecology Journal* 2022; 33 (2): 309–318. doi: 10.1007/S00192-021-04727-9.
6 Chen CCG, Cox JT, Yuan C et al. Knowledge of pelvic floor disorders in women seeking primary care: A cross-sectional study. *BMC Family Practice* 2019; 20 (1). doi: 10.1186/S12875-019-0958-Z.
7 Falvey L, Salameh F, O'Sullivan OE et al. What does your pelvic floor do for you? Knowledge of the pelvic floor in female university students: A cross-sectional study. *Female Pelvic Medicine and Reconstructive Surgery* 2021; 27 (2): E457–E464. doi: 10.1097/SPV.0000000000000962.
8 Rossetti SR. Functional anatomy of pelvic floor. *Archivio Italiano di Urologia e Andrologia* 2016; 88 (1): 28–37. doi: 10.4081/aiua.2016.1.28.
9 Ashton-Miller JA, DeLancey JOL. Functional anatomy of the female pelvic floor. *Annals of the New York Academy of Sciences* 2007; 1101: 266–296. doi: 10.1196/ANNALS.1389.034.
10 Hoare BS, Khan YS. Anatomy, abdomen and pelvis: Female internal genitals. *StatPearls*. Published online March 3, 2020. http://europepmc.org/books/NBK554601. Accessed January 2024.
11 Nguyen J, Duong H. Anatomy, abdomen and pelvis: Female external genitalia. *StatPearls*. Published online October 16, 2019. http://europepmc.org/books/NBK547703. Accessed January 2024.
12 Betschart C, Singer A, Scheiner D. Female pelvic floor: Anatomy and normal function. *Ther Umsch* 2019; 73 (9): 529–534. doi: 10.1024/0040-5930/A001035.
13 Bharucha AE. Pelvic floor: Anatomy and function. *Neurogastroenterology & Motility* 2006; 18 (7): 507–519. doi: 10.1111/J.1365-2982.2006.00803.X.
14 Eickmeyer SM. Anatomy and physiology of the pelvic floor. *Physical Medicine and Rehabilitation Clinics of North America* 2017; 28 (3): 455–460. doi: 10.1016/j.pmr.2017.03.003.
15 Prather H, Dugan S, Fitzgerald C et al. Review of anatomy, evaluation, and treatment of musculoskeletal pelvic floor pain in women. *PM and R* 2009; 1 (4): 346–358. doi: 10.1016/j.pmrj.2009.01.003.

16 Quaghebeur J, Petros P, Wyndaele JJ et al. Pelvic-floor function, dysfunction, and treatment. *European Journal of Obstetrics & Gynecology and Reproductive Biology* 2021; 265: 143–149. doi: 10.1016/J.EJOGRB.2021.08.026.
17 Talasz H, Kremser C, Kofler M et al. Phase-locked parallel movement of diaphragm and pelvic floor during breathing and coughing-a dynamic MRI investigation in healthy females. *International Urogynecology Journal* 2011; 22 (1): 61–68. doi: 10.1007/S00192-010-1240-Z/TABLES/3.
18 Ferla L, Darski C, Paiva LL et al. Synergism between abdominal and pelvic floor muscles in healthy women: A systematic review of observational studies. *Fisioterapia em Movimento* 2016; 29 (2): 399–410. doi: 10.1590/0103-5150.029.002.AO19.
19 Madill SJ, McLean L. Quantification of abdominal and pelvic floor muscle synergies in response to voluntary pelvic floor muscle contractions. *Journal of Electromyography and Kinesiology* 2008; 18 (6): 955–964. doi: 10.1016/J.JELEKIN.2007.05.001.
20 Vesentini G, El Dib R, Righesso LAR et al. Pelvic floor and abdominal muscle cocontraction in women with and without pelvic floor dysfunction: A systematic review and meta-analysis. *Clinics* 2019; 74: e1319. doi: 10.6061/CLINICS/2019/E1319.
21 Junginger B, Baessler K, Sapsford R et al. Effect of abdominal and pelvic floor tasks on muscle activity, abdominal pressure and bladder neck. *International Urogynecology Journal* 2010; 21 (1): 69–77. doi: 10.1007/S00192-009-0981-Z/FIGURES/4.
22 Shaw JM, Hamad NM, Coleman TJ et al. Intra-abdominal pressures during activity in women using an intra-vaginal pressure transducer. *Journal of Sports Sciences* 2014; 32 (12): 1176. doi: 10.1080/02640414.2014.889845.
23 Bo K, Berghmans B, Morkved S et al., eds. *Evidence-Based Physical Therapy for the Pelvic Floor: Bridging Science and Clinical Practice,* 3rd Edition. Elsevier, 2024.
24 Rahn DD, Roshanravan SM. Pathophysiology of urinary incontinence, voiding dysfunction, and overactive bladder. *Obstetrics and Gynecology Clinics of North America* 2009; 36 (3): 463–474. doi: 10.1016/j.ogc.2009.08.012.
25 Keane DP, O'Sullivan S. Urinary incontinence: Anatomy, physiology and pathophysiology. *Best Practice & Research Clinical Obstetrics & Gynaecology* 2000; 14 (2): 207–226. doi: 10.1053/BEOG.1999.0072.
26 Tahra A, Bayrak Ö, Dmochowski R. The epidemiology and population-based studies of women with lower urinary tract symptoms: A systematic review. *Turkish Journal of Urology* 2022; 48 (2): 155. doi: 10.5152/TUD.2022.21325.
27 Altman D, Cartwright R, Lapitan MC et al. Epidemiology of urinary incontinence (UI) and other lower urinary tract symptoms (LUTS), pelvic organ prolapse (POP) and anal incontinence (AI). Published online 2017:1–141. https://researchportal.helsinki.fi/en/publications/epidemiology-of-urinary-incontinence-ui-and-other-lower-urinary-t. Accessed November 2023.
28 Abufaraj M, Xu T, Cao C et al. Prevalence and trends in urinary incontinence among women in the United States, 2005–2018. *American Journal of Obstetrics & Gynecology* 2021; 225 (2): 166. e1–166.e12. doi: 10.1016/J.AJOG.2021.03.016.
29 Milsom I, Gyhagen M. The prevalence of urinary incontinence. *Climacteric* 2019; 22 (3): 217–222. doi: 10.1080/13697137.2018.1543263.
30 Bo K, Frawley HC, Haylen BT et al. An International Urogynecological Association (IUGA)/International Continence Society (ICS) joint report on the terminology for the conservative and nonpharmacological management of female pelvic floor dysfunction. *International Urogynecology Journal* 2017; 28 (2): 191–213. doi: 10.1007/S00192-016-3123-4/FIGURES/9.
31 Abrams P, Andersson KE, Birder L et al. Fourth international consultation on incontinence recommendations of the international scientific committee: Evaluation and treatment of urinary incontinence, pelvic organ prolapse, and fecal incontinence. *Neurourology and Urodynamics* 2010; 29 (1): 213–240. doi: 10.1002/nau.20870.

32 Fritel X, Panjo H, Varnoux N et al. The individual determinants of care-seeking among middle-aged women reporting urinary incontinence: Analysis of a 2273-woman cohort. *Neurourology and Urodynamics* 2014; 33 (7): 1116–1122. doi: 10.1002/NAU.22461.

33 Koch LH. Help-seeking behaviors of women with urinary incontinence: An integrative literature review. *Journal of Midwifery & Women's Health* 2006; 51 (6): e39–e44. doi: 10.1016/J.JMWH.2006.06.004.

34 Dakic JG, Hay-Smith J, Cook J et al. Effect of pelvic floor symptoms on women's participation in exercise: A mixed-methods systematic review with meta-analysis. *Journal of Orthopaedic & Sports Physical Therapy* 2021; 51 (7): 345–361. doi: 10.2519/JOSPT.2021.10200.

35 Aoki Y, Brown HW, Brubaker L et al. Urinary incontinence in women. *Nature Reviews Disease Primers* 2017; 3: 17042. doi: 10.1038/NRDP.2017.42.

36 Baykuş N, Yenal K. Prevalence of urinary incontinence in women aged 18 and over and affecting factors. *Journal of Women & Aging* 2020; 32 (5): 578–590. doi: 10.1080/08952841.2019.1682923.

37 Bodner-Adler B, Alarab M, Ruiz-Zapata AM et al. Effectiveness of hormones in postmenopausal pelvic floor dysfunction—International Urogynecological Association research and development—committee opinion. *International Urogynecology Journal* 2020; 31 (8): 1577–1582. doi: 10.1007/S00192-019-04070-0/TABLES/1.

38 Gandhi J, Chen A, Dagur G et al. Genitourinary syndrome of menopause: An overview of clinical manifestations, pathophysiology, etiology, evaluation, and management. *American Journal of Obstetrics & Gynecology* 2016; 215 (6): 704–711. doi:10.1016/J.AJOG.2016.07.045.

39 Huang H, Ding G, Li M et al. Menopause and stress urinary incontinence: The risk factors of stress urinary incontinence in perimenopausal and postmenopausal women. *Journal of Obstetrics and Gynaecology Research* 2023; 49 (10): 2509–2518. doi: 10.1111/JOG.15742.

40 Bodner-Adler B, Alarab M, Ruiz-Zapata AM et al. Effectiveness of hormones in postmenopausal pelvic floor dysfunction—International Urogynecological Association research and development—committee opinion. *International Urogynecology Journal* 2020; 31 (8): 1577–1582. doi: 10.1007/S00192-019-04070-0/TABLES/1.

41 Dietz HP, Socha M, Atan IK et al. Does estrogen deprivation affect pelvic floor muscle contractility? *International Urogynecology Journal* 2020; 31 (1): 191–196. doi: 10.1007/S00192-019-03909-W/TABLES/2.

42 Miljkovic N, Lim JY, Miljkovic I et al. Aging of skeletal muscle fibers. *Annals of Rehabilitation Medicine* 2015; 39 (2): 155–162. doi: 10.5535/ARM.2015.39.2.155.

43 Rieger M, Duran P, Cook M et al. Quantifying the effects of aging on morphological and cellular properties of human female pelvic floor muscles. *Annals of Biomedical Engineering* 2021; 49 (8): 1836–1847. doi: 10.1007/S10439-021-02748-5/FIGURES/4.

44 Cook MS, Bou-Malham L, Esparza MC et al. Age-related alterations in female obturator internus muscle. *International Urogynecology Journal* 2017; 28 (5): 729–734. doi: 10.1007/S00192-016-3167-5/FIGURES/2.

45 Burnett LA, Cook M, Shah S et al. Age-associated changes in the mechanical properties of human cadaveric pelvic floor muscles. *Journal of Biomechanics* 2020; 98: 109436. doi: 10.1016/J.JBIOMECH.2019.109436.

46 Talar K, Hernández-belmonte A, Vetrovsky T et al. Benefits of resistance training in early and late stages of frailty and sarcopenia: A systematic review and meta-analysis of randomized controlled studies. *Journal of Clinical Medicine* 2021; 10: 1630. doi: 10.3390/JCM10081630.

47 Grgic J, Garofolini A, Orazem J et al. Effects of resistance training on muscle size and strength in very elderly adults: A systematic review and meta-analysis of randomized controlled trials. *Sports Medicine* 2020; 50 (11): 1983–1999. doi: 10.1007/S40279-020-01331-7/FIGURES/6.

48 Meier NF, Lee DC. Physical activity and sarcopenia in older adults. *Aging Clinical and Experimental Research* 2020; 32 (9): 1675–1687. doi: 10.1007/S40520-019-01371-8/TABLES/6.

49 Cacciari LP, Dumoulin C, Hay-Smith EJ. Pelvic floor muscle training versus no treatment, or inactive control treatments, for urinary incontinence in women: A cochrane systematic review abridged republication. *Brazilian Journal of Physical Therapy* 2019; 23 (2): 93–107. doi: 10.1016/J.BJPT.2019.01.002.

50 Radzimińska A, Strączyńska A, Weber-Rajek M et al. The impact of pelvic floor muscle training on the quality of life of women with urinary incontinence: A systematic literature review. *Clinical Interventions in Aging* 2018; 13: 957–965. doi: 10.2147/CIA.S160057.

51 Handa VL, Whitcomb E, Weidner AC et al. Sexual function before and after nonsurgical treatment of stress urinary incontinence. *Female Pelvic Medicine and Reconstructive Surgery* 2011; 17 (1): 30–35. doi: 10.1097/SPV.0B013E318205E263.

52 Kargar Jahromi M, Talebizadeh M, Mirzaei M. The effect of pelvic muscle exercises on urinary incontinency and self-esteem of elderly females with stress urinary incontinency, 2013. *Global Journal of Health Sciences* 2015; 7 (2): 71. doi: 10.5539/GJHS.V7N2P71.

53 Russo E, Caretto M, Giannini A et al. Management of urinary incontinence in postmenopausal women: An EMAS clinical guide. *Maturitas* 2021; 143: 223–230. doi: 10.1016/J.MATURITAS.2020.09.005.

54 Buck ES, Lukas VA, Rubin RS. Effective prevention of recurrent UTIs with vaginal estrogen: Pearls for a urological approach to genitourinary syndrome of menopause. *Urology* 2021; 151: 31–36. doi: 10.1016/J.UROLOGY.2020.05.058.

55 Meister MR, Wang C, Lowder JL et al. Vaginal estrogen therapy is associated with decreased inflammatory response in postmenopausal women with recurrent urinary tract infections. *Female Pelvic Medicine and Reconstructive Surgery* 2021; 27 (1): e39. doi: 10.1097/SPV.0000000000000790.

56 Chang E, Kent L, Prieto I et al. Vaginal estrogen as first-line therapy for recurrent urinary tract infections in postmenopausal women and risk factors for needing additional therapy. *Female Pelvic Medicine and Reconstructive Surgery* 2021; 27 (3): e487–e492. doi: 10.1097/SPV.0000000000000989.

57 Baruch Y, Torella M, De Bastiani S et al. Pre- versus post-menopausal onset of overactive bladder and the response to vaginal estrogen therapy: A prospective study. *Medicina* 2023; 59: 245. doi: 10.3390/MEDICINA59020245.

58 Kagan R, Kellogg-Spadt S, Parish SJ. Practical treatment considerations in the management of genitourinary syndrome of menopause. *Drugs Aging* 2019; 36 (10): 897–908. doi: 10.1007/S40266-019-00700-W/TABLES/3.

59 Piercy KL, Troiano RP, Ballard RM et al. The physical activity guidelines for Americans. *JAMA* 2018; 320 (19): 2020–2028. doi: 10.1001/JAMA.2018.14854.

60 Virtuoso JF, Menezes EC, Mazo GZ. Effect of weight training with pelvic floor muscle training in elderly women with urinary incontinence. *Research Quarterly for Exercise and Sport* 2019; 90 (2): 141–150. doi: 10.1080/02701367.2019.1571674.

61 Marques SAA, Silveira SRB da, Pássaro AC et al. Effect of pelvic floor and hip muscle strengthening in the treatment of stress urinary incontinence: A randomized clinical trial. *Journal of Manipulative & Physiological Therapeutics* 2020; 43 (3): 247–256. doi: 10.1016/J.JMPT.2019.01.007.

62 Steimling M, Roberto M, Steimling M. Running gait retraining in the management of a multiparous runner with chronic stress urinary incontinence: A case study. *Journal of Women's & Pelvic Health Physical Therapy* 2023; 47 (2): 114–121.

63 Giannini A, Russo E, Cano A et al. Current management of pelvic organ prolapse in aging women: EMAS clinical guide. *Maturitas* 2018; 110: 118–123. doi: 10.1016/J.MATURITAS.2018.02.004.

64 Abrams P, Andersson KE, Birder L et al. Fourth international consultation on incontinence recommendations of the international scientific committee: Evaluation and treatment of urinary

incontinence, pelvic organ prolapse, and fecal incontinence. *Neurourology and Urodynamics* 2010; 29 (1): 213–240. doi: 10.1002/nau.20870.
65. Espiño-Albela A, Castaño-García C, Díaz-Mohedo E et al. Effects of pelvic-floor muscle training in patients with pelvic organ prolapse approached with surgery vs. conservative treatment: A systematic review. *Journal of Personalized Medicine* 2022; 12 (5): 806. doi: 10.3390/JPM12050806/S1.
66. Basnet R. Impact of pelvic floor muscle training in pelvic organ prolapse. *International Urogynecology Journal* 2021; 32 (6): 1351–1360. doi: 10.1007/S00192-020-04613-W/TABLES/3.
67. Li C, Gong Y, Wang B. The efficacy of pelvic floor muscle training for pelvic organ prolapse: A systematic review and meta-analysis. *International Urogynecology Journal* 2016; 27 (7): 981–992. doi: 10.1007/S00192-015-2846-Y/FIGURES/5.
68. Sansone S, Sze C, Eidelberg A et al. Role of pessaries in the treatment of pelvic organ prolapse: A systematic review and meta-analysis. *Obstetrics & Gynecology* 2022; 140 (4): 613–622. doi: 10.1097/AOG.0000000000004931.
69. Zeiger BB, da Silva Carramão S, Del Roy CA et al. Vaginal pessary in advanced pelvic organ prolapse: Impact on quality of life. *International Urogynecology Journal* 2022; 33 (7): 2013–2020. doi: 10.1007/S00192-021-05002-7/TABLES/3.
70. Bugge C, Adams EJ, Gopinath D et al. Pessaries (mechanical devices) for managing pelvic organ prolapse in women. *Cochrane Database of Systematic Reviews* 2020; 2020 (11). doi: 10.1002/14651858.CD004010.PUB4/PDF/CDSR/CD004010/CD004010.PDF.
71. Mattsson NK, Karjalainen PK, Tolppanen AM et al. Pelvic organ prolapse surgery and quality of life—a nationwide cohort study. *American Journal of Obstetrics and Gynecology* 2020; 222 (6): 588.e1–588.e10. doi: 10.1016/J.AJOG.2019.11.1285.
72. Belayneh T, Gebeyehu A, Adefris M et al. Pelvic organ prolapse surgery and health-related quality of life: A follow-up study. *BMC Womens Health* 2021; 21 (1): 1–11. doi: 10.1186/S12905-020-01146-8/TABLES/3.
73. Streicher LF. Diagnosis, causes, and treatment of dyspareunia in postmenopausal women. *Menopause* 2023; 30 (6): 635–649. doi: 10.1097/GME.0000000000002179.
74. Franco MM, Pena CC, de Freitas LM et al. Pelvic floor Muscle training effect in sexual function in postmenopausal women: A randomized controlled trial. *Journal of Sexual Medicine* 2021; 18 (7): 1236–1244. doi: 10.1016/J.JSXM.2021.05.005.
75. Phillips NA, Bachmann GA. The genitourinary syndrome of menopause. *Menopause* 2021; 28 (5): 579–588. doi: 10.1097/GME.0000000000001728.
76. Mercier J, Morin M, Lemieux MC et al. Pelvic floor muscles training to reduce symptoms and signs of vulvovaginal atrophy: A case study. *Menopause* 2016; 23 (7): 816–820. doi: 10.1097/GME.0000000000000620.
77. Miles K, Miles S. Low dose, high frequency movement based dilator therapy for dayspareunia: Retrospective analysis of 26 cases. *Sex Medicine* 2021; 9 (3): 100344–100344. doi: 10.1016/J.ESXM.2021.100344.
78. Mercier J, Morin M, Tang A et al. Pelvic floor muscle training: Mechanisms of action for the improvement of genitourinary syndrome of menopause. *Climacteric* 2020; 23 (5): 468–473. doi: 10.1080/13697137.2020.1724942.

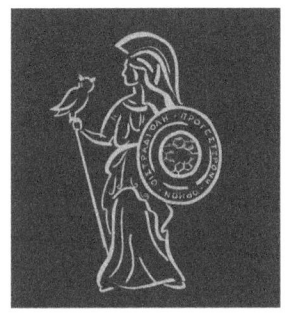

Act 7

Age Group Athletes
Orpheus and Eurydice

Act 7 Age Group Athletes

Orpheus and Eurydice

Dr Nicky Keay

In this Greek myth, Orpheus is a talented musician who manages to overpower the Sirens with his own music when sailing with the Argonauts. On his return, he marries Eurydice and they are very happy together until Eurydice is mortally bitten by a snake. Stricken with grief, Orpheus takes the perilous journey to the underworld to plead for his wife's return to the world of the living by playing music to the king and queen of the underworld, Hades and Penelope. They agree that Eurydice can return to the land of the living by being rowed across the river Styx by the ferryman Charon, provided Orpheus does not look back to check if Eurydice is following him. Unfortunately, Orpheus could not resist a glance back. So, Eurydice stays in the underworld.

Don't look back

As an older exerciser, athlete or dancer, however tempting it might be to look back and want to exercise, dance, train and compete as you did in youth; don't do it. Don't look back with regret. You have progressed through the female hormone odyssey, so the hormones that drive the adaptive changes to exercise have changed. To maintain your health and performance, you need to adapt your approach to exercise, training and competition. This can also be a psychological challenge.

This Act explores how to embrace the changes of hormone choreography in a positive, proactive forward-looking way as an age group athlete.

Scene 1 Relative energy deficiency in sport only happens in young exercisers?!

Dr Nicky Keay

Icarus

In the Greek myth about Icarus, his inventor father Daedalus made him wings using feathers held together with beeswax so he could fly. Daedalus warned his son not to fly too high, lest the sun's heat should melt the wax, nor too low where the feathers might be dampened by the sea. Icarus enjoyed the experience so much that he did not heed the warning and flew too close to the sun. The beeswax melted and he crashed into the sea and drowned.

As you get older, it can be tempting to think like Icarus – that you can continue to push yourself to perform at the highest level in your chosen sport or physical activity without worrying about the physical constraints. After all, relative energy deficiency in sport (REDs) is only something that happens in young exercisers, or is it?

Relative energy deficiency in sport (REDs) describes the syndrome of negative health and performance consequences of a cumulative deficit in energy availability.

The physiological systems in our body that keep us alive compete for energy that we derive from food, often expressed in Calories. The energy required for movement is prioritised over other life processes. From an evolutionary point of view, running away from predators is a top priority for survival. Once energy demand from movement has been met, the residual is known as energy availability. This available energy is used to meet the demands of all our other physiological processes, keeping them ticking over at our resting metabolic rate (RMR). RMR varies between individuals, depending on body composition.

Eating too many calories creates an excess that tends to be stored as fat. Although this is a growing problem of epidemic proportions, more active people, particularly endurance athletes, need to contend with the possibility of going into an energy deficit. If your energy availability is insufficient to meet the needs of your physiological systems, eventually systems that are less essential to staying alive start to shut down.

The ideal situation is to adapt, on a daily basis, the energy content of the food we eat to match the energy requirements of physical activity and our personal RMR. This happy balance is shown in the central panel of Figure 7.1.1. In contrast, the unhappy

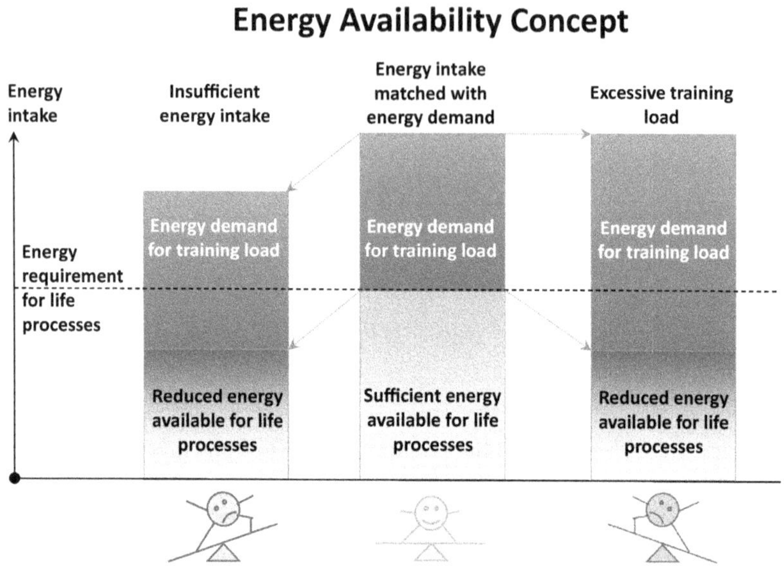

Energy Availability Concept

FIGURE 7.1.1 Energy availability concept. Credit Hormones, Health and Human Potential. Keay 2022. Sequoia books

person on the right has fallen into a state of low energy availability by taking on a higher training load without recognising the need to increase energy intake. This is often a situation of unintentional low energy availability. The distressed person on the left has arrived in low energy availability by a different route. In this case, training has been maintained, but food calories have been intentionally reduced, in the hope and belief that this confers an athletic performance advantage[1].

The body can rebound from a short time of low energy availability. We can comfortably tolerate a delayed meal. However, if an energy deficit is maintained over days, weeks and months, then the body and specifically hormone networks, will have to respond and adapt to "save energy". Cumulative low energy availability results in the syndrome (collection of signs and symptoms) of REDs[2]. REDs encompasses the adverse health and performance consequences of this long-term energy deficit[3].

Myth 1 REDs only happens in elite, competing athletes?

Despite its name, REDs can occur in any level of exerciser and is not limited to those who are participating in competitive sport or athletes at the elite level. I see many individuals with REDs who say that they are not athletes and assume they are not experiencing REDs. Some of these amateurs are training like elite competitive athletes, in addition to the pressures of work and family commitments, but without sufficient energy to cover all these demands.

In fact, amateurs are potentially more at risk of REDs than elite athletes because they lack the support network of physiologists, dieticians, sports nutritionists and coaches enjoyed by top professionals. Furthermore, exercise is not restricted to competitive sport; many people exercise in the gym or dance studio[4]. Although the "s" in REDs refers to sport, the syndrome is not limited to people doing sport.

Myth 2 REDs only occurs in young exercisers?

It is true that teenagers have a higher energy demand than older adults. Active young athletes might be more at risk of running into low energy availability, as it is physically and practically challenging to meet all the energy demands of exercise (in and out of school), growth and development, academic study (the brain takes 20% of energy intake) and other activities. Young people also face increasing social pressures around body shape and weight on pervasive social media platforms. Nevertheless, as adults, we are not immune to these pressures: whether originating from our own internal psychological drivers or triggers from external sources such as social media.

As we have discussed throughout this book, there are physiological reasons why navigating menopause is challenging when it comes to body shape, composition and exercise performance. However, if, like Icarus, you rigidly stick to the same set pattern of nutrition and exercise that served you well 30 years ago, then you run the risk of crashing and burning.

> ***REDs story***
>
> *Monica was a 43-year-old doctor who, in addition to having a busy schedule working in a hospital, was a dedicated cyclist. However, she was struggling with fatigue and felt "lazy" struggling to do her usual training. Monica had noticed that her shape had changed and her cycling performance had dropped, especially when she compared herself with the younger cyclists in the club. This annoyed Monica. She was a hard worker, in both her job and exercise, and she knew that if she set her mind to anything, she would achieve her goal. Monica decided to restrict what she was eating and train more. After a few months, she was frustrated to see this had not helped, so she decided to try harder by restricting her food intake further and training harder. Maybe an extra fasted session before work would help? When we met, Monica reported that her periods had all but stopped, her weight had not changed and if anything, her body fat had increased, not decreased.*

Monica is the typical "high achiever" in work and exercise with the associated psychological traits. These qualities are laudable, and if applied in a flexible way, they can lead to positive outcomes in terms of health and performance, by focusing on nutrition, fuelling appropriately to meet all demands and factoring in sufficient recovery to allow positive training adaptations to occur. However, if these same characteristics are used to restrict calories and train in a rigid way, this can lead to the negative reinforcement of cumulative low energy availability and ultimately REDs[5]. See Figure 7.1.2.

When I discussed this with Monica, I explained that, although it may feel like eating less and training more is a logical approach, in reality, this prevents, and in the long term negates, the positive hormone-driven adaptations to exercise. Rather, the endocrine networks transition into a mode that prioritises survival over performance[6]. This is illustrated in Figure 7.1.3. The hypothalamus, located deep in the brain, is perfectly positioned to act as the neuroendocrine gatekeeper of the endocrine network, alert to all sources of stress: whether from external sources or from low energy availability. If cumulative stressors are registered, then short-range hormone signals are sent from the hypothalamus to the pituitary gland to initiate a "stress response mode", which downregulates hormone networks such as the reproductive and thyroid axes. This has the effect of preserving resources by saving energy on reproduction hormones and by slowing the metabolic rate. The only hormone axis that gets upregulated is the hypothalamic-pituitary-adrenal (HPA) axis, which responds to "stress" by increasing the production of cortisol, thereby favouring the deposition of fat over muscle.

This hormonal adaptation to cumulative low energy availability and other stressors results in the clinical syndrome of REDs. In older exercisers, this is on the backdrop of declining anabolic hormones with increasing age, such as growth hormone and ultimately oestradiol after menopause is reached. In other words, the effects of sustained low energy availability on endocrine networks are compounded by the effects of getting older.

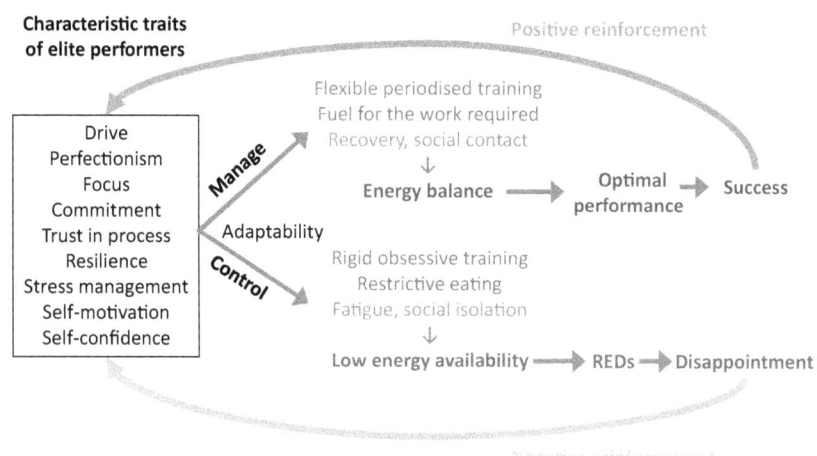

FIGURE 7.1.2 Psychological factors in REDs

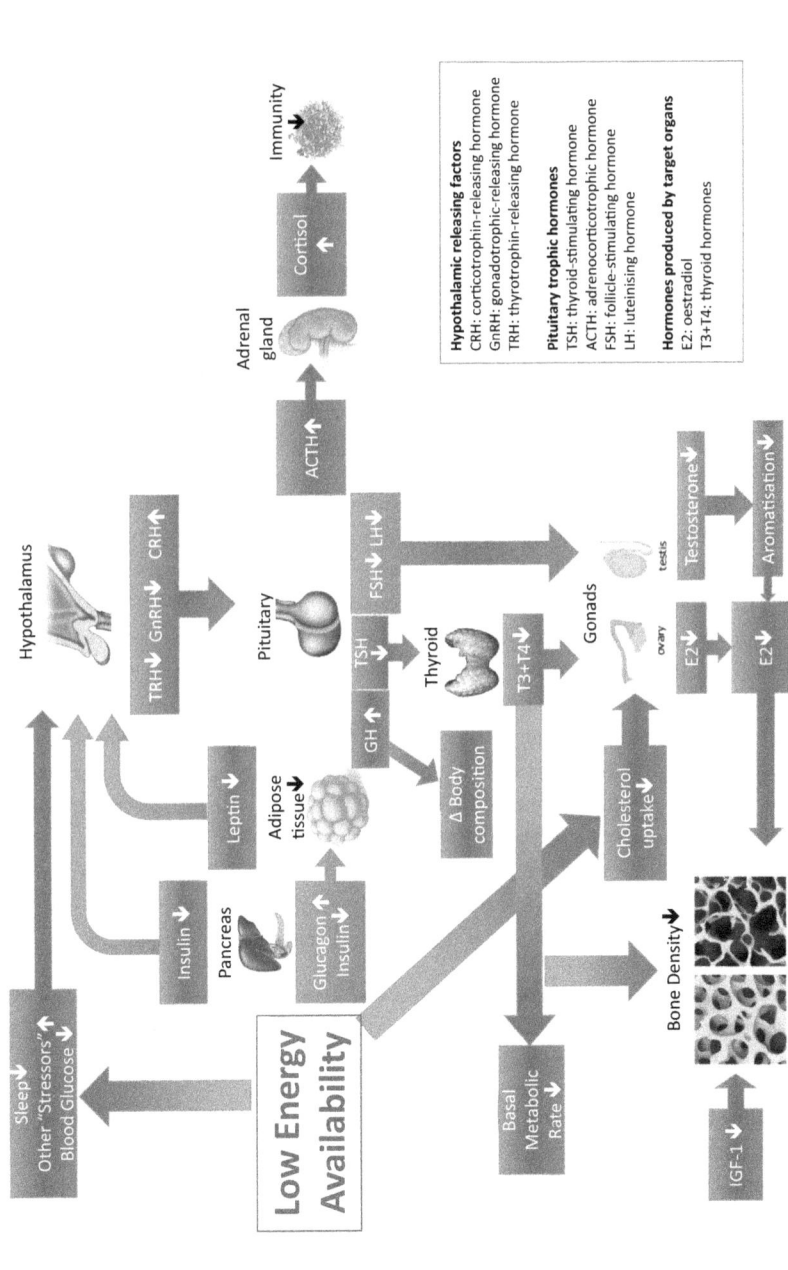

FIGURE 7.1.3 Effects of low energy availability on endocrine systems. Hormones, Health and Human Potential. Keay 2022. Sequoia books

Younger and older exercisers and athletes are the age groups at the highest risk of REDs, but for different reasons. Both age groups share the same psychological drivers, but in younger athletes the endocrine systems should be in full drive, whereas in older age groups some endocrine systems might be winding down, reducing the capacity to adapt. Furthermore, older exercisers might be tempted to restrict food intake to mitigate the potential effects of declining anabolic hormones on body shape.

Myth 3 REDs or perimenopause?

Monica wanted to know whether her symptoms of fatigue and sporadic periods were a result of REDs or perimenopause. How can one distinguish between these two scenarios? As discussed in Act 1, doing a blood test for female hormones cannot be used to diagnose perimenopause, due to the inherent variability of menstrual cycle hormones[7] and the unpredictable, non-linear nature of hormone changes as ovarian response declines during this stage of the female hormone odyssey.

One approach might be to try to calculate energy availability by using a diet diary to assess energy intake and calculate energy expenditure. However, this is known to be fraught with the possibility of error and even if a value could be calculated, it would have to be corrected for lean body mass from a dual X-ray absorptiometry (DXA) scan, as energy availability is defined as Kcal/Kg lean body mass. Then, what does that value mean for Monica? This is only a snapshot. Fortunately, the solution comes in the form of a hormone that reflects energy availability: triiodothyronine (T3) is one of the hormones produced by the thyroid gland that is a primary indicator of low energy availability, according to the IOC consensus statement on REDs[8].

Although it is helpful to have tests and data, a good detective always considers the narrative. Ultimately, the crucial clue lies in Monica's account of her clinical history. Monica described how she had increased her training load and intentionally restricted what she was eating. Although the symptoms and signs of fatigue, irregular cycles and urinary leakage (a recently added symptom in the IOC consensus statement 2023) could, at face value, be due to either perimenopause or REDs, the background information leans in favour of cumulative low energy availability as the underlying cause. Interestingly, although there is an overlap in symptoms of perimenopause and REDs, vasomotor symptoms (VMS) are unique to perimenopause and menopause, as this is thought to be due to a resetting of the central thermostat as described in Act 2.

Ultimately, REDs is a result of adaptive change in hormone networks to chronic low energy availability, whereas perimenopause is due to a physiological change in ovarian function. REDs is reversible, but menopause is not.

Once we had confirmed that long-term low energy availability was the underlying cause of Monica's issues, we agreed on a pattern of eating in a consistent way to meet her demands, combined with a review of her training and recovery. We discussed that quality of training rather than quantity was the priority, including adding strength training. The quality of training is, in turn, dependent on the quality and timing of recovery and nutrition. Training under-fuelled and under-recovered is counterproductive.

We also agreed that as perimenopause could become a factor in the near future, considering hormone replacement therapy (HRT) would be a conversation to revisit once menopausal symptoms emerged. Although HRT is used in women experiencing REDs, this is specifically for bone protection, in combination with addressing exercise and nutritional behaviours simultaneously to redress low energy availability as discussed in Act 5.

Myth 4 What have eating behaviours got to do with hormones?

Our eating behaviours are directed, in part, by our hormones as shown in Figure 7.1.4. Ghrelin, dubbed the "hungry hormone", is released from the gastrointestinal tract, while the "satiety hormone" leptin is secreted from adipose tissue. These hormone messages, together with neuroendocrine signals such as PYY, are brought together in the hypothalamus, the neuroendocrine gatekeeper, to direct our eating behaviours: determining when to seek food, eat and when to stop eating.

It is possible to "override" these neuroendocrine signals. For example, intentionally restricting what you eat either in disordered eating (selective and restricted timing or composition of food intake) or in an eating disorder (diagnosed on clinical criteria). The potential problem of "tuning out" to the neuroendocrine signals that direct eating behaviours is that consequent energy surplus or deficiency forces hormone networks to adapt in an attempt to restore homeostasis. However, this adaptation can become dysregulation with adverse consequences for both health and performance, as shown in

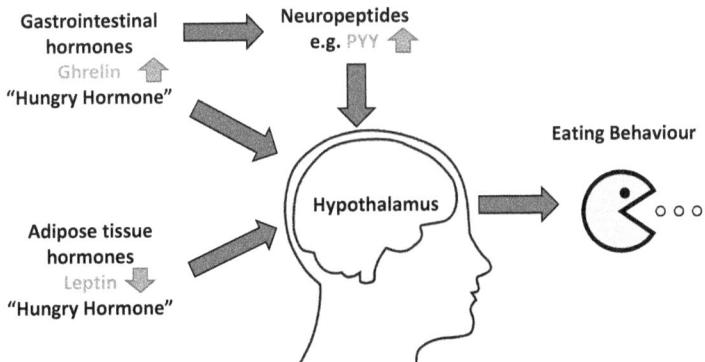

FIGURE 7.1.4 Neuroendocrine control of eating behaviours

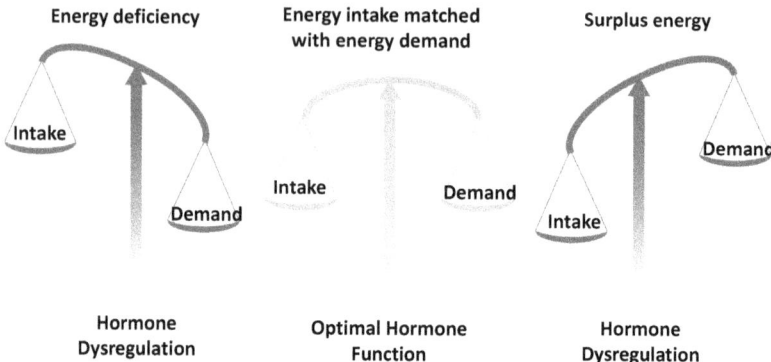

FIGURE 7.1.5 Energy availability and hormone function

Figure 7.1.5. The good news is that this is a potentially reversible situation. Rebalancing behaviours around nutrition, exercise and recovery/sleep allows hormone networks to return back to their homeostatic duties.

> *It is a fallacy that hormones can become "unbalanced" (outside of specific medical endocrine conditions). After millions of years of evolution, hormone networks have become super-efficient and effective in maintaining homeostasis. Claiming that hormones are "out of balance" indicates a failure to understand that the role of hormones is to maintain balance. The real sources of disequilibrium are unbalanced lifestyle behaviours, which force the endocrine system to adapt[9].*

Myth 5 Underactive thyroid, menopause or REDs?

In addition to the possible mistaken identity of REDs and perimenopause, there is another player in the hormone masquerade.

The thyroid gland produces the hormones thyroxine (T4) and triiodothyronine (T3). Production is controlled by thyroid-stimulating hormone (TSH) released by the pituitary gland. Levels of T4 and T3 are maintained in a healthy range through the "classic" negative feedback loop, characteristic of many hormone systems. Sometimes the thyroid gland malfunctions: primary hypothyroidism is where the thyroid gland stops producing T4 and T3, resulting in an elevated TSH signal from the pituitary gland as it attempts to trigger a response from the thyroid. Thus, an underactive thyroid is diagnosed by raised levels of TSH. Although some people use the term "underactive thyroid" loosely, the National Institute for Health and Care Excellence is very clear that you do not have primary hypothyroidism and should not be prescribed thyroxine replacement unless blood tests show "TSH of 10 mIU/litre or higher on 2 separate occasions 3 months apart with concurrent low T4"[10].

The symptoms of primary hypothyroidism include fatigue, heavy periods, low mood and health consequences of weight gain and an increased risk of cardiovascular disease. As warned by NICE, the symptoms and potential health consequences of primary hypothyroidism can be very similar to those associated with perimenopause. Thyroid function tests can distinguish between the underlying cause of these similar symptoms.

REDs is another contender for the symptoms of irregular menstrual cycles, fatigue, low mood, poor bone health and suboptimal lipid profile. Furthermore, thyroid function tests may well indicate low-range levels of T4 and T3. Indeed, the IOC REDs clinical assessment tool version 2 (REDsCAT v2) advises using T3 levels as a primary indicator of low energy availability[8]. However, crucially, TSH will not be raised to a level indicative of primary underactive thyroid. Rather, due to sustained low energy availability, the whole thyroid axis has adapted and downregulated to slow the metabolic rate and "save energy". This is potentially a reversible situation of endocrine adaptation, whereas primary hypothyroidism and menopause are not.

A runner's story

> *Susan was 51 years of age and a keen runner. In the past, she had had an eating disorder, anorexia nervosa, where she lost a lot of weight and her periods stopped. Although she had been declared "recovered", she was still sensitive about food and weight and had suffered stress fractures of the pelvis. Noticing that she had recently gained some weight, she had restricted her complex carbohydrate intake. Susan also noticed that she was really struggling with recovery and generally feeling fatigued. She hadn't had a period for over a year. Susan was concerned as she had been told that her T4 was in the lower range and thought this meant she had an underactive thyroid and needed thyroxine, which she understood would help control weight.*

Did Susan have a primary underactive thyroid? Does she need thyroxine? Susan's blood test showed TSH, T4 and T3 were all in the lower low range. In other words, this indicated that her thyroid axis had adapted and downregulated to slow the metabolic rate to "save energy" as a consequence of low energy availability. Since TSH was not elevated, there was no indication of an underactive thyroid and thyroxine would neither be appropriate nor helpful[11]. Rather fuelling in a way to meet demand would be the best way forward. Susan's bone health was a concern given her stress fractures at "high risk" sites and a DXA scan showed osteoporosis of the lumbar spine (T-score <2.5) with an age-matched Z-score well below −1. Most likely, this reflected previous functional hypothalamic amenorrhoea (FHA) with an eating disorder and current declining ovarian hormones with menopause. As discussed in Act 5, HRT is recommended for bone protection in REDs. This is the recommendation in the updated 2022 National Institute for Health and Care Excellence (NICE) guidelines, which brought the recommendation of HRT over hormonal contraception for women experiencing

FHA[12] in line with earlier Endocrine Society guidelines and the International Olympic Committee (IOC) consensus statement on relative energy deficiency. HRT is also the primary treatment for poor bone health in menopause[13]. So, it is really important to distinguish between three potential situations:

- Primary hypothyroidism (a medical condition requiring thyroxine), which is not reversible.
- Perimenopause/menopause (physiological process of the female hormone odyssey), which is not reversible but does not require thyroxine.
- REDs, which is a result of unbalanced behaviours causing adaptation of hormone networks, which is reversible and does not require thyroxine.

Conclusion

In conclusion, it is certainly possible for REDs to occur, whether intentionally or unintentionally, in older exercisers, masters age group athletes and dancers. It can be challenging to distinguish symptoms of age-related changes in hormone networks with adaptive changes due to cumulative low energy availability. A suitably qualified medical doctor can help avert steering the misguided course of Icarus.

References

1. Keay N, Francis G. Infographic. Energy availability: Concept, control and consequences in relative energy deficiency in sport (RED-S). *British Journal of Sports Medicine* 2019; 53: 1310–1311.
2. Keay N, Rankin A. Infographic. Relative energy deficiency in sport: An infographic guide. *British Journal of Sports Medicine* 2019; 53: 1307–1309.
3. Mountjoy M, Ackerman KE, Bailey DM et al. 2023 International Olympic Committee's (IOC) consensus statement on Relative Energy Deficiency in Sport (REDs). *British Journal of Sports Medicine* 2023; 57: 1073–1098.
4. Keay N, Overseas A, Francis G. Indicators and correlates of low energy availability in male and female dancers. *BMJ Open Sport & Exercise Medicine* 2020; 6: e000906. doi: 10.1136/bmjsem-2020-000906.
5. Keay N. The state of play on relative energy deficiency in sport (REDs) Hormone Psychology Nutrition Exercise. *ResearchGate* March 2024. doi: 10.13140/RG.2.2.13883.02083.
6. Keay N. *Hormones, Health and Human Potential: A Guide to Understanding Your Hormones to Optimise Your Health and Performance*. Sequoia Books, 2022.
7. Francis G, Keay N. Quantitative hormone analysis reveals sources of variability in the menstrual cycle. *Women in Sport and Physical Activity Journal* 2024; 32 (S1): wspaj.2023-0062. https://doi.org/10.1123/wspaj.2023-0062. Accessed April 2024.
8. Stellingwerff T, Mountjoy M, McCluskey WT et al. Review of the scientific rationale, development and validation of the International Olympic Committee Relative Energy Deficiency in Sport Clinical Assessment Tool: V.2 (IOC REDs CAT2)—by a subgroup of the IOC consensus on REDs. *British Journal of Sports Medicine* 2023; 57: 1109–1121.
9. Keay N. Interactions of the female hormone network, exercise training and nature of adaptation. *ResearchGate* June 2023. doi: 10.13140/RG.2.2.28787.71204.

10 Thyroid disease: Assessment and management. NICE guideline [NG145] Published: 20 November 2019 Last updated: 12 October 2023 Accessed April 2024.
11 Keay N. Thyroid function in athletes and dancers. *British Journal of Sports and Exercise Medicine* 2020. https://blogs.bmj.com/bjsm/2020/03/12/thyroid-function-in-athletes-and-dancers/.
12 British Association Sport and Exercise Medicine. 'Concerning' lack of awareness of how best to reduce risk of stress fractures in female athletes and dancers, a year after change in NICE guidelines. 2023. https://basem.co.uk/concerning-lack-of-awareness-of-how-best-to-reduce-risk-of-stress-fractures-in-female-athletes-and-dancers-a-year-after-change-in-nice-guidelines/.
13 Stevenson J. Medical advisory council of the British Menopause Society. Prevention and treatment of osteoporosis in women. *Post Reproductive Health* 2023 Mar; 29 (1): 11–14. doi: 10.1177/20533691221139902. Epub 2022 Nov 10. PMID: 36357006; PMCID: PMC10009319.

Scene 2 Can I maintain athletic effort and performance?

Tenille Hoogland

Myth 1 Eat less to maintain body composition?

Meno-pot. Spare tire. Meno-belly. This is slang used to describe the female body in menopause transition. Add in decades of diet culture, body-shaming and the pervasive image of the photo-shopped, thin (usually white) and young athletic body, pressures many women in the menopause transition to target unwanted weight gain with eating less, seeking diet fads or supplement-based quick fixes.

For decades athletes in endurance sports have been told that the best way to get fast and improve power, measured as force times velocity, is to lose weight. But getting the optimal power to weight ratio emphasises weight loss rather than increases in strength or force. To add more frustration, body composition change can feel like it happens overnight. The exercise effort feels the same, eating has not changed, but the layer around the midsection builds.

The response of many women: eat less, train more. These two actions may bring a sense of control at a time when hormone change feels out of control and certainly unpredictable. This response can end however, in frustration, injury, mood change and sadly, more weight gain.

Body composition change in the menopause transition can be due to several factors, many of which are impacted by the change of hormones, namely the decline of oestradiol and progesterone. Figure 7.2.1 shows some factors and possible actions that can positively impact body composition change in the menopause transition.

When all the factors of body composition change are considered, prioritising actions to support the body through change is important. First, establish health fundamentals: sleep, nutrition and exercise. Then, optimise athletic performance. Let's dig into the health fundamentals.

> *"To have rhythm, to be in sync, is to be healthy. But not just any rhythm will do."*
>
> Dr Satchin Panda[1]

Sleep is the foundation of health and our ability to manage stress and physiological change. Sleep enhances our ability to learn, memorise and make logical decisions and choices. We can better navigate social and psychological challenges[2]. Specific to body

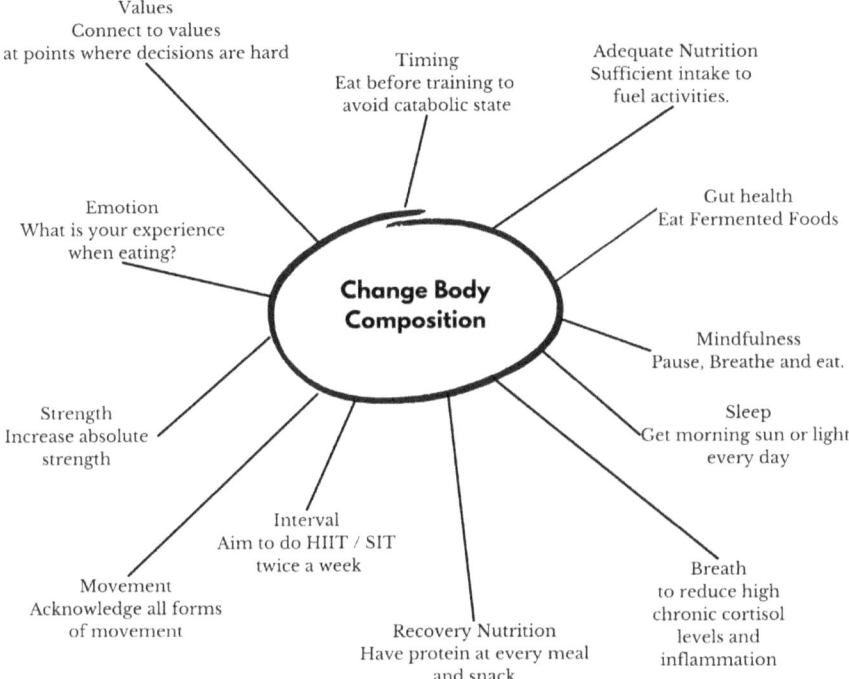

FIGURE 7.2.1 Factors that positively change body composition

composition, sleep fine-tunes the balance of insulin and circulating glucose. It supports the regulation of appetite through hormones such as leptin and insulin and is important for a healthy gut microbiome[3]. Finally, it is intimately connected to cardiovascular fitness and lowering blood pressure. If you don't sleep, the body will break down eventually and body composition change is just one of many negative health consequences.

The reality, however, is that many women in the menopause transition struggle with sleep. They suffer from hot flushes which disrupt sleep patterns. They wake in the early hours and are not able to fall back asleep.

So, what can we do?

In addition to improving sleep hygiene, there is strong research that demonstrates that timing nutrition intake and adhering to exercise can promote circadian alignment[4,5,6]. Circadian alignment means that that physical (e.g. digestion, hormone secretion, metabolism), mental and behavioural changes that are experienced over 24-hour cycle rhythms are optimised. While more research is needed on circadian rhythms and the fluctuation and/or reduction of hormones such as oestrogen, progesterone, melatonin and cortisol, creating a consistent routine around eating and exercise can support sleep and hormone health.

One specific action could be to time dinner at least 3 hours before sleep. This promotes digestion and signals to the body preparation to sleep. If you find yourself waking in the night, experiment with trying a small protein snack with fibre and/or fat (e.g. cottage cheese with blueberries or nuts with apple) to even out the blood-sugar response through the night. Establishing the optimal time of exercise during the day is complex and influenced by several variables (e.g. entrained waking time, circadian phenotype, mode and duration/intensity of exercise and meal timing)[7]. More important than getting the timing right is that we get in the movement when it works for us.

Eat to support all our activities so our bodies can function optimally, with energy and in health.

In simplest terms, the body response to low energy availability is one of preservation. The body slows the rate for which energy is used so primary body functions like digestion and breathing can continue. When additional physical stress is induced, catabolism, the breakdown of tissue occurs. Because the body does not have the energy available to adapt and respond optimally to the stress, chronic inflammation occurs. Over time the ability to reach performance targets in exercise is diminished despite strong efforts. The result is a lower overall expenditure of energy. The best method to counter low energy availability is to support exercise with eating before and after the effort and sometimes during depending on length and intensity. During exercise, the body is primed to use energy. After exercise, the body is primed to adapt and respond to the stress. By timing nutrition to support your activities, we can reap the benefits of our hard work.

When it comes to exercise and supporting body composition, do hard things for less time rather than lots of things for longer times.

The third priority action that is important for body composition is doing activity that supports maintenance of muscle mass and strength. Maintaining muscle supports healthy metabolism, bone health, preventing injury and glucose control to name a few. Oestrogen has an anabolic (growth) effect on muscle primarily by lowering the protein turnover (i.e. breakdown) and enhancing sensitivity to resistance training[8]. Oestrogen also influences how carbohydrates and fats are utilised during exercise[9]. As oestrogen decreases in the menopause transition, women must continue to create a strong stimulus or stress to the muscle in order to keep it. This is most effectively done two ways: resistance and intensity exercise.

When it comes to resistance exercise, lifting weights is new for many women and requires attention to form. Fear of bulking up is one concern of women when they consider lifting heavy weights. The reality is that to actually increase overall muscle mass through resistance training, particularly in peri- or postmenopause, requires significant diligence and intention to methodology and nutrition support. The critical points to completing resistance exercise effectively and safely are as follows:

1. Make it challenging.
2. All challenge(s) must be completed with good form.

Completing sets with lower repetitions (e.g. 3–5 sets of 5 repetitions) increases the strength of the muscle and is particularly beneficial for bone health. Completing sets with higher repetitions (e.g. 3–5 sets of 10–15 repetitions) increases strength endurance and muscle mass. Both have benefits and are positive methods to work towards maintaining muscle and body composition goals.

High-intensity exercise is typically understood as an exercise that brings your heart rate to above 85% of maximum[10]. High Intensity Interval Training (HIIT) and Sprint Interval Training (SIT) are highly effective for recreational to elite athletes aiming to improve body composition and health goals. In particular, HIIT training has shown improvements in $\dot{V}O_2$ maximum, which has been correlated to reduce all-cause and disease-specific mortality[11].

We have both actions and inaction that can support body composition goals. Actions can be timing nutrition around activities or adding more protein to your diet. Necessary inaction may include taking a rest day or only doing light movement after a poor night's sleep. What remains important is that both support the health fundamental of sleep, sufficient energy and keeping your skeletal and heart muscle strong. Also remember that, when no amount of kale, perfect sleep hygiene or hitting the gym helps achieve health fundamentals, menopause hormone therapy is an option to smooth out the challenges.

Myth 2 Is the number of birthdays a limiting factor?

In general, there is a linear decline of performance in sports up until the age of 70, when the decline of speed and power accelerates. The decline is relatively consistent between males and females although research on females is limited due to sample size[12]. While it may seem obvious that we all will slow down and lose strength, the reasons for decline go beyond how fit or strong we are. We tend to use the same training or exercise methodologies as we did when we were younger which can contribute to our decline in performance. Here we break the myth that the number of birthdays is our limiting factor. We first examine what performance markers show a clear decline and then determine what we can do about it.

Aerobic Capacity and Age: Your $\dot{V}O_2$ max

Cardiorespiratory fitness, measured by maximum aerobic capacity or $\dot{V}O_2$ max, is inversely associated with long-term mortality. Remarkably, there is no observed upper limit of benefit[13]. In the St James Women Take Heart Project, researchers found that this finding is greater in women than men[14]. $\dot{V}O_2$ max is also a variable, along with lactate threshold and skill, associated with endurance performance[15]. Essentially, women with a higher $\dot{V}O_2$ max will live longer and be faster.

With the exception of one incredible man who demonstrated that even at 103 years old we can improve our $\dot{V}O_2$ max, it generally declines with age[16]. The decline of $\dot{V}O_2$ max is less in sedentary females than in endurance-trained females. The reason suggested is that athletes, as they age, may be doing relatively less volume and intensity exercise to their previous levels in comparison to their sedentary counterparts. When women already have low fitness, there is less room to fall. The loss of muscle mass is another variable in the age-associated decline of $\dot{V}O_2$ max[17]. Regardless of the relative decline, approximately 9–10% per decade, $\dot{V}O_2$ max remains overall higher in active populations than in sedentary populations.

Maximum Heart Rate

Another measure that declines with age is maximum heart rate. In general, one can see a reduction of 5.6–6 beat per minute per decade regardless of $\dot{V}O_2$ max[18,19]. Dr Meagan Wasfy, Sports Cardiologist at Mass General Brigham and Harvard Medical School, explains that a lower maximum heart rate can be explained by likening the heart to a house. A house has doors, an electrical system and plumbing. With age, the structure of the house stiffens and loses efficiency. Using nutrition and exercise we slow the rate of decline by working to prevent blockages in our pipes (i.e. coronary arteries) and by keeping circuits working (i.e. muscle contractions)[20].

Muscular Power and Strength

The old adage – if you don't use it, you lose it – rings true for muscle mass as we age. Sarcopenia is the loss of muscle mass and quality. Declining levels of hormones, and particular oestrogen, impacts the structure and function of musculoskeletal tissues such as muscle, tendons and ligaments. While actual prevalence of sarcopenia is difficult to establish due to varying definitions, some research states that from the age of 30, muscle mass can decrease up to 8% each decade and that this accelerates after the age of 60[21,22].

Physiologically it does seem that we will get slower and less strong as we age.

And yet, what I see is that female athletes are getting faster, stronger and fitter as they age.

In my work with recreational female athletes in their 40s, 50s or 60s, I see the women getting faster and stronger. The reason is because the methodology of training I use accounts for female physiology and hormone change.

Let's start with $\dot{V}O_2$ max.

$\dot{V}O_2$ max can change when a significant enough stress is applied to the cardiovascular system. As discussed in the previous myth, in recent years HIIT has gained significant popularity in its effectiveness to improve aerobic fitness, cardiac function and insulin resistance[23,24]. This type of training, of which Tabata is one type, is typically short in overall duration and follows a general pattern of eight times 20–30 seconds at near maximal effort, 10–15 seconds very easy, repeated a number of times with sufficient rest in between. Other interval sets such as one minute on, one minute easy, can also fall into the HIIT category of training. There are two reasons for its success in raising $\dot{V}O_2$ max. One is that the stress applied is significant enough to signal mitochondrial adaptations in the skeletal muscle. Mitochondria is the energy powerhouse of a cell. In simplest terms, with significant stress, mitochondria function is improved to adapt to that stress. The other reason why $\dot{V}O_2$ max is improved is that pushing to a maximal effort for 30 seconds at a time, compared to four minutes, can be easier to take on.

The second critical shift in training to improve $\dot{V}O_2$ max is the recognition that more recovery time between exercise sessions is needed for females as they age. The loss of oestrogen results in a higher level of oxidative stress and systemic inflammation generally[25,26]. If the chronic stress load of hormone change, work, familial responsibilities, coupled with training stress is not considered, higher levels of inflammation can result. This takes a toll on our ability to show up consistently, in strength and with power. Without sufficient time between sessions there is insufficient training stress for cardiovascular adaptations resulting in a lower $\dot{V}O_2$ max.

The take-home: Work less often, but keep it hard.

I established that your maximum heart rate will lower as we age. What can change is your ability to tolerate a higher threshold heart rate. Threshold heart rate can be defined as the highest heart rate we are able to sustain for durations from 10 minutes to one hour. When we repeat hard sessions, we establish belief in ourselves that we can do hard things. We increase the confidence that we can handle the intensity safely and without injury. The result: we tolerate a faster pace or power for longer.

For decades women have shied away from the weight room for fear of bulking up. Getting strong was a thing guys did. This is changing. In the previous myth, we discuss the two ways to get stronger: (1) hypertrophy training (i.e. higher number of repetitions with less weight) and (2) muscular strength (i.e. lower repetitions with heavy weight). Type II muscle fibres, also known as fast twitch, are activated with heavy and explosive movements. They fatigue quickly. Type I muscle fibres, also known as slow twitch, keep us going all day long and are slow to fatigue. As we age, there is a switch of muscle fibre type from fast to slow twitch. If we do not use the fast twitch muscle fibres, they will die or become a slow twitch fibre. It is fast twitch muscle fibres that are more susceptible to muscle atrophy (decrease) and possibly sarcopenia[27]. So like with HIIT training, the strength of the stimulus or stress becomes important to staying strong.

Historically, women were not encouraged to participate in sport. It remains unknown if differences observed in older athletes reflect biological mechanisms versus less lifetime access to sports in females[28]. At one time, it was regarded as unsafe for women to ride a bike for fear of bicycle-face. Symptoms included "usually flushed, but sometimes pale, often with lips more or less drawn, and the beginning of dark shadows under the eyes, and always with an expression of weariness" as well as a "hard, clenched jaw and bulging eyes"[29]. While this now seems laughable, the result was young girls missing out on hopping curbs on a bike, lifting heavy and being on start lines. Research on female athletes across the age-span is still in its infancy. Recreational female athletes have the largest opportunity to actually get faster and stronger as they age. Age is not our limiting factor.

Myth 3 Is Effort the barometer of success?

You're running into the finish line with everything you have. People on either side of the finish chute cheer you on. Your legs are heavy and tired, but oh, just a few more steps. Your heart's beating right out of your chest. And then you cross. It's over. You did it. Bent over, hands on your thighs, you stop. You have nothing left. You feel immensely proud. Your endorphins are flowing.

A few hours pass and the excitement settles. Despite you telling yourself how hard you worked, you start to doubt your accomplishment. You are slower than last year. Your friend beat you by more than she usually does. She's the same age!

Comparison zaps you of joy. In its place is a feeling of being less than. What you just did is somehow diminished. All that work is simply not enough.

In the last myth, we learnt about the effects of ageing and how age is not your limiting factor. In this myth, we tackle the need to keep up. We address the desire to strive for an outcome that is not within our control and we explore the power of effort.

Comparison is "the crush of conformity from one side and competition from the other – it's trying simultaneously to fit in and stand out. Comparison says, 'Be like everyone else but better'".[30] Being an athlete has comparison and competition woven into it. For many athletes, the competition is the point of a race, tournament or event. We compare how we did *against* others. We compare what they did, what they look like, what they have or what we don't have. If we replace against with *with* then the negative power of comparison lessens. We find the commonality of showing up and ready to do our best.

In general, there are two comparisons that the athletic female in perimenopause makes. The first is to slimmer, stronger, faster body they had. The second comparison is to everyone else's body; also slimmer, stronger and faster.

Reality Check One: The body we once knew is gone.

Dr Nicky Keay, in Act 2 of her book *Hormones, Health and Human Potential* connects how hormone function change at different stages of life create physiological changes[31]. At the highest level, we are never in the body we once knew. It is always changing. Body composition change, menstrual cycle timing and flow, body temperature regulation, headaches, new aches and pains, brain fog, itchy skin are just a snapshot of possible symptoms. With such challenges there's no doubt why we'd want the body we once knew! If only we appreciated it back then.

Dina Bell-Laroche supports Olympians and Paralympians who move through grief after their careers have ended, sometimes to devastating injury, sometimes to disastrous or lacklustre results. The first step, she suggests, is to acknowledge what is lost. For elite athletes the loss they grieve may be the camaraderie and/or singular life purpose[32]. For recreational athletes it may be the inability to do the epic adventures. It could be that you can't do the sport you love because one twist of the knee could take you out of movement completely. Your body has changed and you have to change with it. There is loss.

Our society celebrates a push-through and a never-give-up mentality. This mindset likely has been a critical component of your success. Work hard, put in the effort and get results. Dig in your heels and keep going. This is what it takes to reach your goals. Instead of honouring the body in change and finding new ways to access strength, fitness and enjoyment of movement, you fight against it. Effort equals hard work. In this way, effort is singular in dimension and limited in scope. There is only one way.

Acknowledgement of loss is not the same as settling for being less strong, fast or able to do hard things. Effort must include a new way of being and a new sense of self. It requires expansive ways of looking at ourselves, our abilities and our strengths.

Reality Check Two: Everyone else is slimmer, stronger and faster. Or not.

Sadly, comparison is a human trait that we'll never be rid of. As such, we can only change our reaction when we enter into comparison[33]. There is one question that may help when we start spiralling down the comparison vortex. Would I take every aspect of the life of the person I covet to be in their shoes at this very moment?

In general, we arrive here, in the present based on past actions. Our body tells a story of our life and even the lives of those before us[34]. That woman beside you, her body, has a story. She may have been a professional athlete in the past. She may be in a position now to focus entirely on sport with a professional coach to guide her. Alternatively, she may have come from a family that was never active or had goals in sport. She may have only realised that she was "an athlete" late in life and is trying to learn what her best actually is! When we race or participate *with* the person beside us, we look at them in their whole human experience. We celebrate the choices they made to arrive where they are. Effort is based on the starting point for which we begin our own personal journey. It is not based on the starting point of someone else's. What is effort? Where does it reside in the human spirit? It is related to having a growth mindset. Dr Carol Dweck, the foremost authority and creator of growth mindset, defines it as a belief that construes intelligence as malleable and improvable[35]. Students with a growth mindset are likely to learn by a mastery approach, embracing challenges and putting in the effort to learn. Effort is not singular based on one dimension of work. Effort is looking at the problem from every angle. Effort can even count twice as we aim for mastery. First we have talent times effort = skill. Then skill times effort = achievement. Without effort all the talent in the world will not go anywhere. Without effort, no matter how skilled you are, you will not find achievement[36].

There is one more physiological aspect to effort that we benefit from: Dopamine.

Dopamine is a neurotransmitter involved in reward and motivation[37]. It can enhance our depth of focus and lower our threshold for taking action toward specific goals. Dopamine is guided by an intricate balance we have to pleasure and pain[38]. If we continuously seek a reward (e.g. Facebook likes, performance bests, besting our competitor) then the intricate balance of pleasure and pain is upset. We will want more and more of the reward, but it feels further and further away because dopamine is not regenerated. This is called addiction. One method to re-establish balance is to actually seek out the pain of effort itself[39]. Pain of effort is to delve into the friction of challenge. The reward becomes secondary to the process.

Effort is grit. Effort is curiosity. Effort is the process of moving towards the goals that inspire you with others. Engaging in the very friction of effort is the barometer of success.

References

1 Panda S. *The Circadian Code. Lose Weight, Supercharge Your Energy, and Transform Your Health from Morning to Night.* Rodale Publishing, 2018.
2 Walker M. *Why We sleep: Unlocking the Power of Sleep and Dreams.* Scribner, 2017.
3 Keay N. *Hormones, Health and Human Performance: A Guide to Understanding Your Hormones to Optimise Your Health and Performance.* Sequoia Books, 2022.
4 Challet E. The circadian regulation of food intake. *Nature Reviews Endocrinology* 2019; 15 (7): 393–405.
5 Gabriel BM, Zierath JR. Circadian rhythms and exercise — re-setting the clock in metabolic disease. *Nature Reviews Endocrinology* 2019; 15: 197–206. doi: 10.1038/s41574-018-0150-x.
6 Kravitz HM, Kazlauskaite R, Joffe H. Sleep, health, and metabolism in midlife women and menopause: Food for thought. *Obstetrics and Gynecology Clinics of North America* 2018 Dec; 45 (4): 679–694. doi: 10.1016/j.ogc.2018.07.008. Epub 2018 Oct 25. PMID: 30401550; PMCID: PMC6338227.
7 Parr EB, Heilbronn LK, Hawley JA. A time to eat and a time to exercise. *Exercise and Sport Sciences Reviews* 2020; 48 (1): 4–10. doi: 10.1249/JES.0000000000000207.
8 Hansen M, Kjaer M. Influence of sex and estrogen on musculotendinous protein turnover at rest and after exercise. *Exercise and Sport Sciences Reviews* 2014 Oct; 42 (4): 183–192. doi: 10.1249/JES.0000000000000026. PMID: 25062001.
9 D'Eon T, Braun B. The roles of estrogen and progesterone in regulating carbohydrate and fat utilization at rest and during exercise. *Journal of Women's Health & Gender-Based Medicine* 2002 Apr; 11 (3): 225–237. doi: 10.1089/152460902753668439. PMID: 11988133.
10 Ito S. High-intensity interval training for health benefits and care of cardiac diseases – The key to an efficient exercise protocol. *World Journal of Cardiology* 2019 Jul 26; 11 (7): 171–188. doi: 10.4330/wjc.v11.i7.171. PMID: 31565193.
11 Mandsager K, Harb S, Cremer P et al. Association of cardiorespiratory fitness with long-term mortality among adults undergoing exercise treadmill testing. *JAMA Network Open* 2018; 1 (6): e183605. doi: 10.1001/jamanetworkopen.2018.3605.
12 Ganse B, Ganse U, Dahl J et al. Linear decrease in athletic performance during the human life span. *Frontiers in Physiology* 2018 Aug 21; 9: 1100. doi: 10.3389/fphys.2018.01100.

13 Mandsager K, Harb S, Cremer P et al. Association of cardiorespiratory fitness with long-term mortality among adults undergoing exercise treadmill testing. *JAMA Network Open* 2018; 1 (6): e183605. doi: 10.1001/jamanetworkopen.2018.3605.
14 Gulati M, Pandey DK, Arnsdorf MF et al. Exercise capacity and the risk of death in women. *Circulation* 2003; 108 (13): 1554–1559. doi: 10.1161/01.CIR.0000091080.57509.E9.
15 Bassett DR Jr, Howley ET. Limiting factors for maximum oxygen uptake and determinants of endurance performance. *Medicine & Science in Sports & Exercise* 2000 Jan; 32 (1): 70–84. doi: 10.1097/00005768-200001000-00012. PMID: 10647532.
16 Billat V, Dhonneur G, Mille-Hamard L et al. Case studies in physiology: Maximal oxygen consumption and performance in a centenarian cyclist. *Journal of Applied Physiology* 1985 2017 Mar 1; 122 (3): 430–434. doi: 10.1152/japplphysiol.00569.2016. Epub 2016 Dec 29. PMID: 28035015.
17 Fleg JL, Lakatta EG. Role of muscle loss in the age-associated reduction in VO_2 max. *Journal of Applied Physiology* 1988; 65: 1147–1151.
18 Valenzuela PL, Maffiuletti NA, Joyner MJ et al. Lifelong endurance exercise as a countermeasure against age-related VO_2 max decline: Physiological overview and insights from masters athletes. *Sports Medicine* 2020; 50: 703–716.
19 Tanaka H, Desouza CA, Jones PP et al. Greater rate of decline in maximal aerobic capacity with age in physically active vs. sedentary healthy women. *Journal of Physiology* 1997. https://doi.org/10.1152/jappl.1997.83.6.1947https://journals.physiology.org/doi/full/10.1152/jappl.1997.83.6.1947.
20 Wasfy M, Hoogland T. Interview on heart health in perimenopause and beyond. *Youtube* 2023. https://youtu.be/x-qYVyDW6VM.
21 Purcell SA, Mackenzie M, Barbosa-Silva TG et al. Sarcopenia – Prevalence using different definitions in older community-dwelling Canadians. *Journal of Nutrition, Health and Aging* 2020; 24: 783–790. doi: 10.1007/s12603-020-1427-z.
22 Buckinx F, Aubertin-Leheudre M. Sarcopenia menopausal women: Current perspectives. *International Journal of Women's Health* 2022 Jun 23; 14: 805–819. doi: 10.2147/IJWH.S340537. PMID: 35769543; PMCID: PMC9235827.
23 Hwang CL, Yoo JK, Kim HK et al. Novel all-extremity high-intensity interval training improves aerobic fitness, cardiac function and insulin resistance in healthy older adults. *Experimental Gerontology* 2016; 82: 112–119.
24 Klonizakis M, Moss J, Gilbert S et al. Low-volume high-intensity interval training rapidly improves cardiopulmonary function in postmenopausal women. *Menopause* 2014; 21 (10): 1099–1105. doi: 10.1097/GME.0000000000000208.
25 Doshi SB, Agarwal A. The role of oxidative stress in menopause. *Journal of Mid-life Health* 2013 Jul; 4 (3): 140–146. doi: 10.4103/0976-7800.118990. PMID: 24672185; PMCID: PMC3952404.
26 Geraci A, Calvani R, Ferri E et al. Sarcopenia and menopause: The role of estradiol. *Frontiers in Endocrinology* 2021; 12: 682012–682012.
27 Arthur ST, Cooley ID. The effect of physiological stimuli on sarcopenia; impact of Notch and Wnt signaling on impaired aged skeletal muscle repair. *International Journal of Biological Sciences* 2012; 8 (5): 731–760.
28 Petek Bradley J, Chung Eugene H, Kim Jonathan H et al. Impact of sex on cardiovascular adaptations to exercise: JACC review topic of the week. *Journal of the American College of Cardiology* 2023; 82 (10): 1030–1038. ISSN 0735-1097. doi: 10.1016/j.jacc.2023.05.070.
29 Nicole, Toronto Reference Library Blog. *"Bicycle Face!" Women and Cycling in the Victorian Age*. https://torontopubliclibrary.typepad.com/trl/2015/08/bicycle-face-women-and-cycling-in-the-victorian-age-.html. Accessed February 2024.

30 Brown B. *Atlas of the Heart: Mapping Meaningful Connection and the Language of Human Experience*. Random House, 2021.
31 Keay N. *Hormones, Health and Human Performance: A Guide to Understanding Your Hormones to Optimise Your Health and Performance*. Sequoia Books, 2022.
32 Bell-Laroche D. The risk of not reconciling grief – A different way for sport leaders to integrate loss. *Sportlaw*. https://sportlaw.ca/the-risk-of-not-reconciling-grief-a-different-way-for-sport-leaders-to-integrate-loss/. Accessed January 2024.
33 Brown B. *Atlas of the Heart: Mapping Meaningful Connection and the Language of Human Experience*. Random House, 2021.
34 This refers to the research of epigenetics. Epigenetics is the study of how your behaviors and environment can cause changes that affect the way your genes work.
35 Brown B. *Atlas of the Heart: Mapping Meaningful*.
36 Duckworth A. *Grit: The Power of Passion and Perseverance*. Collins, 2016.
37 Speranza L, di Porzio U, Viggiano D et al. Dopamine: The neuromodulator of long-term synaptic plasticity, reward and movement control. *Cells* 2021 Mar 26; 10 (4): 735. doi: 10.3390/cells10040735. PMID: 33810328; PMCID: PMC8066851.
38 Lembke A. *Dopamine Nation: Finding Balance in the Age of Indulgence*. Penguin Random House, 2021.
39 Huberman A. Tools to manage dopamine and improve motivation & drive. *Huberman Lab*. https://www.hubermanlab.com/newsletter/tools-to-manage-dopamine-and-improve-motivation-and-drive. Accessed February 2024.

Scene 3 Not always an injury?!

Nicole Oh

Myth 1 My performance as a competitive cyclist is going to decline now that I have hit menopause

Ageing is inevitable, but a decline in the health and performance of female athletes and active women due to hitting menopause is not necessarily so.

As we know, during perimenopause and menopause, the ovaries start to wind-down their production of eggs and hormones. It is this decline in hormones, particularly in oestrogen, that is responsible for many of the unfavourable changes that occur in our body during this period.

In terms of performance, the changes that worry us most are a loss of muscle mass and strength, and undesirable changes to body composition. There is also an increased risk of injury due to declining bone health and changes to our ligaments and tendons. Disruption of sleep and psychological issues can be more far-reaching.

Some masters athletes may feel even more disadvantaged if they continue to compete at an elite level against much younger athletes who have yet to experience hormonal-related decline.

So how do these changes affect us as masters athletes and active women?

Muscle mass in women tends to decrease gradually after 30 years of age, then shows an accelerated decline after 50. Low muscle mass and strength is known as sarcopenia. A paper in 2022[1] states that during the menopausal transition lean body mass decreased by 0.5% per year, whilst fat mass increased by 1.7% per year. The loss of oestradiol (the most potent and abundant type of oestrogen) is believed to be the most important contributor to menopause-associated loss of muscle mass. The decline in free testosterone could also play a role in the accelerated muscle mass loss with menopause.

Since muscle mass is more metabolically active than fat mass, a loss of lean muscle mass and a subsequent increase in fat mass can affect body composition. Furthermore, increased levels of cortisol (the stress hormone) have been associated with menopausal symptoms, and one of the side effects of chronically elevated cortisol is an increase in fat storage. Less muscle and more fat mass can negatively affect the power-to-weight ratio, which is of concern to competitive cyclists in particular.

It is understandable that some women may start to restrict calorie (and carbohydrate) intake in an attempt to mitigate these changes. However, low-calorie diets can also increase cortisol levels due to under-fuelling, making it harder to lose weight.

Low levels of oestrogen significantly increase bone resorption over formation due to the loss of restraint and control that oestrogen has over mediators of bone resorption, thus inducing accelerated bone loss. This loss of bone mineral density puts menopausal women at increased risk of osteopenia and osteoporosis, which predisposes them to fractures.

Declining bone health may be of particular concern for cyclists and runners. Unlike other menopausal symptoms, which are more apparent, there is little indication of what your bone density is like unless you have a fracture, perhaps a bony stress fracture or one resulting from a crash or fall.

Hormone-related sleep disturbances present another challenge. Whilst adequate sleep is important for everyone, it is particularly important for athletes to allow the body to recover sufficiently and adapt to the training undertaken during the day. The production and regulation of hormones such as growth hormone, cortisol and leptin occur during sleep, all of which play an important role in keeping us strong, lean and healthy.

Finally, a number of psychological changes are associated with the menopause transition. Some commonly reported symptoms are low mood, decreased motivation and confidence, and anxiety. If this is coupled with a performance drop, it can lead to a vicious cycle of demoralisation and helplessness.

Perimenopause cyclist story

"Liz has been a competitive cyclist for 10 years, with a background in triathlon and running. A few years ago, Liz recalls losing '100 watts overnight' with an' associated decline in her cycling performance, whilst at the same time, she started to experience perimenopausal symptoms such as irregular periods and hot flushes. On looking back at her training data, there appears to be a dramatic and sudden drop in her maximum 5-second and 1 minute power over this period, whilst her longer duration powers (10-minute, 20-minute, 60-minute) remained fairly consistent. This was despite continuing with her usual training programme, including strength training three times a week. She just accepted this as a 'normal' part of the ageing process and did not seek any assistance.

More recently, Liz was encouraged to have a DEXA (dual X-ray absorptiometry) scan to check her bone density, as she was still training and competing in local and Masters level bike racing. This proved to be within normal ranges, perhaps due to her running and strength training background. She decided to consult her GP anyway about starting HRT to offset any further declines and address her menopausal symptoms".

Since a decline in oestrogen is largely responsible for most menopausal changes and symptoms, hormone replacement therapy (HRT) is an effective treatment option supported by an increasing amount of research. However, the issues that athletes and active women experience can also be addressed with exercise, nutrition and lifestyle changes.

Heavy resistance strength training should be of high priority. This should involve lifting heavy weights at low repetitions and ideally include some plyometrics for speed and impact loading. This is particularly important for cyclists as cycling is largely a non-weight-bearing sport. Strength training will help to preserve muscle mass and slow bone loss by providing a mechanical stimulus for both muscle and bone. Strength and power should also improve, which will enhance performance.

Prioritising more high-intensity interval training (HIIT) and sprint interval training (SIT) over long endurance training is recommended. This type of training, which involves short bursts of hard exercise with relatively short recovery periods, has been shown to have significant metabolic benefits, helping your body to process insulin efficiently, to control blood glucose levels and make you less prone to insulin resistance and weight gain. It has also been shown to reduce abdominal and visceral fat in menopausal women.

Dietary changes can play an important role, not only what you eat but also when you eat it. The needs of your body change as you hit menopause, with your body becoming more sensitive to insulin and carbohydrates and needing fewer carbohydrates overall. This needs to be balanced with ensuring you still eat enough to fuel the training you do, reducing the risk of Relative Energy Deficiency in Sport (REDs) and increased cortisol response. You will also benefit from increased protein intake for muscle protein synthesis and recovery.

The recommended daily intake (RDI) of protein for all ages is 0.8 g/kg body weight per day. For female athletes (premenopausal), it is more like 1.2–2.0 g/kg. Some authors have recommended as much as 1.8–2.4 g/kg for menopausal athletes depending on the type of activity and training undertaken that day. For a 60 kg woman, this equates to 108–144 g of protein. It is suggested that this should be spread out throughout the day in 30–40 g portions.

The timing of protein intake is also crucial and it is imperative to consume protein (as well as carbohydrates) immediately after training to facilitate the muscle-building (anabolic) stimulus of exercise. This will allow for the building and maintenance of muscle and recovery for subsequent sessions.

Taking in some protein before sleep can also support muscle formation by increasing overnight muscle protein synthesis rate. Casein protein (found in milk), characterised by its slow digestion, may be a good choice.

You should also ensure that you are getting enough vitamin D and calcium, both of which have a positive effect on muscle and bone. Vitamin D helps to absorb and retain calcium (important for bone building) as well as playing a major regulating role in muscle function. Vitamins and minerals are best obtained from dietary sources; however, supplementation may be required if this is inadequate. Vitamin D is also produced by our body in response to sun exposure.

Finally, prioritising sleep and recovery will enable us to function at our best, both physically and mentally. It is well known that sleep is important for both optimal health and performance. However, a lack of adequate sleep seems to be an eternal problem of modern society, especially for mid-life athletes with the competing demands of work and family.

Myth 2 I'm experiencing more aches and pains since menopause and seem to be getting injured more often

Joint and musculoskeletal pain is one of the lesser-known symptoms of menopause but can still affect a large number of women. A study in 2020[2] has estimated that its prevalence can be as high as 71%. It is not uncommon for people suffering from increasing aches and pains to attribute them to simply "getting old", when in fact they may have more to do with declining levels of hormones.

It is also feasible that female masters athletes and active women assume these pains are due to some form of musculoskeletal injury, perhaps related to their training load, technique or biomechanical factors, rather than to their hormones.

Furthermore, studies[3] have shown that underlying joint conditions such as osteoarthritis (OA), are more commonplace in women of menopausal age, far more than their male counterparts of equivalent age. If you have an underlying joint condition, it can be difficult to tell the difference between aches and pains from menopause and those from arthritis.

It is important to distinguish between the likely causes of these aches and pains so that they can be managed effectively. It is essential to know when and whom to ask, for more help, advice and treatment.

An overuse or musculoskeletal injury will commonly only involve a single joint. There may have been some trauma or a preceding incident or a buildup of load prior to the pain starting. It is largely mechanical in nature, meaning it will vary depending on movement and load. There are usually activities and positions that aggravate the issue and ones that ease it (including rest). There could perhaps be changes on investigative scans, such as magnetic resonance imaging (MRI) or ultrasound, if some degree of tissue damage is present. If an actual injury is suspected, it is important to seek appropriate management from a medical doctor, physiotherapist or other healthcare practitioner.

There are other causes of aches and pains that need to be identified, as they would also benefit from medical investigation, diagnosis and treatment. Inflammatory arthritis (e.g. rheumatoid arthritis, psoriatic arthritis, ankylosing spondylitis), other autoimmune disorders, postviral syndrome and chronic fatigue are just a few other conditions that can manifest as joint pain. These are more likely to involve multiple joints, stiffness (especially first thing in the morning) and systemic symptoms such as dry eyes and mouth, skin rashes, fatigue and other organ involvement (heart, lung, bowels).

So, what happens when the physiotherapist and medical team are not able to find any evidence of underlying injury or illness? These aches and pains could in fact be due to menopause, particularly if the woman is also suffering from other menopausal symptoms.

Joint symptoms experienced are similar to inflammatory arthritis, often involving more than one joint, with some associated stiffness. Oestrogen and progesterone have anti-inflammatory properties, and as levels of these hormones drop during menopause, it can lead to increased inflammation and joint discomfort.

A reduction in oestrogen also results in changes to tendons, ligaments and cartilage through decreased collagen synthesis. This reduces tensile strength (tension under load) and negatively effects healing. We already know declining oestrogen levels result in decreased bone density and muscle loss.

A lack of support from muscles and connective tissue surrounding joints due to these changes can contribute to joint pain. Weakening of these musculoskeletal structures makes them more susceptible to injury. Therefore, during menopause, women are at increased risk of muscle tears, bony stress injuries and tendinopathies, to name a few.

OA is a degenerative joint disease and is the most common form of arthritis. There have been many papers looking into the relationship between menopause and OA. OA and OA-related pain, regardless of the joint, are experienced by up to twice as many women as men, and this difference is amplified during menopause[3]. The presence of oestrogen receptors in joint tissues suggests that oestrogen could have a protective role in the development of OA[4]. However, all aches and stiff joints are not necessarily indicative of radiological OA[5].

If aches and pains are largely due to menopause rather than any specific condition, there are a number of things that can be done to address them. As mentioned previously, restoring hormone levels through HRT is a recommended treatment for menopausal symptoms, including joint pain. The same strategies that build muscle mass and bone density (strength training, protein intake, vitamin D and calcium) will also help by providing more support to joints.

General exercise, particularly mobility work, will also help to manage joint pain and stiffness. This includes dynamic stretching, foam rolling, Pilates or yoga, and whole body aerobic exercise such as swimming, walking and dance, which will also help to manage weight, and hence place less load and stress on joints.

Finally, pain relief in the form of analgesic and anti-inflammatory medication, ice or heat, and massage may be effective. It will also help you keep moving and enable you to continue to exercise.

Sally, cyclist, menopause story

"Sally is a physiotherapist and competitive cyclist, competing at elite and national levels. She had been on the combined contraceptive pill for more than 10 years, which she decided to stop after forgetting to take it for a few days at the age of 45, and never regained her period. Around this time, she started to notice some menopausal symptoms such as hot flushes, sleep disturbances, poor memory, and most notably, joint stiffness and aching of her hands, wrists, elbows, knees and spine. It was hard to distinguish whether these aches and pains were due to the high load of training and/or her occupation, from overuse injury or from other causes.

She was concerned about both her lack of period and joint aching, and whether they might indicate systemic issues such as REDs or some form of arthritis or autoimmune disorder. Her GP sent her for some blood tests to investigate, including rheumatoid markers, thyroid function, vitamin D, full blood count and hormone levels, as well as a DEXA scan.

The blood tests were all essentially normal. However, all her hormones were at a menopausal level (low oestrogen and progesterone, and high follicle-stimulating hormone [FSH] and luteinising hormone [LH]). Bone density was now of concern, having appeared to have hit menopause at a young age, and the high risk of crashing during bike races. Her DEXA scan showed that she was osteopenic. This was in comparison to a DEXA scan 5 years earlier, which showed above-average bone density.

She decided to start HRT immediately, mainly to prevent further bone loss, but also to assist in maintaining muscle mass to remain competitive as a cyclist, as well as manage some menopausal symptoms."

In conclusion, there are challenges in progressing into the masters ranks, especially if your age group includes "youngsters" who have not yet reached perimenopause and menopause. As youngsters, we hope to be the oldest in a particular age group, but the reverse applies when moving into masters ranks. It can become complicated when it takes time to realise that "aches and pains" might not be due to injury but rather associated with hormone changes occurring around menopause. However, once the connection has been made, it becomes easier to plan moving forward with a combination of modifications in training, nutrition and recovery and consideration of HRT.

References

1 Buckinx F, Aubertin-Leheudre M. Sarcopenia in menopausal women: Current perspectives. *International Journal of Women's Health* 2022; 14: 805–819. doi: 10.2147/IJWH.S340537.
2 Lu C, Liu P, Zhou Y et al. Musculoskeletal pain during the menopausal transition: A systematic review and meta-analysis. *Neural Plasticity* 2020. doi: 10.1155/2020/8842110.
3 Pang H, Chen S, Klyne D et al. Low back pain and osteoarthritis pain: A perspective of estrogen. *Bone Research* 2023; 11: 42. doi: 10.1038/s41413-023-00280-x.
4 Xiao Y, Tian F, Dai M et al. Are oestrogen-related drugs new alternatives for the management of osteoarthritis? *Arthritis Research & Therapy* 2016; 18: 15. doi: 10.1186/s13075-016-1045-7.
5 Szoeke C, Cicuttini F, Guthrie J et al. The relationship of reports of aches and joint pains to the menopausal transition: A longitudinal study. *Climacteric* 2008; 11 (1): 55–62. doi: 10.1080/13697130701746006.

Scene 4 Strength training for performance and health

Dr Richard C Blagrove

Introduction

Women experience many physiological changes during menopause, including several that affect musculoskeletal health, which can impact quality of life and risk of disease. Despite these physical changes, menopause should not be viewed as a sign of inevitable decline in health and performance. There is clear evidence that regular participation in physical activity and exercise programmes, which includes strength training, can offset the physical decline associated with menopause. Furthermore, for many women, menopause can represent a 'window of opportunity' where motivation is high to make positive lifestyle modifications[1]. This may include trying new and challenging forms of exercise, such as strength training!

For women who are already physically active and/or participate in sport(s) after menopause, the decline in musculoskeletal health is likely to be slower, but not completely halted. Participating in strength training alongside other types of exercise and sport is therefore important and is likely to reduce the risk of developing an injury. The aim of this scene is to outline the main changes that occur to muscle and bone in the postmenopausal years and explain how strength-based exercise can be beneficial during this stage of a woman's life. The scene also addresses common myths related to strength training and includes recommendations on basic strengthening exercises and prescription.

Postmenopausal changes to muscle and bone

With ageing and particularly after menopause, women experience reductions in the circulating levels of several important hormones responsible for regulating muscle mass and bone health status. Progressive reductions in muscle and bone mass have important implications for health, physical fitness and risk of disease; therefore, they represent a significant problem for postmenopausal women. if left unchecked.

From around 30 years of age, muscle mass begins to decline (a process known as 'atrophy') by 3–8% per decade. After menopause, muscle loss begins to accelerate, and above age 70, the decreases in muscle are ~0.7% per year in women[2]. Alongside a loss of muscle, ageing is also associated with a loss of function (collectively known as 'sarcopenia'), which can compromise daily living and is associated with frailty and disability.

In postmenopausal women, decreasing levels of oestrogen result in greater bone breakdown than bone formation/repair, which can lead to reductions in bone health and eventually osteoporosis. The rate of bone loss is around 1–2% per year in postmenopausal women, with maximum losses typically occurring 5–7 years after menopause[3]. Due to the fragility in bones, osteoporosis is associated with a high incidence of fractures, particularly in the spine and hip[4]. These fractures are often caused by minimal trauma and falls, with the risk exacerbated in those with reduced muscular strength and function. In postmenopausal women, with reduced muscle mass and bone health, the risk of falling is twice as high and risk of sustaining a fracture is 2.7 times greater, compared to women who maintain their muscle mass[5]. Low oestrogen levels in postmenopausal years also accelerates the rate of cartilage degeneration in joints, which can cause inflammation and eventually osteoarthritis[6]. This condition is associated with pain, swelling and joint stiffness, making everyday movements difficult.

Muscle is an energetically active tissue; therefore, a loss in muscle mass often results in gains in fat mass, which is linked with metabolic diseases, such as type 2 diabetes[7]. On average, women gain approximately 0.7 kg (1.5 lbs.) per year during their 5th and 6th decades of life, independent of initial body size or race/ethnicity[8]. In particular, for postmenopausal women, a decrease in oestrogen can lead to a redistribution of fat to visceral (deeper) areas around the abdomen, which increases the risk of cardiovascular disease[9]. Typically, visceral fat increases from 5–8% of total body fat during premenopausal years to 15–20% of total body fat in postmenopausal years[10].

Benefits of strength training

The postmenopausal years are clearly associated with many health-related challenges for women. In older individuals, deteriorations in health are also exacerbated by a sedentary lifestyle and physical inactivity. Consistent long-term engagement in a variety of different types of exercise and sports has been shown to confer numerous health benefits in menopausal and postmenopausal women, that can reduce disease risk and frailty and improve quality of life[11,12]. Although the modality of exercise or sport that women choose to participate in is influenced by personal preference and accessibility, it is well-established that different types of exercise bring about different physiological benefits[13]. Specifically, aerobic-based exercise (e.g. jogging/running, cycling and swimming) is important for maintaining and improving cardiorespiratory fitness, whereas strength training (e.g. resistance training, ballistic exercise and high-impact/plyometric exercises) is important for offsetting the declines in muscle mass, strength and bone and joint health. In this regard, including a combination of both exercise types appears to be most beneficial as a therapeutic strategy for combating health risks in postmenopausal women..

More specifically, strength training activities are imperative to include as part of a holistic and well-rounded approach to healthy living in postmenopausal women, for the reasons summarised in Figure 7.4.1.

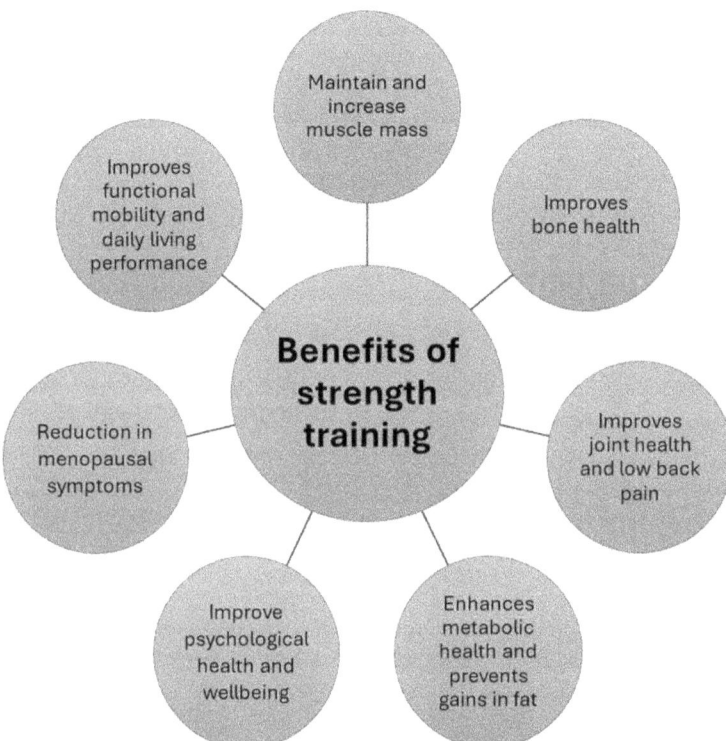

FIGURE 7.4.1 Summary of the main benefits associated with strength training for menopausal and postmenopausal women

Maintain and increase muscle mass

Resistance training is a highly effective stimulus for promoting muscular strength and offsetting the loss of muscle mass[14]. Specifically in postmenopausal and elderly women, numerous scientific studies have shown that engaging in a programme of resistance training can actually increase muscle mass, particularly in those who have not engaged with this form of exercise before[15]. By stimulating muscle growth through resistance training, postmenopausal women can increase strength and functional capacity, ultimately improving their overall health and quality of life.

Improves bone health

Physical inactivity is a major risk factor for osteoporosis and osteoarthritis, with resistance training and high-impact jump training being highlighted as the most effective types of exercise to maintain or improve bone and joint health[16]. By strengthening bones, resistance training reduces the risk of fractures and osteoporosis, allowing women to stay active and continue exercising safely.

Improves joint health and low back pain

Strengthening the muscles around the joints, particularly the trunk muscles, can provide better support and stability to the joints, including those in the lower back. This support can help reduce stress on the joints and alleviate pain[17]. In particular, resistance training that includes exercises targeting the 'posterior chain muscles' (i.e. gluteals, back extensors and hamstrings) are more effective than general exercise for addressing joint stiffness and low back pain[18].

Enhances metabolic health and prevents gains in fat

Muscle is metabolically active tissue, meaning it burns more calories at rest compared to other tissues in the body. By maintaining or increasing muscle mass through resistance training, postmenopausal women can boost their metabolic rate and potentially mitigate age-related weight gain[12].

Improves psychological health and well-being

Exercise stimulates the release of neurotransmitters in the brain, such as endorphins, serotonin and dopamine. These chemicals play a key role in alleviating depression and elevating mood and well-being[19]. Regular strength training exercise also decreases levels of cortisol, the body's primary stress hormone. Lower cortisol levels are associated with reduced feelings of stress and anxiety[20]. Achieving fitness goals and making progress with a strength training programme can also provide a sense of accomplishment and improve self-confidence[21].

Reduction in menopausal symptoms

A high proportion of women experience menopausal symptoms, which are unique to each person. Hormonal therapy is often prescribed to help manage symptoms; however, exercise can be an effective alternative to help manage severity in some women[22]. Hot flushes and night sweats are two of the most common symptoms and strength training can help regulate hormone levels, including oestrogen, thereby alleviating some of these symptoms. Participating in regular exercise can also improve circulation, which may help regulate body temperature and reduce the frequency or severity of hot flushes. The endorphin release that is associated with exercise also provides natural pain relief, which may help reduce the discomfort associated with these symptoms.

Improves functional mobility and daily living performance

While declines in physical performance with ageing can be attributed to a variety of factors, the relationship between muscle capacity measures and physical function is well-established. For example, leg muscle strength is associated with maximum walking/running speed[23], and older women with the lowest knee extension strength are 6 times more likely to report impairments in daily living activities compared to the strongest women[24]. In older women, falls can be catastrophic, often resulting in fracture, serious injury, chronic pain and disability. Resistance training, particularly exercises that have an element of instability, has been shown to reduce the risk of falls in older individuals[25,26].

Myths associated with strength training in postmenopausal women

Many barriers to strength training exercise in older women have been previously documented[27], with several of these perceived challenges linked to myths associated with strength-based exercise. These include a fear of injury or worsening pain with strength training, health beliefs associated with different exercise modalities, a lack of support and lack of access to appropriate facilities.

Myth 1 Postmenopausal women cannot increase muscle mass because of low hormone levels

Important hormones that have anabolic (tissue-building) effects (e.g. oestrogen, testosterone) show a decline with ageing, which has a detrimental effect on skeletal muscle mass and functionality. It could therefore be assumed that women are unable to maintain or increase muscle mass during their postmenopausal years; however, this is not the case. There is clear evidence that significant improvements in lean muscle mass are possible in postmenopausal women[15,28], and oestrogen levels are not associated with muscle mass or function after the menopause[29]. Although female sex hormones play a minor role in stimulating an increase in muscle mass with resistance training, there is consensus that mechanical tension (i.e. a high load imposed on muscle fibres) and metabolic stress (i.e. rapid use of energy in muscles during high-effort exercise) are more important for producing a hypertrophy (muscle building) response[30]. Importantly, these factors are unrelated to ageing; therefore, women should feel confident they can make meaningful improvements in strength and muscle mass in their later years.

Myth 2 Strength-based exercises are risky and dangerous at my age

It is often assumed that lifting heavy weights carries a high risk of injury; however, there is barely a shred of evidence to support this assertion. There is overwhelming agreement that strength training activities are safe and beneficial for postmenopausal women when performed under the guidance of a qualified practitioner. In fact, there is no scientific evidence that shows that progressive strength training carries any greater risk in older adults compared to younger individuals. The risk of an adverse medical event, including an injury, in older women participating in strength training is very low[16,31], and injuries that do occur tend to be due to inappropriate training behaviours, such as poor technique or progressing too quickly. Recommendations for strength training in older individuals do tend to follow a cautious approach, which certainly helps reduce the risk of injury further. However, data from studies that have taken an aggressive approach to loading intensity in postmenopausal women unaccustomed to exercise have shown this type of exercise is remarkably safe and only provides benefits to participants[32].

Myth 3 Why can't I get the same results as I used to from exercise?

Although there are inevitable age-related declines in physical function and musculoskeletal health, these can be substantially offset by consistent engagement with exercise. In active women and competitive master athletes who habitually engage in strength training exercise, it is likely that with ageing, a higher dose of weekly loading compared to young individuals is required to maintain or increase muscle mass long-term[33]. However, strength in long-term exercisers remains well-preserved and above levels of untrained adults[34]. In peri- and postmenopausal women who commence strength training for the first time, or after a long period of disengagement, improvements in strength-related qualities and performance are likely to be large. Indeed, increases in muscle mass following a period of resistance training appear to be similar in old versus young individuals, as do the improvements in the underlying neuromuscular and skeletal adaptations[35].

Myth 4 Other types of exercise are a higher priority than strength training

The British Menopause Society, as well as other prominent health organisations[36], recommend that ageing women participate in both cardiorespiratory (aerobic) exercise, for example, walking/running and strength-based exercise several times per week. Continuous prolonged exercise at a moderate intensity improves cardiorespiratory and metabolic health and fitness and is therefore important to include as part of a well-rounded exercise routine. However, strength training offers a broad range of benefits to musculoskeletal health, including the positive effects described in this chapter, which cardiorespiratory exercise cannot provide.

Individual preferences and barriers to some exercise modalities can make engagement with both aerobic and strength training difficult to achieve for many women. There is, however, an emerging body of evidence showing that resistance training appears to be equally as effective as aerobic endurance exercise in improving cardiometabolic health and reduces risk of several chronic diseases in those who are less active[37,38]. Indeed, it is recognised that engaging in higher-intensity (high relative 'physical effort') exercise is the most impactful type of training to reduce risk of disease, with strength training falling into this higher effort-based paradigm of activity[38].

Myth 5 I need to join a gym to do strength training

Although public gyms or fitness centres offer a range of different equipment and classes that women can use to improve their strength, it is not necessarily essential to pay for a membership. For those who are new to strength training and are unsure about correct technique and prescription, it is highly advisable to speak to a qualified fitness professional who can guide you through a programme. Thereafter, particularly in the early stages of a programme, many strength training exercises can be performed in a home-based environment against bodyweight or with minimal equipment such as resistance bands or light free weights (e.g. barbells, dumbbells, kettlebells). Examples of these types of exercises are shown later in this chapter. Furthermore, there is a strong argument that 'ballistic exercises', which aim to develop explosive power, and high-impact jump training are the most important types of strength training for older individuals. These types of exercises require virtually no equipment, so a gym facility is not essential.

Should any women be cautious or seek medical advice before commencing strength training?

Older women with frailty, osteoporosis, arthritis, cardiometabolic disease or other chronic conditions may be limited with the exercise testing and prescription they are able to safely perform. However, there is clear evidence that almost all older individuals can benefit from increasing their levels of physical activity, which includes strength-based exercise[39]. It is important for those with an existing chronic health condition to initially consult with their medical doctor/physician, and preliminary risk stratification should be conducted based on the risk for cardiovascular incidents or other adverse events[40]. In general, strength training is well-tolerated by older women with chronic health conditions[39]; however, exercise professionals should ensure that prescriptions are individualised based on recommendations from a medical doctor/physician. For women who are currently exercising and are asymptomatic, preparticipation screening is not required and presents an unnecessary barrier to beginning and maintaining an exercise programme[41].

Resistance training has been associated with safety concerns for older adults with hypertension (high blood pressure) and cardiovascular disease. Unstable hypertension is a contraindication to resistance training exercise; thus, it is advised that clinical stability in blood pressure is reached in these individuals prior to commencing a strength training programme[42]. In women with medically diagnosed hypertension that is under control, resistance training is effective for improving outcomes related to blood pressure and cardiovascular health; however, blood pressure response and symptoms should be monitored closely during exercise. Older women with cardiovascular disease who have obtained medical clearance to perform resistance training should commence exercises at a relatively low intensity, progress slowly and avoid breath-holding techniques, that is, the Valsalva manoeuvre[39].

For women with frailty, a lower load should initially be selected, and progressive overload should be gradual. Those with mobility limitations may also benefit more from exercise in a seated position. For older women with mild cognitive impairments or dementia, simple exercises should be selected, and clear instructions should be provided. Strength training performed under close supervision in osteoporotic women has been linked with very few adverse effects and no vertebral fractures, thus is considered safe and appropriate[16]. In women with osteoporosis, exercises to improve muscle strength in the back muscles are recommended to improve posture and support the spine; however, movements that involve sustained, repeated or end-range spinal flexion or hyperextension should be avoided, especially under-load[16].

Strength training exercises

Strength training activities broadly fall into three main categories: resistance training, ballistic exercises and high-impact (or plyometric) exercises. Each type of strength training offers slightly different, but equally important, benefits for musculoskeletal health, functional living and reduced risk of disease.

Resistance training

Resistance training involves moving a load (your bodyweight and/or external load) through a defined movement pattern. These movement patterns could be dictated by a resistance machine, for example, a leg press or chest press machine; however, research suggests that more 'functional' training exercises are more beneficial for several important health reasons and transfer better to daily living tasks[39]. These 'functional' exercises tend to be multi-joint dynamic skills that involve individuals supporting their own bodyweight (plus external load where appropriate). It is best to think about, and progress, these exercises within six main categories that target different movement patterns and muscle groups:

- Squat
- Hip hinge
- Step-up
- Lunge
- Push
- Pull

In simple terms, selecting one exercise from each of these categories as part of a resistance training session offers a well-rounded approach to improving muscular strength in different body parts. It is also a good idea to include an exercise that targets muscles that 'brace' (or stiffen) and rotate your trunk. Examples of these exercises in both a home-based and gym setting are described in the next section.

Ballistic exercises

Muscular power represents a particularly important target for strength training interventions as it declines with ageing sooner and more rapidly compared to maximal strength[43]. Muscle power also has important implications for tasks involving rapid application of force, such as preventing falls and any sports skills. Although traditional resistance training can improve muscular power to a small extent, it is important to include some 'ballistic' exercises in a long-term strength programme. Ballistic training involves movements without a deceleration phase, performed as fast and explosively as possible with only bodyweight or a light external load.

High-impact (plyometric) exercise

Plyometric training uses jumping and hopping exercises that involve 'bouncing' from one repetition to the next. The aim of the exercises is to 'bounce' or jump/hop high whilst also ensuring the foot spends a short time in contact with the ground. Like ballistic training, these exercises benefit muscular power, but importantly, they involve relatively high-impact landing forces that are a potent stimulus for improving bone health. For those with osteoporosis, or new to this type of training, it is important to start with lower-intensity impact exercises before gradually increasing the intensity.

Strength training prescription

A summary of the recommendations for prescribing the three main types of strength training is shown in Table 7.4.1. It is important that these general guidelines are adapted for an individual's level of experience, personal preferences and chronic health conditions.

Home-based resistance training

Squat

1. Stand with feet slightly wider than hip width with toes turned out at 5-to-1 on a clockface (Figure 7.4.2a).
2. Raise arms in front at shoulder height (Figure 7.4.2b).
3. Bend at the knees and hips, keeping feet flat on the ground and back straight. Squeeze knees outwards along the line of the big toes.

TABLE 7.4.1 Strength training recommendations for menopausal and postmenopausal women relatively new to strength training[16,39]. *Exercises could be part of a resistance training session; 1RM = maximum load that can be lifted just once; GCT = ground contact time

	Resistance training	Ballistic exercises	High-impact (plyometric) exercises
Frequency (per week)	2–3	2–3	Most days
Number of exercises per session	5–8	2*	2–3
Sets per exercise	3	2–3	2–3
Repetitions per set	6–12	6	10
Repetitions per session	120–200	24	50–80
Intensity	80–85% 1RM or effort of 8 out of 10	40–60% 1RM; maximal effort or intent to move fast	Short GCT; large height/distance
Inter-set recovery	2–3 min	2–3 min	~2 min

4. Descend until thighs are roughly parallel to the ground or the spine begins to flex (Figure 7.4.2c).
5. Push through the heels and lead with the chest to return to a standing position.

Progression: Stand on a resistance band, ensuring you grip the band in a position where there is no slack in the bottom position of the movement (Figure 7.4.2d).

Glute bridge

1. Lie on your back with your knees bent and feet flat on the floor, hip-width apart.
2. Fold your arms across your chest (Figure 7.4.3a).
3. Engage your trunk muscles to maintain a neutral spine position. throughout the movement.
4. Push through your heels as you lift your hips towards the ceiling, forming a straight line from your shoulders to your knees (Figure 7.4.3b).
5. Squeeze your glutes at the top of the movement and hold for a moment.
6. Lower your hips back down to the starting position under control, avoiding any arching or overarching of the lower back.

Progression: Place the ends of a resistance band around your feet and the middle part of the band across your hips (Figure 7.4.3c).

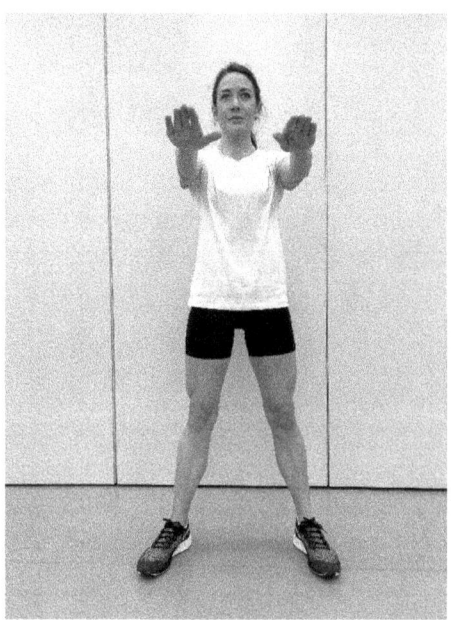

FIGURE 7.4.2A Squat start position (front view)

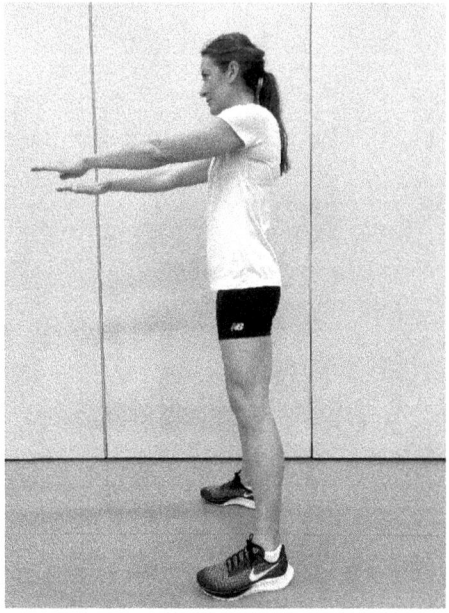

FIGURE 7.4.2B Squat start position (side view)

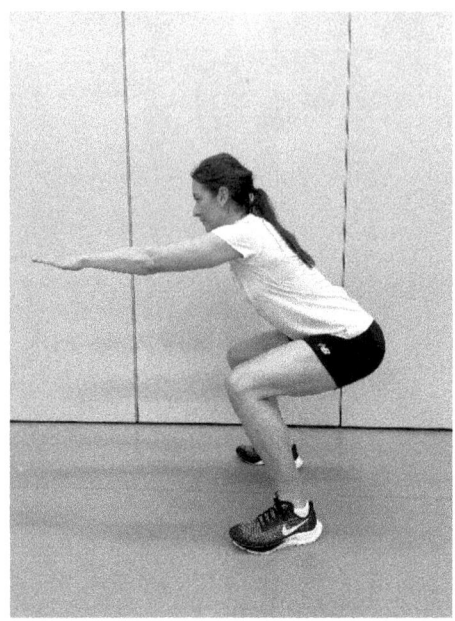

FIGURE 7.4.2C Squat bottom position

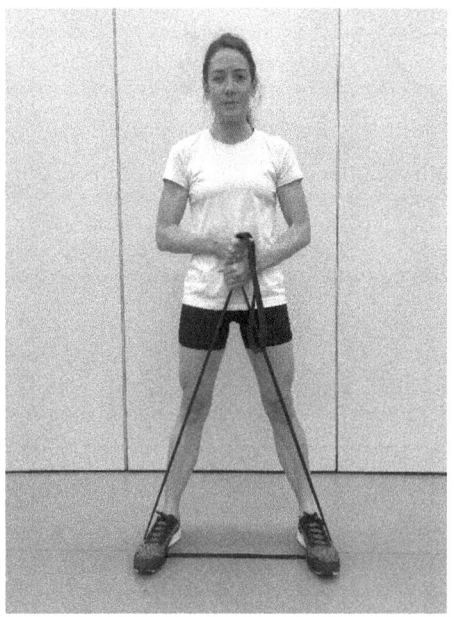

FIGURE 7.4.2D Squat with resistance band

Age Group Athletes

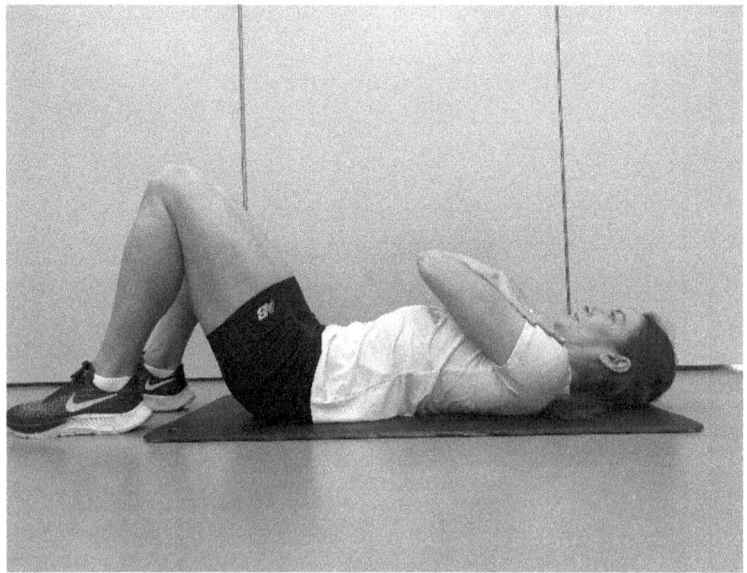

FIGURE 7.4.3A Glute bridge start position

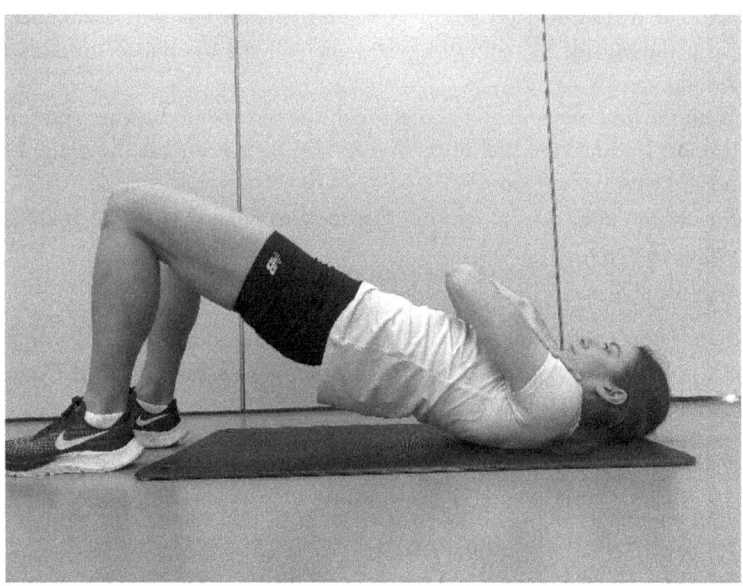

FIGURE 7.4.3B Glute bridge top position

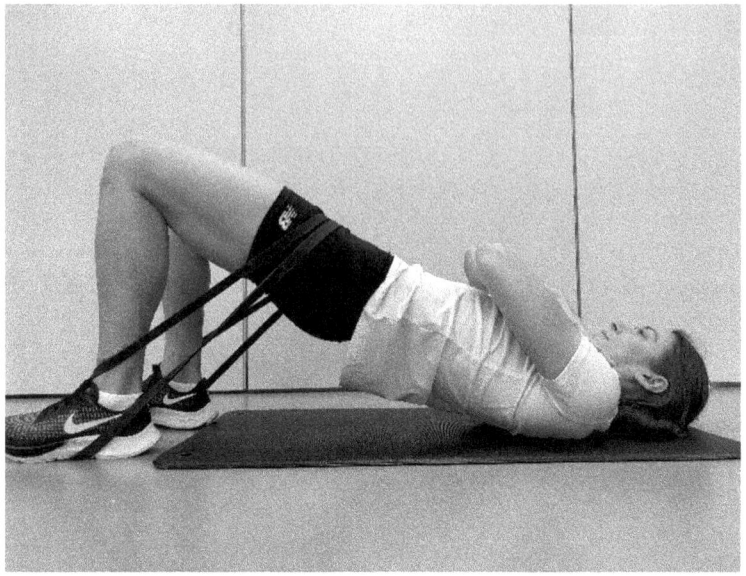

FIGURE 7.4.3C Glute bridge with resistance band

Dead-leg step-up

1. Stand on one leg on a low box or step with arms raised in front at shoulder height.
2. Keep the outside leg completely straight and the toe pulled upwards (Figure 7.4.4a).
3. With the heel remaining in contact with the step, bend the knee and hip of the support leg until the heel of the outside leg lightly touches the ground slightly behind your body (Figure 7.4.4b).
4. Ensure the knee on the standing leg remains aligned with the ankle and hip (Figure 7.4.4c).
5. Push through the heel of the support leg to return back to standing.

Progression: Loop a resistance band around the standing foot and ensure you grip the band in a position where there is no slack in the bottom position of the movement (Figure 7.4.4d).

Split squat

1. Take an exaggerated stride forward so the back heel rises off the ground (Figure 7.4.5a).
2. With the torso in a vertical position, bend the front and back knees so the hips lower vertically downwards.
3. Lower down until the back knee is only just above the ground (Figure 7.4.5b).
4. Push through the front leg to return to a split standing position.

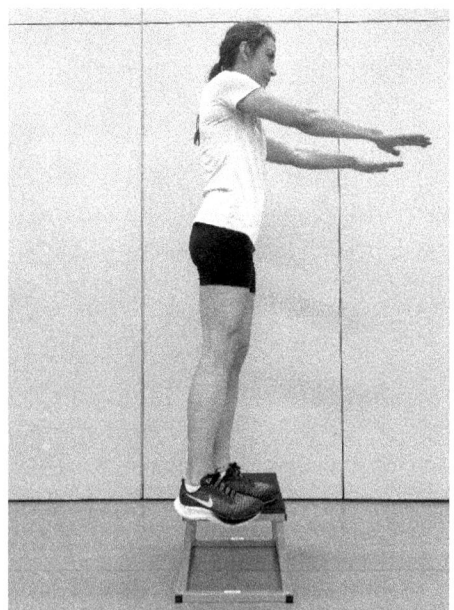

FIGURE 7.4.4A Dead-leg step-up start position

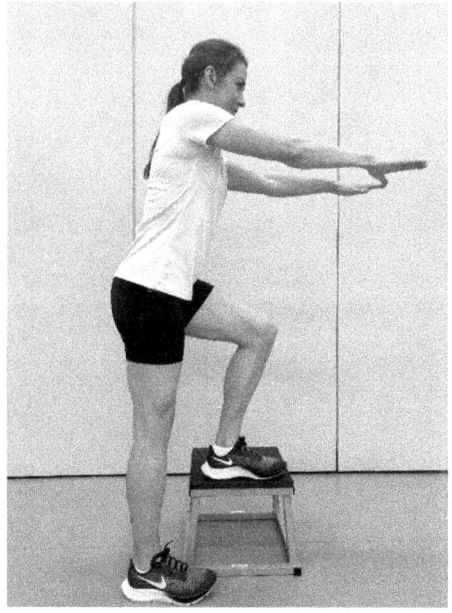

FIGURE 7.4.4B Dead-leg step-up bottom position (side view)

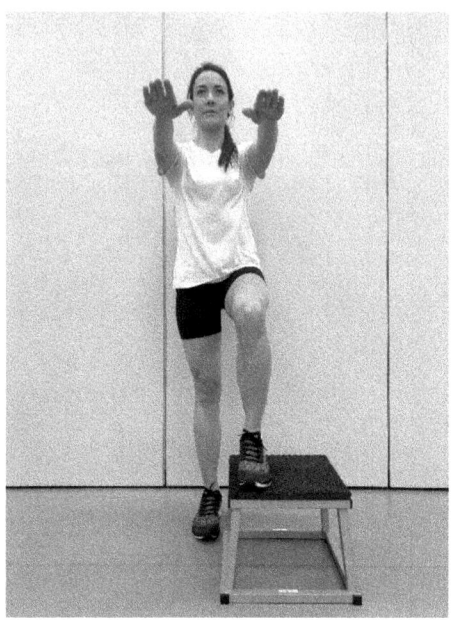

FIGURE 7.4.4C Dead-leg step-up bottom position (front view)

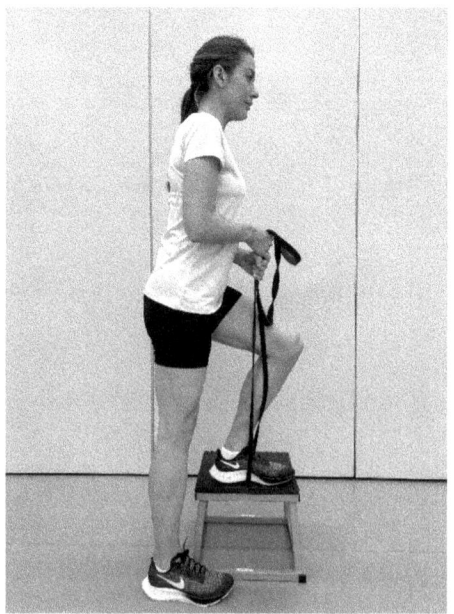

FIGURE 7.4.4D Band resisted dead-leg step-up

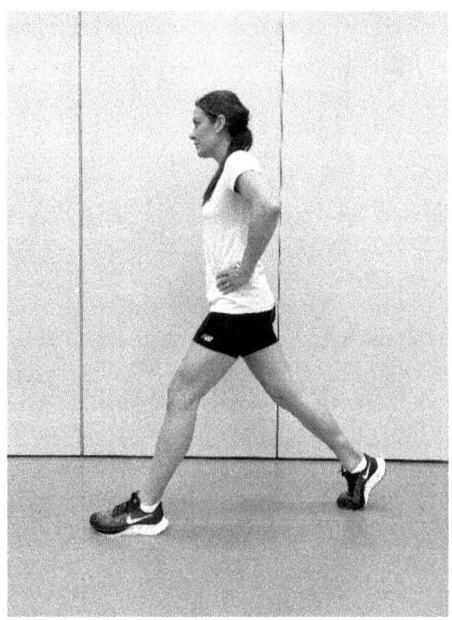

FIGURE 7.4.5A Split squat start position

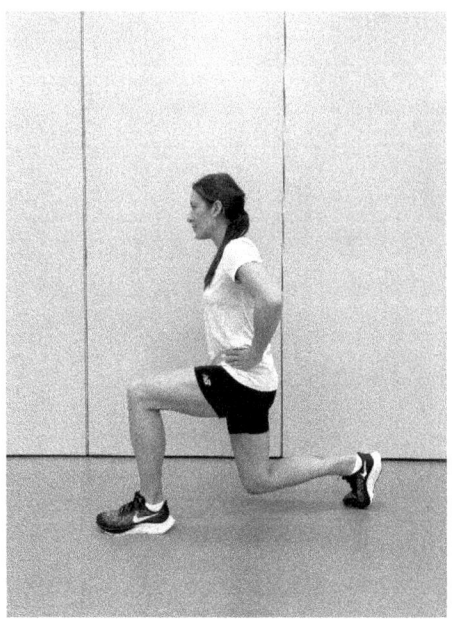

FIGURE 7.4.5B Split squat bottom position

Progression: Perform a reverse lunge by standing on one leg (Figure 7.4.5c) and lunging backwards with the free leg, until you reach the bottom position of a split squat (Figure 7.4.5d). Push off the front leg to return to a standing position.

Kneeling press-up

1. Adopt a press-up position with feet hip-width apart and hands directly under the shoulders.
2. Place knees on the ground so there is a straight line from knees to shoulders (Figure 7.4.6a).
3. Stiffen the trunk so the back remains straight and fix your gaze slightly in front.
4. Bend your elbows to lower your chest until it is slightly above the ground; elbows should remain relatively close to the body (Figure 7.4.6b).
5. Push against the ground to straighten your elbows and return to the start position.

Progression: Perform the exercise from your feet, without the knees on the ground (Figures 7.4.6c and 7.4.6d).

Kneeling band row

1. Tether a resistance band around a fixed, immovable object, such as the handle of a closed door.
2. Remove the slack from the band and kneel down, gripping the band at chest height (Figure 7.4.7a).

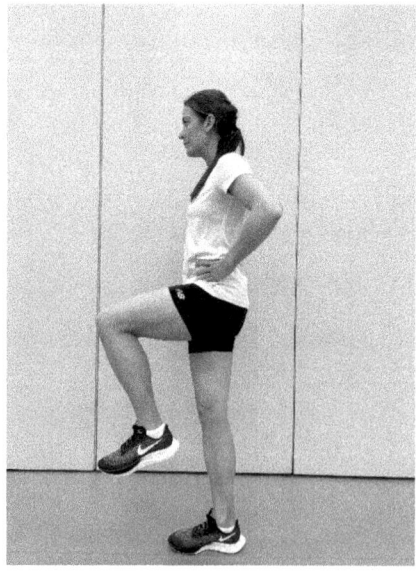

FIGURE 7.4.5C Reverse lunge start position

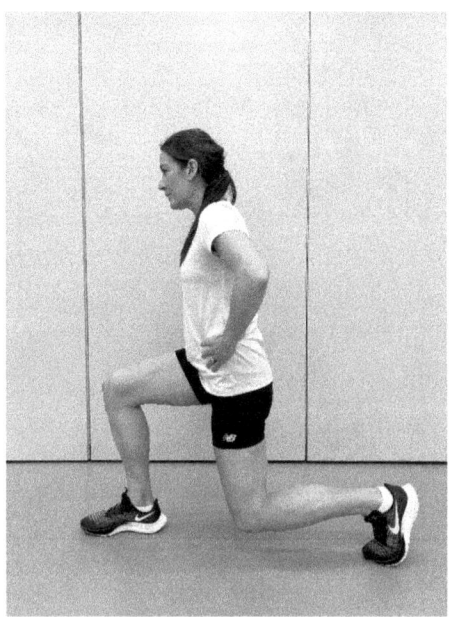

FIGURE 7.4.5D Reverse lunge bottom position

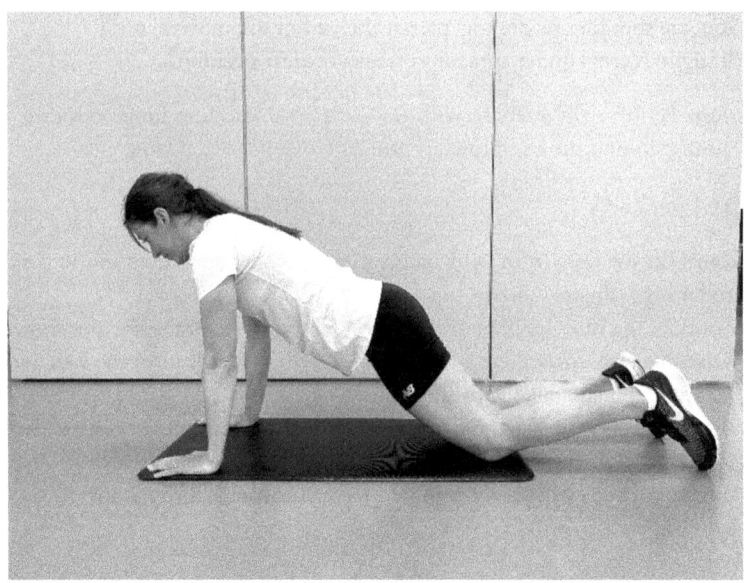

FIGURE 7.4.6A Kneeling press-up start position

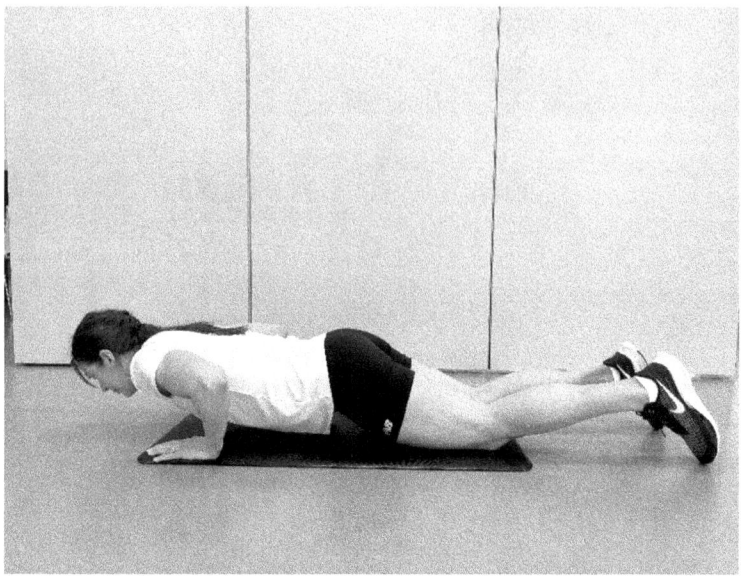

FIGURE 7.4.6B Kneeling press-up bottom position

3. Maintaining torso position and without leaning back, pull the band towards the chest (Figure 7.4.7b).
4. Squeeze shoulder blades together at the end of the movement.
5. Straighten arms under control to return to start position.

Progression: Perform the exercise with one arm in a kneeling lunge position (Figure 7.4.7c) aiming to pull the band to your arm-pit.

Superman from knees

1. Kneel on the floor with your hands directly under shoulders and knees directly under hips (Figure 7.4.8a)
2. Contract the muscles in your trunk to maintain a neutral spine position.
3. Raise one arm upwards and the opposite leg backwards until the arm and upper leg are roughly parallel with the ground.
4. Slowly sweep your leg and arm in and out, brushing the ground at the end of each repetition.
5. Your spine and head position should remain constant throughout the set (Figure 7.4.8b).

Progression: Raise the support-side knee slightly off the ground so you are only supported by one hand and one foot.

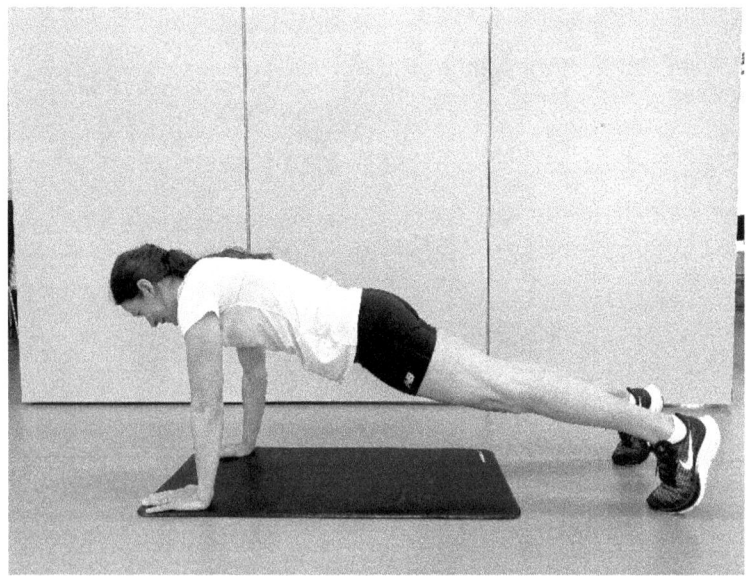

FIGURE 7.4.6C Press-up from feet start position

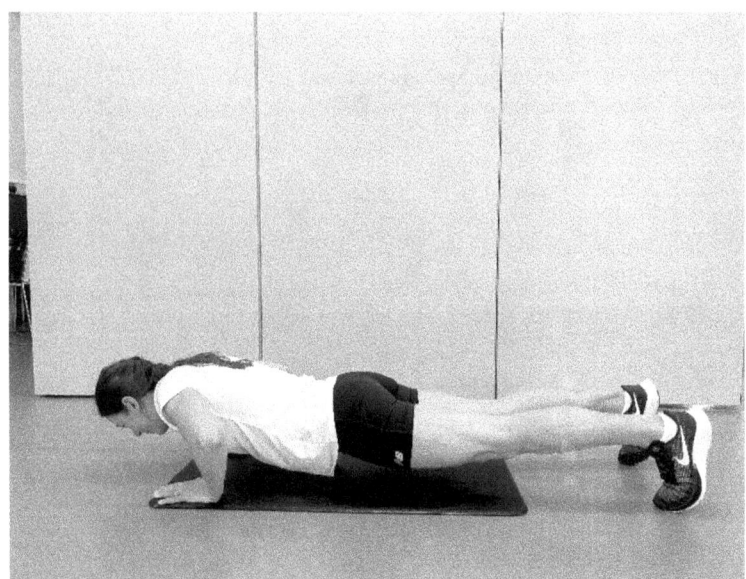

FIGURE 7.4.6D Press-up from feet bottom position

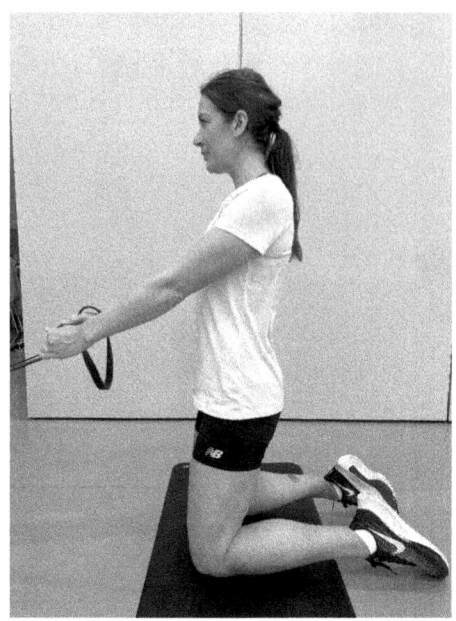

FIGURE 7.4.7A Kneeling band row start position

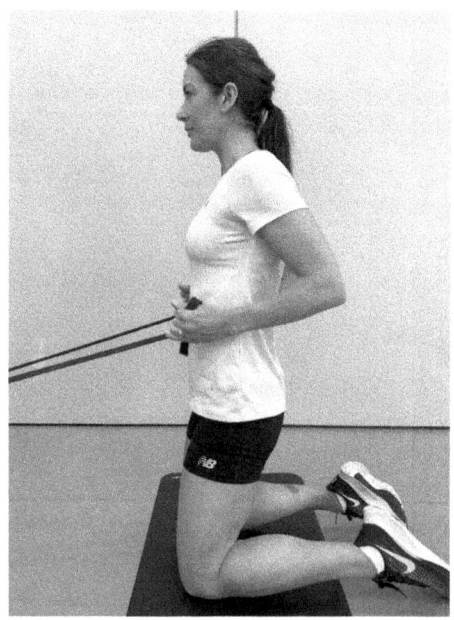

FIGURE 7.4.7B Kneeling band row end position

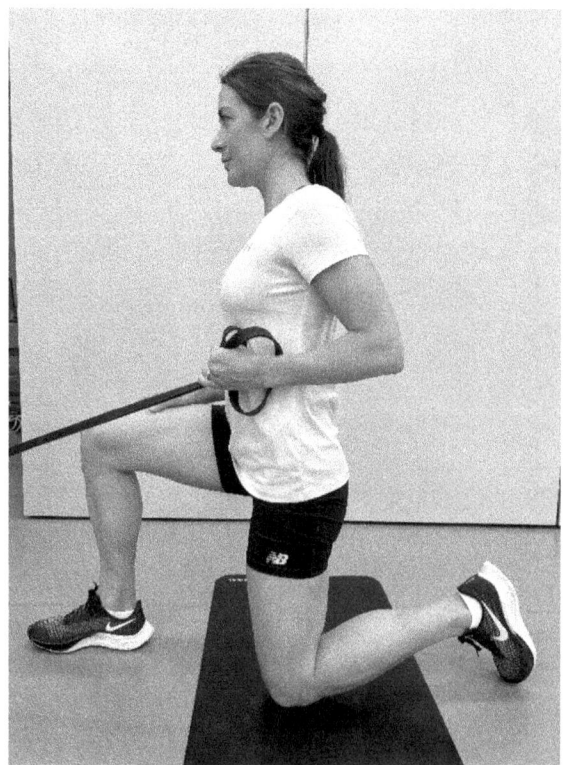

FIGURE 7.4.7C Single-arm kneeling band row

Gym-based resistance training

Back squat

1. Using a squat stand/rack, set up the J-hooks/supports just below shoulder height.
2. Place a barbell in the J-hooks of the squat stand.
3. Facing the stand, grip the barbell evenly and position the centre of the barbell on the muscles of the upper back with shoulder blades squeezed together (Figure 7.4.9a).
4. Standing under the bar in a slightly squatted position, stand up and take one step backwards away from the stand (Figure 7.4.9b).
5. Use the same technique described above for a 'squat' to complete the movement (Figure 7.4.9c).
6. At the end of the set, take a step forward and slowly lower the barbell back into the J-hooks/supports.

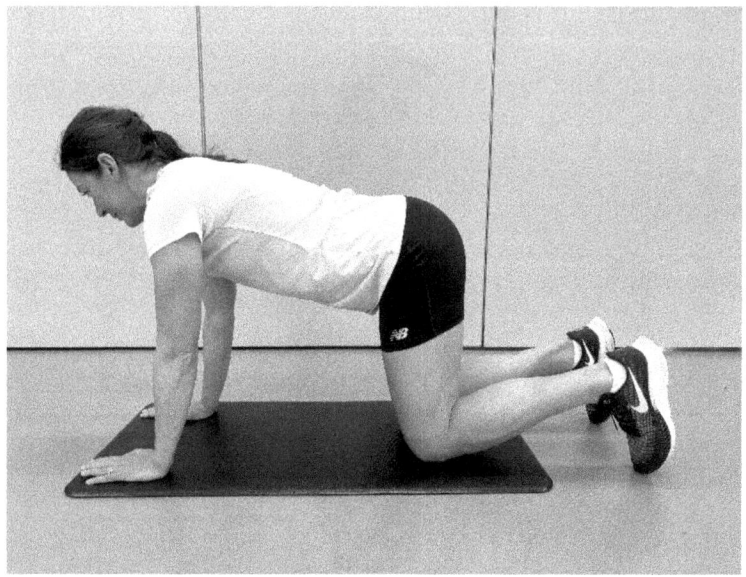

FIGURE 7.4.8A Superman start position

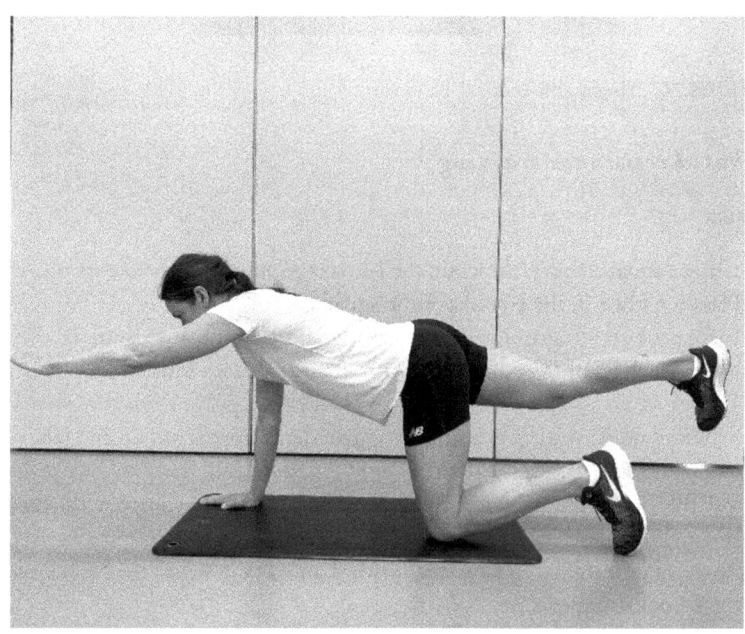

FIGURE 7.4.8B Superman top position

Age Group Athletes

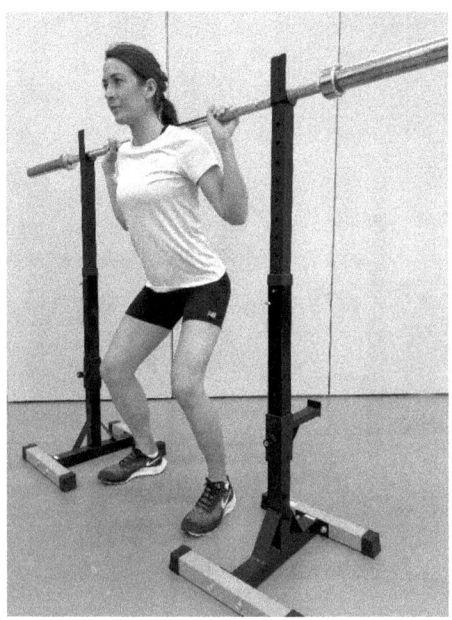

FIGURE 7.4.9A Positioning of the barbell and preparing to perform a back squat

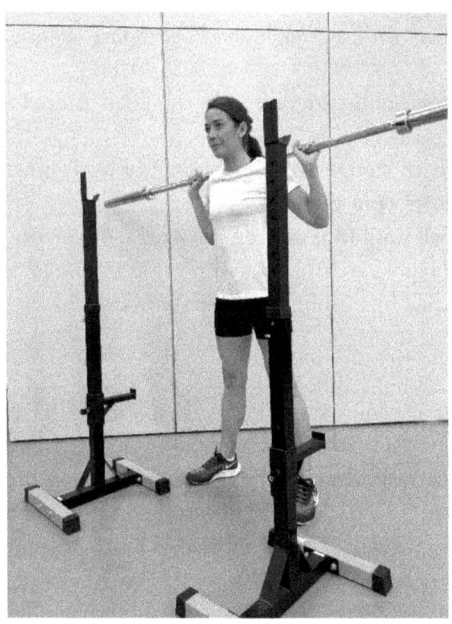

FIGURE 7.4.9B Start position of a back squat

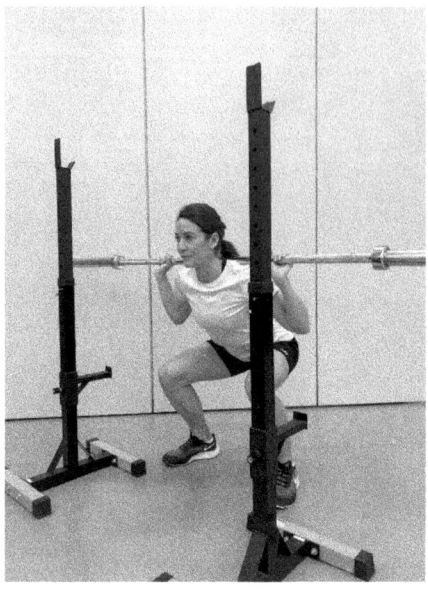

FIGURE 7.4.9C Bottom position of a back squat

Romanian deadlift

1. Pick up a barbell with a straight back, gripping slightly wider than shoulder width.
2. Bend your knees slightly, squeeze your shoulder blades together and stiffen the muscles in the trunk (Figure 7.4.10a).
3. Keeping your back straight and knees slightly bent, hinge from the hip so the barbell slides down your thighs.
4. Lower the barbell until it passes your kneecaps, or you can no longer maintain a straight back (Figure 7.4.10b).
5. Return to standing by pushing your hips forward.

Barbell step-up

1. Set up a barbell in a squat stand/rack as described for a back squat previously.
2. Position a low box/step two steps in front of the squat stand.
3. Approach the barbell facing the box/step and position the barbell on the upper back as described for a back squat previously.
4. Take one step forward so you are positioned just in front of the box/step (Figure 7.4.11a).
5. Place your right foot on the box and push hard through the heel of the right foot, ensuring the knee on the right leg remains aligned with the ankle and hip (Figure 7.4.11b).

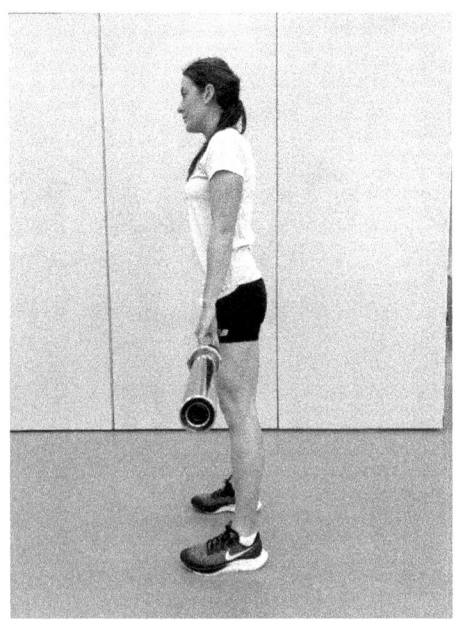

FIGURE 7.4.10A Romanian deadlift start position

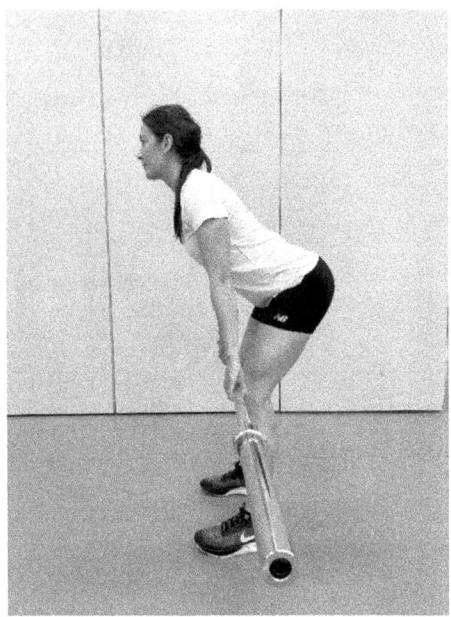

FIGURE 7.4.10B Romanian deadlift bottom position

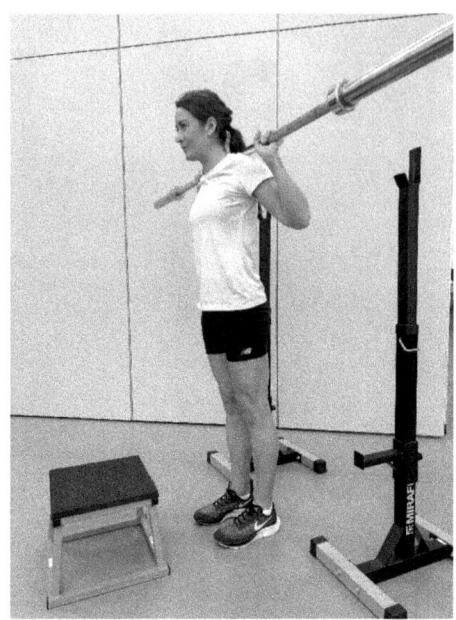

FIGURE 7.4.11A Barbell step-up start position

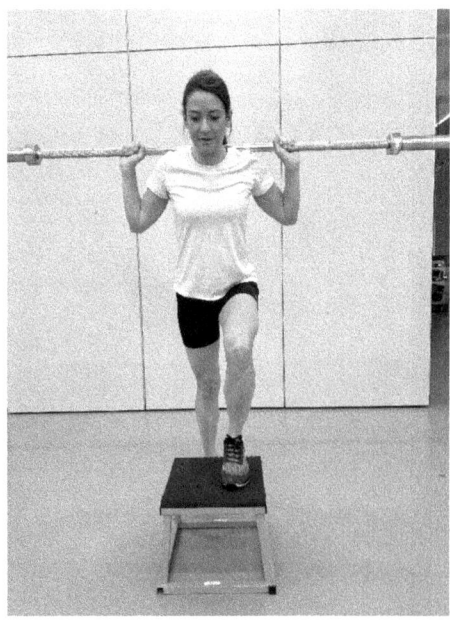

FIGURE 7.4.11B Barbell step-up maintaining knee alignment during push-upwards

Age Group Athletes

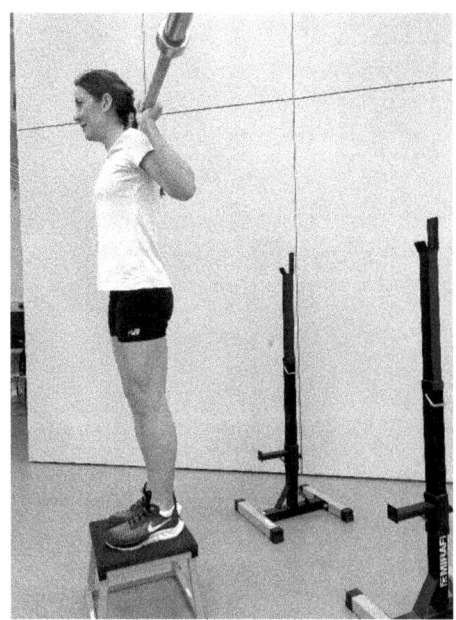

FIGURE 7.4.11C . Barbell step-up finish position

6. Finish with both feet parallel on the box (Figure 7.4.11c).
7. Step down by leading with the left leg first.
8. Complete the prescribed number of repetitions leading with the right leg before switching to the left leg lead.

Dumbbell split squat

1. Pick up two dumbbells and perform a split squat as described previously (Figures 7.4.12a and 7.4.12b).

Barbell press

1. Set up a barbell in a squat stand/rack as described for a back squat previously.
2. Facing the stand, grip the barbell evenly across the upper chest with elbows pointing slightly forward and down.
3. Standing under the bar in a slightly squatted position, stand up and take one step backwards away from the stand (Figure 7.4.13a).
4. Maintaining torso position and without leaning back, push the barbell overhead, being careful not to hit your chin!
5. The barbell should finish over the crown of the head (Figure 7.4.13b).
6. Lower the barbell back down to the upper chest under control.

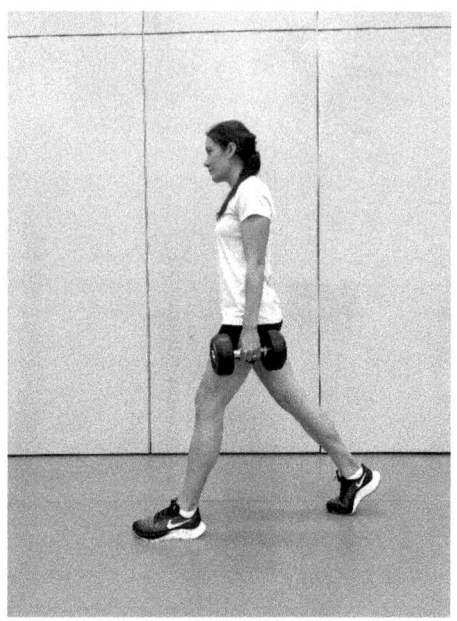

FIGURE 7.4.12A Dumbbell split squat start position

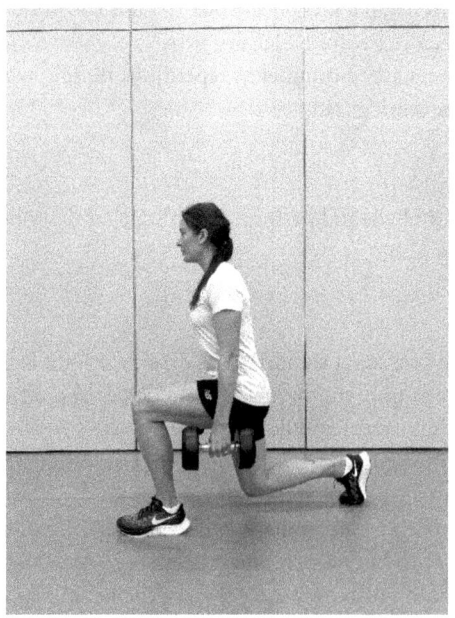

FIGURE 7.4.12B Dumbbell split squat bottom position

Age Group Athletes

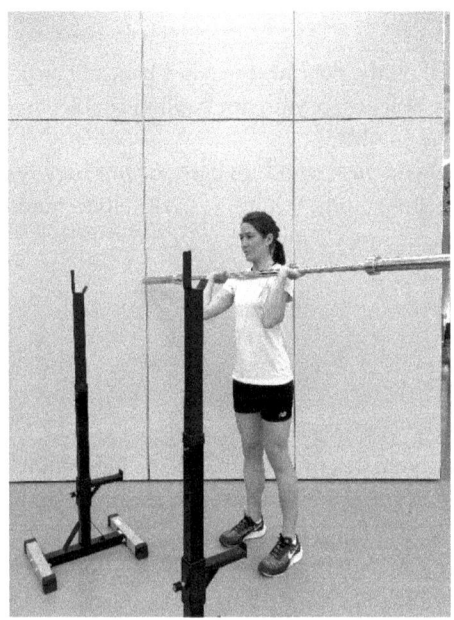

FIGURE 7.4.13A Barbell press start position

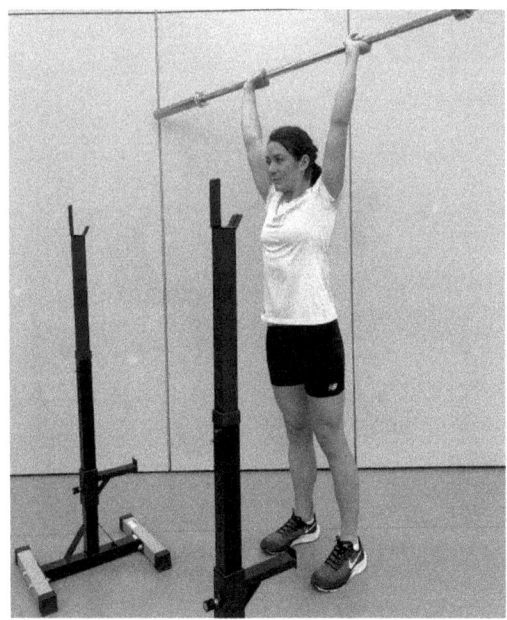

FIGURE 7.4.13B Barbell press top position

Single arm row

1. Place a dumbbell on the floor next to a low bench or step.
2. Crouch over the bench/step, with one hand in contact for support and the other hand holding the dumbbell.
3. Bend your knees and push your hips back so your back is flat (Figure 7.4.14a).
4. Pull the dumbbell vertically, leading with the elbow, until it reaches the armpit and shoulder blades squeeze together (Figure 7.4.14b).
5. Lower the dumbbell down under control.

Ballistic exercises

Squat jump

1. Using only your body weight or holding some light dumbbells or a barbell, start by standing with feet hip-width apart, in a natural jump position.
2. With feet flat on the floor, bend your knees and hips rapidly to a semi-squat position (Figure 7.4.15a), before switching direction and jumping as explosively and high as possible (Figure 7.4.15b).
3. Land under control and ensure knees remain aligned with ankles and hips.

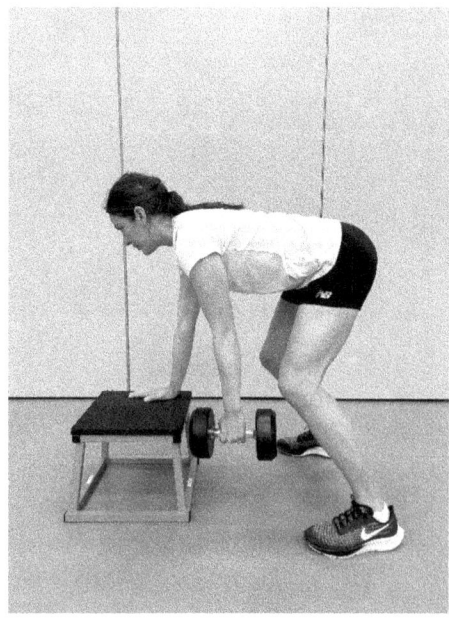

FIGURE 7.4.14A Single arm row start position

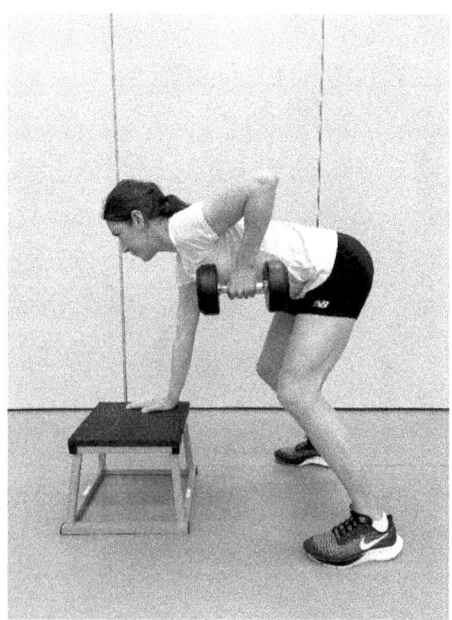

FIGURE 7.4.14B Single arm row top position

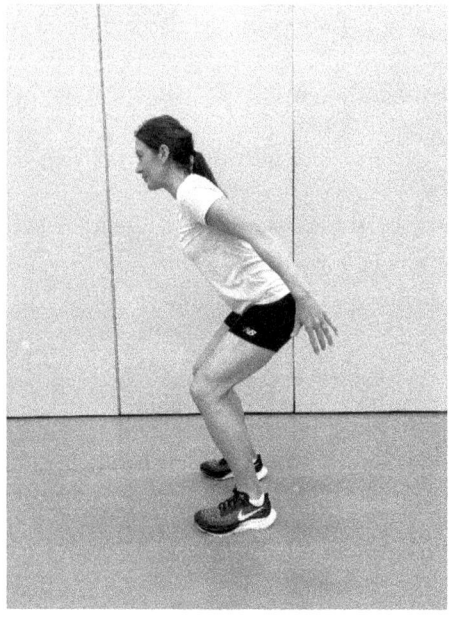

FIGURE 7.4.15A Squat jump bottom of 'dip' or downward phase

Myths of Menopause

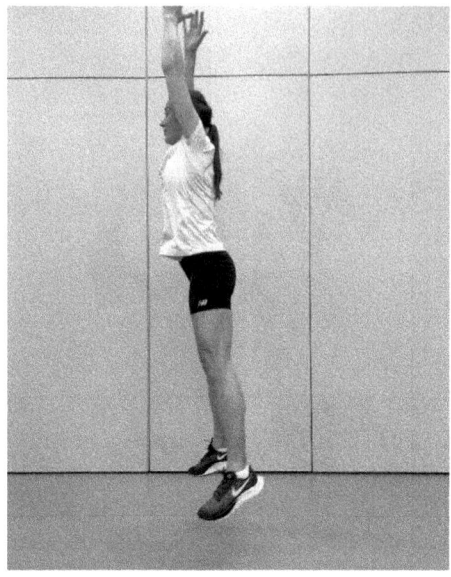

FIGURE 7.4.15B Squat jump as high as possible

Split jumps

1. Stand in a staggered position with right foot forward and left foot backward (Figure 7.4.16a)
2. Bend your knees and hips rapidly before jumping upwards and switching your legs in the air (Figure 7.4.16b)
3. Land back on the same spot but with your left foot forward and right foot backward (Figure 7.4.16c)
4. Once you have mastered the leg switch and are jumping as high as possible, progress to a continuous action by bouncing between repetitions with a short time on the ground.

High-impact (plyometric) exercises

Pogo jumps

1. Perform repeated jumps on the spot, spending as little time in contact with the ground as possible while jumping/bouncing as high as possible (Figure 7.4.17a).
2. Each landing should involve a small bend at the knees and hips while arms swing back and down (Figure 7.4.17b)
3. Ensure that knees point forward and remain aligned with ankles and hips. on every landing (Figure 7.4.17b)

Age Group Athletes

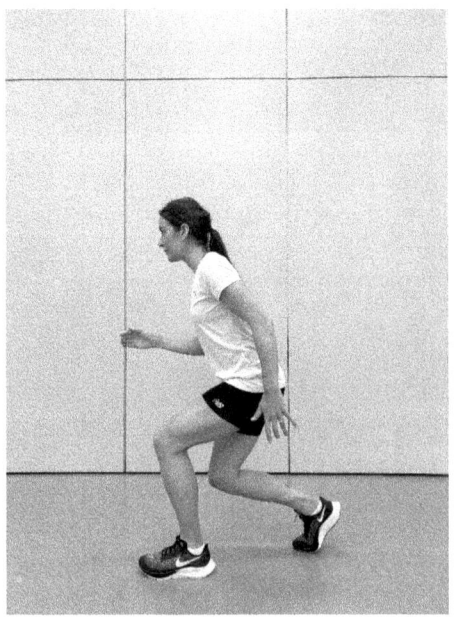

FIGURE 7.4.16A Split jumps start position

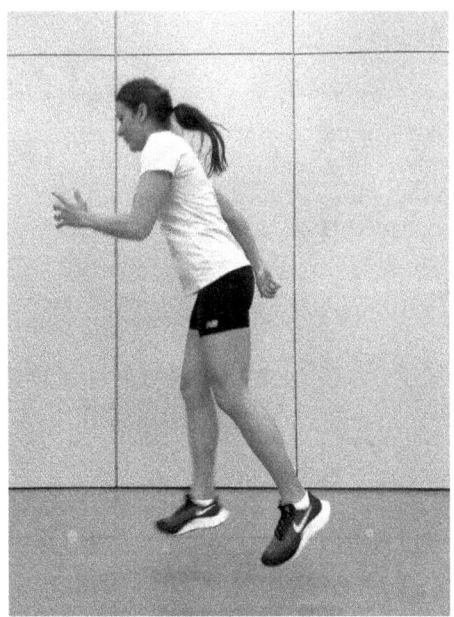

FIGURE 7.4.16B Split jumps mid-air leg switch

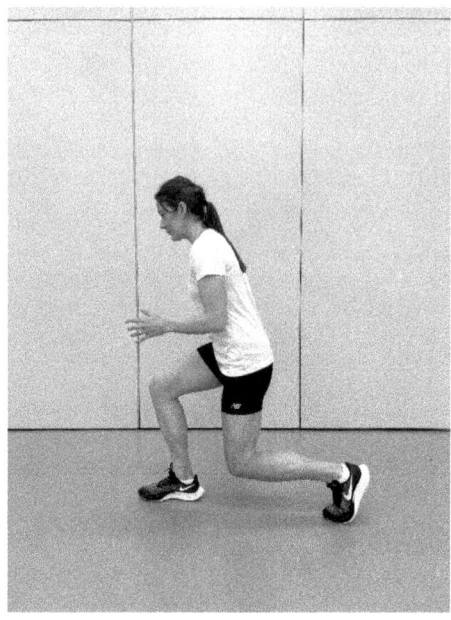

FIGURE 7.4.16C . Split jumps end position

Skater steps

1. Stand on one leg.
2. Flex your knee and hip rapidly and leap side-ways/laterally in the direction of your free leg (Figure 7.4.18a).
3. Land on the opposite leg under control, ensuring knee points forward and remains aligned with the ankle and hip (Figure 7.4.18b).
4. Once you have mastered the balance and coordination of a side-ways step, progress to bouncing from one leg to the next, spending a short time on the ground between steps.

Hopping

1. Stand on one leg
2. Flex your knee and hip and rapidly perform a hop forward (Figure 7.4.19a)
3. Land on the same leg you started on with a small bend at the knee and hip (Figure 7.4.19b)
4. Ensure your knee points forward and remains aligned with the ankle and hip (Figure 7.4.19c)
5. Once you have mastered the balance and coordination of landing from a hop, progress to bouncing forward between each hop, spending a short time on the ground between hops.

Age Group Athletes

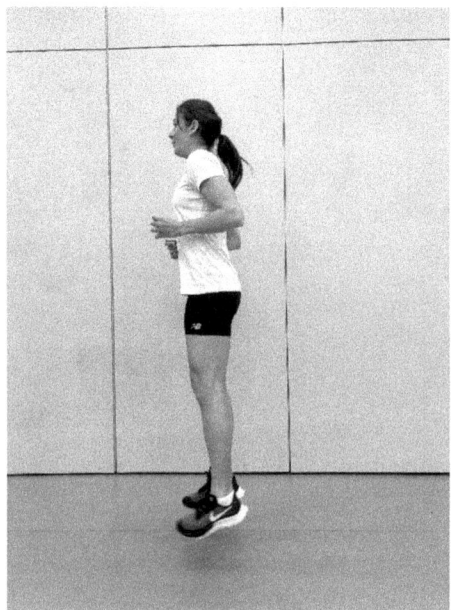

FIGURE 7.4.17A Pogo jumps – jump/bounce as high as possible

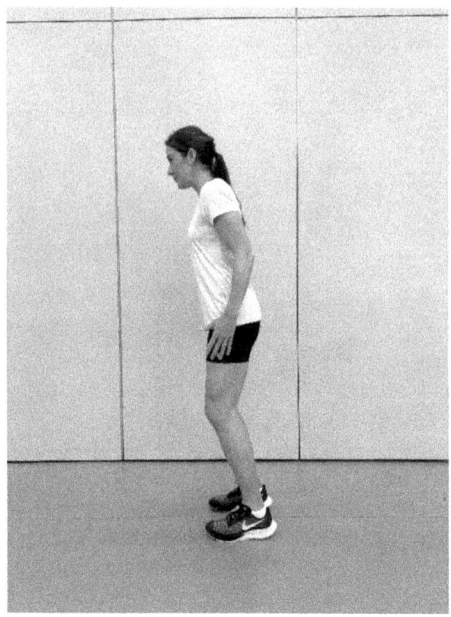

FIGURE 7.4.17B Minimal knee and hip flexion on landing during pogo jumps

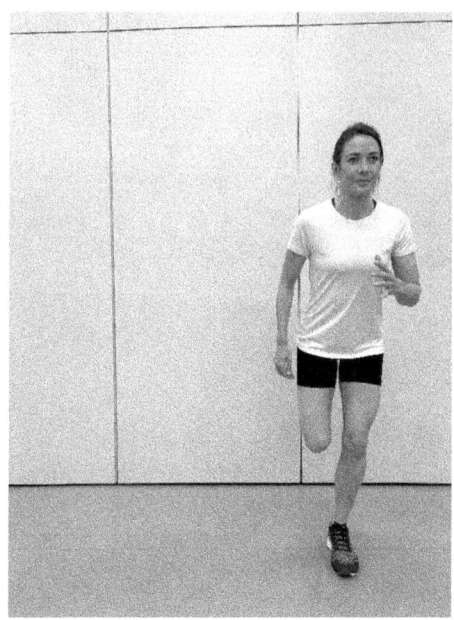

FIGURE 7.4.18A Skater step start position

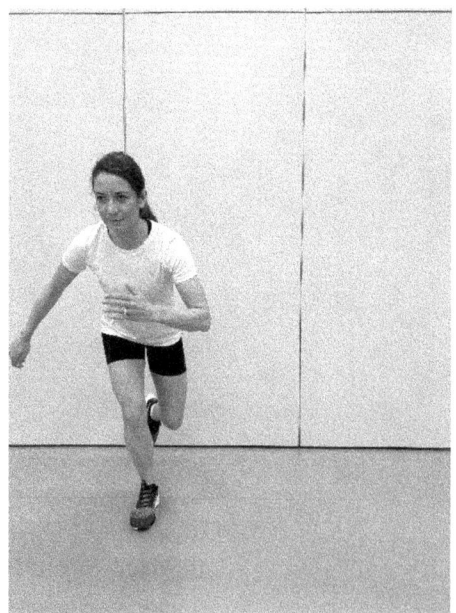

FIGURE 7.4.18B Skater step landing position

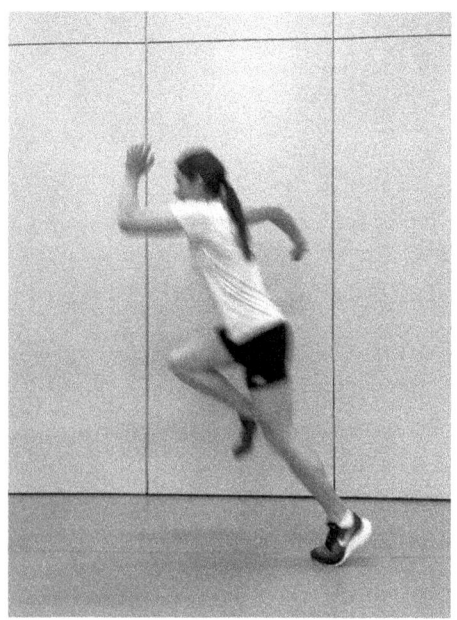

FIGURE 7.4.19A Hop forward push-off movement

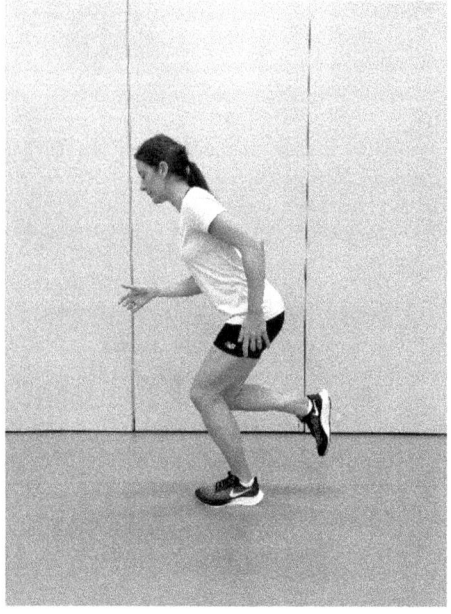

FIGURE 7.4.19B Hopping landing position

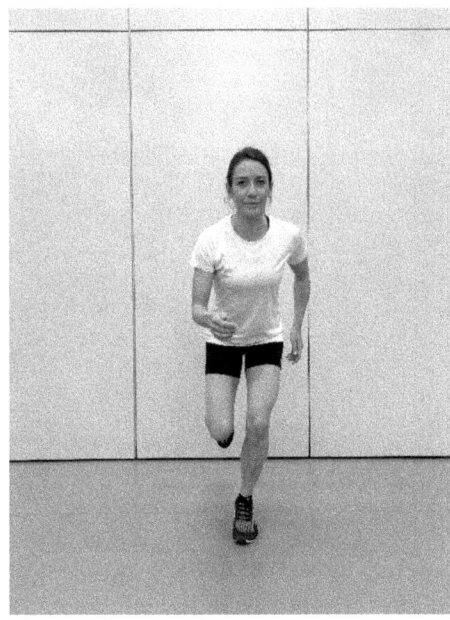

FIGURE 7.4.19C Maintaining knee alignment during hopping landing

References

1. Moilanen JM, Aalto AM, Raitanen J et al. Physical activity and change in quality of life during menopause -an 8-year follow-up study. *Health and Quality of Life Outcomes* 2012; 10 (1): 8. doi: 10.1186/1477-7525-10-8.
2. Buckinx F, Aubertin-Leheudre M. Sarcopenia in menopausal women: Current perspectives. *International Journal of Women's Health* 2022; 14 (null): 805–819. doi: 10.2147/IJWH.S340537.
3. Finkelstein JS, Brockwell SE, Mehta V et al. Bone mineral density changes during the menopause transition in a multiethnic cohort of women. *Journal of Clinical Endocrinology and Metabolism* 2008; 93 (3): 861–868. doi: 10.1210/jc.2007-1876.
4. Sözen T, Özışık L, Başaran NÇ. An overview and management of osteoporosis. *European Journal of Rheumatology* 2017; 4 (1): 46–56. doi: 10.5152/eurjrheum.2016.048.
5. Sjöblom S, Suuronen J, Rikkonen T et al. Relationship between postmenopausal osteoporosis and the components of clinical sarcopenia. *Maturitas* 2013; 75 (2): 175–180.
6. Mühlen D, Morton D, von Muhlen C et al. Postmenopausal estrogen and increased risk of clinical osteoarthritis at the hip, hand, and knee in older women. *Journal of Women's Health & Gender-Based Medicine* 2002; 11: 511–518. doi: 10.1089/152460902760277868.
7. Sartori R, Romanello V, Sandri M. Mechanisms of muscle atrophy and hypertrophy: Implications in health and disease. *Nature Communications* 2021; 12 (1): 330. doi: 10.1038/s41467-020-20123-1.
8. Wing RR, Matthews KA, Kuller LH et al. Weight gain at the time of menopause. *Archives of Internal Medicine* 1991; 151 (1): 97–102.
9. Kodoth V, Scaccia S, Aggarwal B. Adverse changes in body composition during the menopausal transition and relation to cardiovascular risk: A contemporary review. *Women's Health Reports* 2022; 3 (1): 573–581. doi: 10.1089/whr.2021.0119.

10 Karvonen-Gutierrez C, Kim C. Association of mid-life changes in body size, body composition and obesity status with the menopausal transition. *Healthcare* 2016; 4 (3). doi: 10.3390/healthcare4030042.
11 Asikainen TM, Kukkonen-Harjula K, Miilunpalo S. Exercise for health for early postmenopausal women. *Sports Medicine* 2004; 34 (11): 753–778. doi: 10.2165/00007256-200434110-00004.
12 Tan A, Thomas RL, Campbell MD et al. Effects of exercise training on metabolic syndrome risk factors in post-menopausal women – A systematic review and meta-analysis of randomised controlled trials. *Clinical Nutrition* 2023; 42 (3): 337–351. doi: 10.1016/j.clnu.2023.01.008.
13 Khalafi M, Sakhaei MH, Rosenkranz SK et al. Impact of concurrent training versus aerobic or resistance training on cardiorespiratory fitness and muscular strength in middle-aged to older adults: A systematic review and meta-analysis. *Physiology & Behavior* 2022; 254: 113888.
14 Yoo SZ, No MH, Heo JW et al. Role of exercise in age-related sarcopenia. *Journal of Exercise Rehabilitation* 2018; 14 (4): 551–558. doi: 10.12965/jer.1836268.134.
15 Thomas E, Gentile A, Lakicevic N et al. The effect of resistance training programs on lean body mass in postmenopausal and elderly women: A meta-analysis of observational studies. *Aging Clinical and Experimental Research* 2021; 33 (11): 2941–2952. doi: 10.1007/s40520-021-01853-8.
16 Brooke-Wavell K, Skelton DA, Barker KL et al. Strong, steady and straight: UK consensus statement on physical activity and exercise for osteoporosis. *British Journal of Sports Medicine* 2022; 56 (15): 837–846. doi: 10.1136/bjsports-2021-104634.
17 Messier SP, Mihalko SL, Beavers DP et al. Effect of high-intensity strength training on knee pain and knee joint compressive forces among adults with knee osteoarthritis: The START randomized clinical trial. *JAMA* 2021; 325 (7): 646–657. doi: 10.1001/jama.2021.0411.
18 Tataryn N, Simas V, Catterall T et al. Posterior-chain resistance training compared to general exercise and walking programmes for the treatment of chronic low back pain in the general population: A systematic review and meta-analysis. *Sport Medicine - Open* 2021; 7 (1): 17. doi: 10.1186/s40798-021-00306-w.
19 Mahindru A, Patil P, Agrawal V. Role of physical activity on mental health and well-being: A review. *Cureus* 2023; 15 (1): e33475. doi:10.7759/cureus.33475.
20 Corazza DI, Sebastião É, Pedroso RV et al. Influence of chronic exercise on serum cortisol levels in older adults. *European Review of Aging and Physical Activity* 2014; 11 (1): 25–34. doi: 10.1007/s11556-013-0126-8.
21 Dionigi R. Resistance training and older adults' beliefs about psychological benefits: The importance of self-efficacy and social interaction. *Journal of Sport and Exercise Psychology* 2007; 29 (6): 723–746.
22 Liu T, Chen S, Mielke GI et al. Effects of exercise on vasomotor symptoms in menopausal women: A systematic review and meta-analysis. *Climacteric* 2022; 25 (6): 552–561. doi: 10.1080/13697137.2022.2097865.
23 Rantanen T, Guralnik JM, Izmirlian G et al. Association of muscle strength with maximum walking speed in disabled older women. *American Journal of Physical Medicine & Rehabilitation* 1998; 77 (4): 299–305. doi: 10.1097/00002060-199807000-00008.
24 Barbat-Artigas S, Rolland Y, Cesari M et al. Clinical relevance of different muscle strength indexes and functional impairment in women aged 75 years and older. *Journals of Gerontology Series A* 2013; 68 (7): 811–819. doi: 10.1093/gerona/gls254.
25 Alvarez KJ, Kirchner S, Chu S et al. Falls reduction and exercise training in an assisted living population. *Journal of Aging Research* 2015; 2015: 957598. doi:10.1155/2015/957598.
26 Sousa N, Mendes R, Silva A et al. Combined exercise is more effective than aerobic exercise in the improvement of fall risk factors: A randomized controlled trial in community-dwelling older men. *Clinical Rehabilitation* 2017; 31 (4): 478–486. doi: 10.1177/0269215516655857.

27 Burton E, Farrier K, Lewin G et al. Motivators and barriers for older people participating in resistance training: A systematic review. *Journal of Aging and Physical Activity* 2017; 25 (2): 311–324. doi: 10.1123/japa.2015-0289.

28 Grgic J, Garofolini A, Orazem J et al. Effects of resistance training on muscle size and strength in very elderly adults: A systematic review and meta-analysis of randomized controlled trials. *Sport Medicine* 2020; 50 (11): 1983–1999. doi: 10.1007/s40279-020-01331-7.

29 Critchlow AJ, Hiam D, Williams R et al. The role of estrogen in female skeletal muscle aging: A systematic review. *Maturitas* 2023; 178: 107844. doi: 10.1016/j.maturitas.2023.107844.

30 Lim C, Nunes EA, Currier BS et al. An evidence-based narrative review of mechanisms of resistance exercise-induced human skeletal muscle hypertrophy. *Medicine & Science in Sports & Exercise* 2022; 54 (9): 1546–1559. doi: 10.1249/MSS.0000000000002929.

31 Liu CJ, Latham N. Adverse events reported in progressive resistance strength training trials in older adults: 2 sides of a coin. *Archives of Physical Medicine and Rehabilitation* 2010; 91 (9): 1471–1473. doi: 10.1016/j.apmr.2010.06.001.

32 Watson SL, Weeks BK, Weis LJ et al. High-intensity resistance and impact training improves bone mineral density and physical function in postmenopausal women with osteopenia and osteoporosis: The LIFTMOR randomized controlled trial. *Journal of Bone and Mineral Research* 2018; 33 (2): 211–220. doi: 10.1002/JBMR.3284.

33 Bickel CS, Cross JM, Bamman MM. Exercise dosing to retain resistance training adaptations in young and older adults. *Medicine & Science in Sports & Exercise* 2011; 43 (7): 1177–1187. doi: 10.1249/MSS.0b013e318207c15d.

34 Suominen H. Ageing and maximal physical performance. *European Review of Aging and Physical Activity* 2011; 8 (1): 37–42. doi: 10.1007/s11556-010-0073-6.

35 Lambert CP, Evans WJ. Effects of aging and resistance exercise on determinants of muscle strength. *Journal of the American Aging Association* 2002; 25 (2): 73–78. doi: 10.1007/s11357-002-0005-0.

36 World Health Organization. *World Report on Ageing and Health*. World Health Organization, 2015.

37 Mcleod JC, Stokes T, Phillips SM. Resistance exercise training as a primary countermeasure to age-related chronic disease. *Frontiers in Physiology* 2019; 10: 441213.

38 Steele J, Fisher J, Skivington M et al. A higher effort-based paradigm in physical activity and exercise for public health: Making the case for a greater emphasis on resistance training. *BMC Public Health* 2017; 17: 1–8.

39 Fragala MS, Cadore EL, Dorgo S et al. Resistance training for older adults: Position statement from the National Strength and Conditioning Association. *Journal of Strength & Conditioning Research* 2019; 33 (8). https://journals.lww.com/nsca-jscr/fulltext/2019/08000/resistance_training_for_older_adults__position.1.aspx.

40 Liguori G, Medicine AC of S. *ACSM's Guidelines for Exercise Testing and Prescription*. Lippincott Williams & Wilkins, 2020.

41 Riebe D, Franklin BA, Thompson PD et al. Updating ACSM's recommendations for exercise preparticipation health screening. *Medicine & Science in Sports & Exercise* 2015; 47 (11): 2473–2479. doi: 10.1249/MSS.0000000000000664.

42 Fleg JL, Cooper LS, Borlaug BA et al. Exercise training as therapy for heart failure: Current status and future directions. *Circulation: Heart Failure* 2015; 8 (1): 209–220. doi: 10.1161/CIRCHEARTFAILURE.113.001420.

43 Metter EJ, Conwit R, Tobin J et al. Age-associated loss of power and strength in the upper extremities in women and men. *Journals of Gerontology Series A: Biological Sciences and Medical Sciences* 1997; 52 (5): B267–B276. doi: 10.1093/gerona/52a.5.b267.

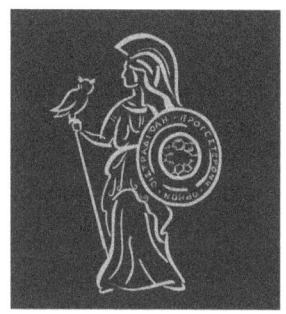

Act 8

Experiencing Menopause
Discord and harmony

Act 8 Experiencing Menopause
Discord and harmony

Dr Nicky Keay

Navigating menopause can feel like being in the realm of Eris, the goddess of discord and strife. You can feel dissonant not only with yourself but with those around you, out of step with colleagues, friends and even family. This is a challenging time of adjustment as you search for the way of Harmonia, to rediscover harmony with yourself and others.

My grandmother and mother are my role models. We shared passions for dancing and hard work. Although I freely confided in them and discussed any topic, I regret never asking my grandmother about how she experienced menopause.

This act explores why society has been reluctant to discuss menopause, even within close-knit families. Experts in this field discuss how our individual life experiences and backgrounds influence the way we experience our female hormone odyssey, with particular focus on the graduation to menopause and beyond.

Scene 1 Am I losing my mind?

Professor Aimee Spector

I was chairing an online meeting during COVID, managing a research project on dementia. I asked my colleagues to share their thoughts on a matter and then attempted to summarise. "*There are two key themes here,*" I said, starting by summarising the first. "*The second is . . . .*" Blank. Not a "*tip of my tongue"* blank, but what I could only describe as a black hole. I felt so ashamed: "*What would they think of me?*"

I'd experienced a similar 'black hole' earlier that week, when a friend had asked me what film I'd watched the previous night. It wasn't even a case of vaguely remembering an actor, the theme or how it made me feel . . . just nothing.

It was something I'd noticed happening more and more regularly. On a personal level, this felt shameful, and as a professor of dementia, particularly sensitive. I reluctantly shared my concerns with colleagues, who looked slightly awkward and tried to reassure me. I went to my GP, who appeared concerned and asked me to come back in three months for a review. At this point, I was close to requesting a dementia assessment and starting to Google things like, 'symptoms of brain tumour'. It was only when a friend asked if I'd had my hormones checked that it even occurred that this could be anything to do with perimenopause. I was 46, with regular periods and no hot flushes. A few months on, some blood tests and hormone replacement therapy (HRT), however, and the 'light bulb' switched back on – like magic. No more embarrassing absences or 'black holes'. Why was this so, and why did nobody, including my GP and colleagues (many being health professionals) work out the menopause link sooner?

Brain fog in perimenopause

Despite nobody knowing what it was, I was astounded to find that there were several published research studies, some from as early as 2009, showing that up to or around 60% of people report what is becoming increasingly known as 'brain fog' in menopause transition: the period between someone's normal reproductive life, and a year following their final period. There have also been several large, published studies confirming that 'verbal learning' and verbal memory are the cognitive domains most affected by menopause. Put simply, this means the learning and recall of words, short stories and other verbal material.

Less affected are working memory or attention, which refers to the ability to hold information in short-term memory, such as keeping a name in mind while writing an email. Research tells us that women **are better at these skills than men**, possibly contributing to the impact when such abilities become impaired. Studies have found that for some people, concerns about failing memory correlate with poorer scores on standardised memory tests, such as tests of immediate and delayed memory of words. A problem lies in the quality of this research. For example, many of the tests used are not fit for purpose. Some are designed to detect early cases of dementia but are not sensitive enough to pick up changes in people who only have subtle cognitive decline. Also, tests are generally developed in Western samples and not adapted for different languages and cultures. Therefore, whilst some studies indicate that the cognitive changes may differ between cultures and contexts, it is hard to reach definitive conclusions.

But the thing that I couldn't quite believe is that approximately 1 in 10 women experience a 'clinically significant' decline in objective cognition in the menopause transition, meaning that their scores on memory tests demonstrate a true impairment in what they can do[1]. Translating worldwide, this amounts to 1 in 20 (5%) of the entire world population experiencing this clinically significant decline. Why had these figures not reached the attention of health professionals working closely with women going through menopause? With two-thirds of UK medical schools still not having mandatory menopause education and women's health often being at the bottom of the policy agenda, it is hardly surprising that the effect of cognitive problems in perimenopause are not recognised by most GPs.

What causes brain fog?

Oestrogen plays a key role in brain functioning by stimulating glucose uptake and energy production. The brain is excellent at adapting to change, so once the transition to menopause is complete, neurons adapt to the absence of oestrogen and create new pathways. But in the perimenopausal period, levels of oestrogen fluctuate hugely throughout the cycle and from cycle to cycle. This yo-yo effect means that brain cells are periodically deprived of oestrogen, but not for long enough to forge the pathways needed to adapt to life without it. This explains the decline in cognition, those frustrating 'black holes', and us suddenly being unable to remember for the life of us, for example, what we went upstairs for.

Following this logic, one would assume that HRT would play a clear role in improving cognitive problems during menopause transition, yet results of research are mixed and inconclusive. Why is this?

One of the reasons is the imbalance of research, with so much focus on the postmenopausal period, at which point the brain has already adapted to losses of oestrogen. This in itself is largely due to the perimenopause period being poorly defined. There is a lack of awareness, as well as not much prescribing of HRT for cognitive problems alone.

Second, as discussed shortly in the next chapter, the menopause transition is a biopsychosocial period, with multiple factors likely to interact and exacerbate all problems, including brain fog. A model developed by Zhu and colleagues[2] (Figure 8.1.1) proposed

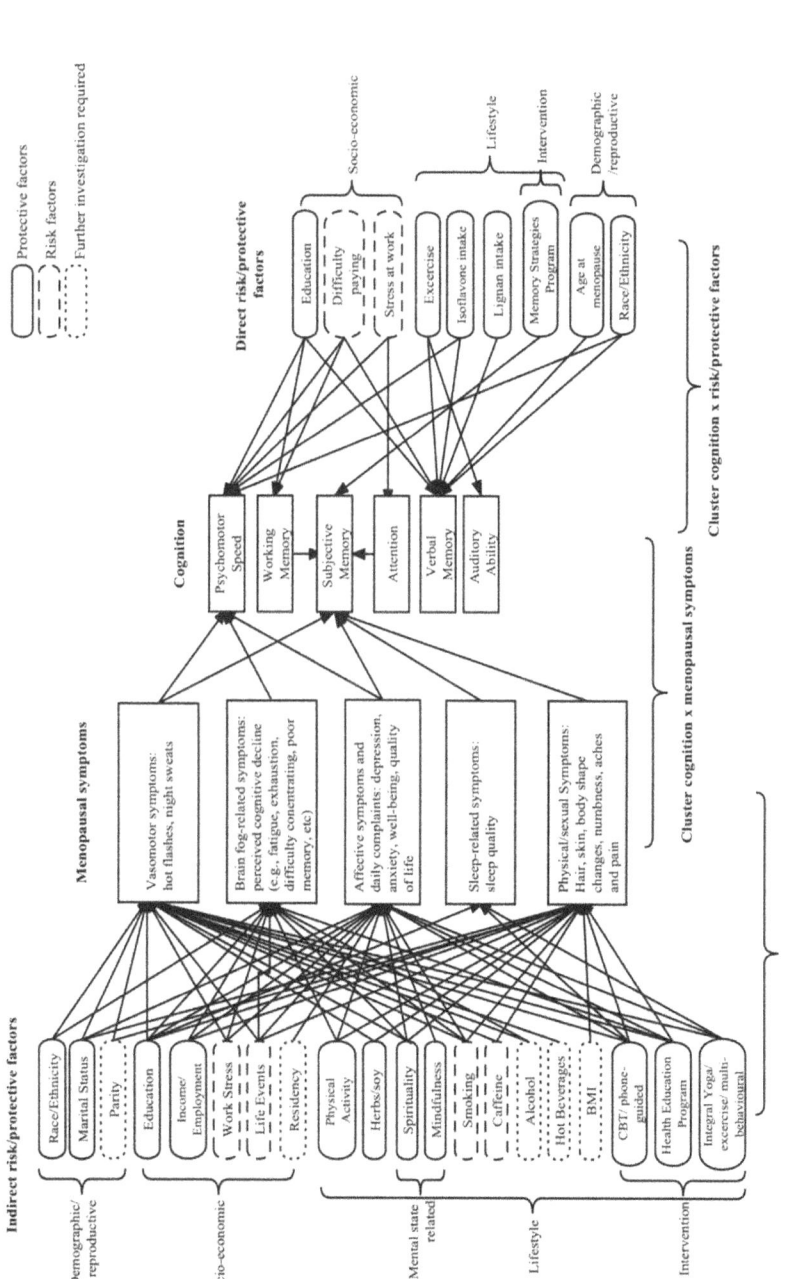

FIGURE 8.1.1 Indirect and direct influences on cognition in menopause (courtesy of Zhu et al., 2022)

a number of both indirect and direct risk and protective factors for cognition: the indirect resulting in menopausal symptoms (such as VMS and mood changes), which may subsequently affect cognition, and others having a direct impact on cognition.

Perimenopause story: Nahid

Nahid is a 47-year-old single mother of two children (aged 10 and 8) and carer for her mother (aged 66), who has early-onset dementia. She was born in India and moved to the United Kingdom as a child. Nahid works full-time in a Human Resources department at a large bank. For the past year, she has made several errors at work. These are mainly around forgetting employees' names and mixing up their paperwork. At her recent appraisal, her manager asked if she was 'coping okay', which has led to catastrophic fears of being fired and not being able to cope financially. Nahid has had irregular periods for 8 months and frequently suffers from insomnia, often caused by worries about her performance at work. She tries to manage this by drinking a large glass of wine before bed and has joined a gym, although she is usually too tired to go. She has not told anyone about her memory struggles, for fear that people will question her ability to be a good mother, carer and worker. She has avoided informing her GP, for fear of being labelled as 'mentally unfit'.

There are several cognitive risk factors for Nahid. Being in the perimenopausal phase, Nahid's hormones are likely to be in a state of flux, which may be impacting both directly on her brain's ability to function and indirectly, for example, through causing problems sleeping, which then makes it harder to function at work. But she also has a huge amount on her plate including two young children and a mother to care for. Being the sole breadwinner, there are likely to be financial pressures and a huge reliance on her income, with constant worries about her performance increasing the likelihood that she makes errors at work. Whilst we may be quick to label her symptoms as 'brain fog', it is important to consider her genetic risk of dementia given her mother's condition; this is likely to cause additional concern for Nahid. It is also important to consider cultural beliefs and expectations. It seems that Nahid is avoiding potential sources of support, such as talking to friends or her GP. Drinking wine before bed may be negatively impacting her sleep, which in turn is reducing her ability to exercise – a missed protective factor.

Impact of cognitive problems

Diminished cognition inevitably will have an impact on all areas of life, an important one for this age group being work. We can expect that up to 47% of the UK workforce, in other words all female workers, to experience menopause transition during their working lives. Multiple studies have found a negative relationship between menopausal symptoms and performance at work, and if this is more pronounced, the more severe the symptoms become. Some maintain that menopause results in millions of days lost through absenteeism and that, when faced with employers' lack of understanding and poorly developed menopause policies, many women choose to leave employment rather than tackle their employers.

The worry, often accompanied by stigma and shame, about brain fog; can result in a vicious cycle whereby, for example, the panic that we might forget a name causes us to forget the name. The lack of awareness about normal cognitive changes during menopause transition results in many women becoming concerned that they have dementia, which, of course causes further anxiety and distress.

What treatments have been developed so far?

The short answer is – not many at all, with only two interventions identified in the research that have been specifically designed to tackle the management of cognitive problems.

The first adapted an intervention used in healthy older people, the LaTCH memory strategies programme, which included information about memory change in menopause, emotional reactions to memory changes and memory strategies[3]. The group sessions included cognitive-behavioural techniques, with the rationale that changing beliefs about memory symptoms would make them less problematic. A significant issue was that the majority (26 of 37) were postmenopausal, at which point it seems that memory problems have often declined or disappeared. Nonetheless, there were some promising trends in how people felt about changes in their memory and positive feedback, for example, around the importance of normalising memory problems.

The other study again involved group sessions that focused on psychoeducation, cognitive compensatory strategies and lifestyle modification[4]. Results were promising, with significant improvement in how confident people *felt* about their memory following the groups (despite an absence of actual cognitive change). However, they had a very high dropout rate of 44%, with many stating that this was due to scheduling difficulties.

Whilst both studies were limited due to small sample sizes and high dropout, both teach us the importance of sharing experiences with others in the same position, normalising symptoms and developing compensatory strategies; the three potential 'key ingredients' to any future intervention. However, given how busy most women are in this life stage, offering a flexible range of ways to access help, for example, through online platforms and apps as well as face-to-face interventions, is preferable.

What can I do?

(1) Reading this chapter and accessing further resources around cognition in menopause is the first important step. Understanding that these symptoms

TABLE 8.1.1 Compensatory strategies

Avoid distractions	Eliminate visual clutter, turn phone and email alerts off when engaging in tasks.
Optimising scheduling	Avoid back-to-back appointments and schedule cognitively demanding tasks at your optimal time of day (e.g. first thing).
Visual association	Create visual images to remember words or names. For example, remembering the name Cara by visualising her driving a car.
Use of compensatory memory aids	Diaries, mobile phones, setting timers

are most likely normal and will settle over time, I hope will reduce the anxiety you hold around them – it certainly did for me. I also think that awareness needs to increase more generally, so that others understand this too and respond with support, compassion and (if needed), humour! Important routes to this are educating professionals, for example ensuring that all medical schools have mandatory menopause training and increasing and improving workplace menopause policies (see Act 9).

(2) Finding support networks. This may be through friends, family, religious or spiritual groups or workplace colleagues – the key thing is that you find a space where you can talk about your problems and share experiences, if you want to. For some of us, we tend to internalise more and find our own ways of managing, for example, through exercise. Search social media and the internet for local support, such as menopause cafes or online forums.

(3) Compensatory strategies. Having a few tricks 'up your sleeve' and strategies that work for you is a great idea. Don't worry if you need to write everything down; it doesn't matter. We wrote a lot more down when we were trying to learn and remember things at school, yet have unrealistic expectations that as adults our brain can manage everything. This is not the case! Table 8.1.1 summarises some useful strategies gathered from research in the area.

(4) Hormonal or other treatment, which may directly or indirectly (e.g. through improving sleep by reducing night sweats) impact cognition.

In summary – are you losing your mind? The most likely answer is *no*!

References

1 Maki PM, Weber MT. A research primer for studies of cognitive changes across the menopause transition. *Climacteric* 2021; 24 (4): 382–388.

2   Zhu C, Thomas N, Arunogiri S et al. Systematic review and narrative synthesis of cognition in perimenopause: The role of risk factors and menopausal symptoms. *Maturitas* 2022; 164: 76–86.
3   Unkenstein AE, Bei B, Bryant CA. Enhancing memory self-efficacy during menopause through a group memory strategies program. *Menopause* 2017; 24 (5): 574–581.
4   Ballantyne EC, King JP, Green SM. Preliminary support for a cognitive remediation intervention for women during the menopausal transition: A pilot study. *Frontiers in Global Women's Health* 2021; 2: 741539.

Scene 2 Why do each of us experience menopause differently?

Dr Helen Donovan, Professor Myra Hunter, Nora Bahhar, Professor Aimee Spector

The menopause inevitably happens to all of us who have periods and the good fortune to live beyond the stage of midlife. For the majority the menopause transition occurs naturally – a reduction of hormones triggers changes in the menstrual cycle until the point where periods cease altogether. At the present time, the United Nations estimate that around one billion women across the globe are postmenopausal; that is 12 months or more beyond their last period.

Although a common global occurrence with a core biological process, the experience of the menopause transition varies greatly between individuals and cultures. Some women navigate this transitional stage of life largely uneventfully, whereas others hit difficulties, experiencing moderate or severe symptoms that affect their daily lives, and may seek support and treatment. There is variation in biology which will account for some of this, such as the severity and frequency of physical symptoms; and some women have menopause early while for others menopause may be induced by surgery or medical treatments. However, we also know from research that there are many individual and wider contextual factors that can impact on people's individual experience of this life stage.

There's ongoing debate amongst experts – some argue that the menopause is a largely under-treated condition of chronic hormone deficiency, while others view the menopause as a natural phase of life which is influenced by psychological, social and cultural as well as hormone changes. If menopause is seen as a deficiency akin to a disease, this may lead to unnecessarily negative expectations both about and by women as they enter their menopause transition.

The biopsychosocial model is a conceptual framework for understanding different factors that contribute to health. It considers the impact of psychological, social and cultural dimensions in addition to a person's biology, as well as the dynamic interaction between the various factors. There is now much more research that supports the 'biopsychosocial model' of menopause as opposed to a purely 'biological' model[1]. The aim of using this model is to hold a more holistic and nuanced understanding of health issues, as well as identifying a wider range of potential factors for change or treatment alongside hormonal treatment. We suggest that thinking about the experience of the menopause in this way provides a balanced perspective in the menopause debate. It can also help women to better understand the factors contributing to their own unique experience, and find helpful ways to deal with challenges and identify positives to build on.

Given that the menopause transition (also known as perimenopause) typically takes place over a period of years, most women negotiating the perimenopause are also dealing with a range of other changes and challenges at the same time. Many are supporting children through to adolescence and/or young adulthood, caring for ageing parents, perhaps progressing or considering a change in a demanding career and possibly dealing with other changes in their health. On top of that, the past several years have been some of the most socially turbulent times many of us have seen in our lifetimes – the pandemic, financial crises and social and political instability. That is a lot to deal with while also navigating and making sense of changes in our bodies.

In this chapter, we will summarise what the research tells us about some of the most common factors which impact on the experience of menopause. We will then pose some questions which may help you to think about your unique experience and create your own biopsychosocial model. We will finish by offering some suggestions about potential changes you might make depending on the challenges you identify. In discussing common menopause experiences in this chapter, we predominantly refer to women in the midlife stage. For those experiencing menopause at an earlier life stage and those of a different gender, the biopsychosocial model is adaptable to each individual, so we invite you to engage with those parts of the chapter which feel helpful in making sense of your experience.

But first, we are going to look at two very different but important historical influences that can shape our understanding of the menopause. We will start by looking at why we have menopause from an evolutionary perspective, and then we will consider how science and medicine in the past has influenced thinking about and management of the menopause.

Why do we have the menopause?

The menopause occurs in all human societies; however, only a few other species experience this transition. Females of most species continue to reproduce up until or very close to the end of their natural lifespan – even those that live a similarly long life, such as elephants. Until very recently, only a few species of toothed whales had been identified as having a menopause like humans. In late 2023, the first research paper was published reporting menopause in another primate – a group of long-studied wild chimpanzees in Uganda[2] – but otherwise other primates including other groups of chimpanzees have not been found to have a significant postreproductive period in females.

Evolutionary biologists have spent time trying to understand the 'why' of menopause as a rare phenomenon. In evolutionary theory, the main consideration is whether a particular trait or characteristic has come about through adaptive or non-adaptive forces. Non-adaptive forces are random such as mutation or genetic drift, whereas adaptive forces systematically select traits that provide a survival advantage which are then passed on genetically.

The main non-adaptive theory of menopause assumes that there is no survival advantage to the menopause and stopping reproduction earlier than the end of the lifespan, as this reduces the opportunities for reproduction. It suggests the menopause has come about as an accidental by-product of the combination of (a) females being born with a finite supply of eggs which stop being viable for reproduction after a certain timespan, and (b) the relatively recent and rapid increase in average lifespan due to medical and social advances. However, although it is the case that the average life expectancy has roughly doubled in the past couple of centuries, this is largely due to dramatic reductions in rates of infant and childhood mortality. In terms of the population who survived into adulthood and reproduced, there has likely always been a sizeable proportion living beyond their middle-age years.

There are also adaptive theories which have been researched in both humans and other species that experience menopause. The mother theory emphasises the increased risks associated with childbirth as we age together with the need for a prolonged period of care in humans due to our unusually extended period of child development and dependency. Stopping reproduction prior to a long postreproductive period reduces the risks of a mother dying during childbirth and increases the length of time available to care for her last child for the many years until they have reached maturity.

Another theory which has gained support in recent research is the grandmother theory, which historian Susan Mattern details in her 2019 book *The Slow Moon Climbs: The Science, History, and Meaning of Menopause*[3]. In this theory, postreproductive grandmothers support the survival of their grandchildren through assisting with childcare and gathering and providing food, allowing their daughters to have more children closer together. This theory also emphasises the reduction of competition for resources which would occur if grandmothers and mothers were both continuing to reproduce at the same time. Mattern suggests that the availability of postreproductive grandmothers provided a higher ratio of adults cooperating to provide care and resources for dependent children, and this provided an evolutionary advantage over other early human species such as Neanderthals. There is current evidence to support this theory, with better survival rates for children with a living grandmother in the Hadza people (a hunter-gatherer population in Tanzania, living most similarly to our distant ancestors of current humans). In killer whales, a better survival rate has also been found for those with a postreproductive grandmother, and having a postreproductive mother present is also associated with fewer socially inflicted injuries in adult sons. These ideas tie in with recent wider thinking in evolutionary theory about survival of the friendliest, where our capacity for social bonds and cooperation rather than competition is viewed as key to the success of the human species.

Aside from academic interest, the understanding of why we have menopause is likely to shape women's feelings and expectations as they move into and beyond their midlife. Non-adaptive theories reinforce the stereotype of older women being 'past their expiration date', while adaptive theories of menopause emphasise the valuable role that postreproductive women play in families and communities.

Menopause in medical history

Western medicine and science have not been known historically for progressive views about women; past writings by men are littered with negative assumptions and theories about women and their bodies, including menstruation, reproduction and hormones. Although many of these ideas seem extreme now and we have thankfully moved on from them, these beliefs have shaped medical discussion and management of menopause, and likely continue to exert subtle influence within the medical profession and in wider society which looks to medicine for advice and treatment.

In her 2023 book *Revolting Women: Why midlife women are walking out and what to do about it*[4], Lucy Ryan provides a brief history of some of the ways in which the female body has been pathologised over time, upholding an assumption of male superiority and normality. While medical discussion and writing of menopause specifically is relatively recent, philosophical and scientific discussion in Ancient Greece conceptualised women's reproductive organs as an inferior and inverted version of the superior male organs. In the Age of Enlightenment in the eighteenth-century women's smaller skulls and wider pelvis were used as justification for their place in the home due to assumed lesser reasoning ability and greater suitability for reproduction and nurturance – not so enlightened regarding women, then! In the Victorian era with the professionalisation of medicine, women were excluded from their long-held traditional role of midwives, and women's bodies were again viewed as irrational and unstable due to female hormones and organs.

A recent paper describes the twentieth-century development of medical views and treatment of menopause[5]. Rather than being understood as a natural life stage, the loss of oestrogen began being described as harmful to both individuals and society, and in the early 1900s hormones extracted from animals began to be injected into women to treat the perceived deficiency. By the 1960s, Hormone Replacement Therapy (HRT) was the most commonly prescribed medication for women aged 50–64, reflecting the growing opinion that menopause should be viewed and treated as a universal deficiency. While it may be understandable that this theory arose, a medical paper in 1963 describing the *"untold misery of alcoholism, drug addiction, divorce and broken homes caused by these unstable, estrogen-starved women"* highlights a strong undercurrent of misogyny clouding scientific impartiality and rigour[6]. Although the language has thankfully moved on, the debate of whether menopause represents a natural and normal phase of life versus a disease of hormone deficiency continues to be discussed.

In the early 2000s, the use of HRT in the United Kingdom sharply declined following publication of a study reporting increased risk of breast cancer and stroke. These risks continue to be researched and recent years has seen the development of safer forms of HRT (Menopausal Hormone Therapy; MHT). In 2020–2022, a dramatic increase was observed again in the prescription of MHT, particularly in women from most affluent areas of the United Kingdom. Reasons for this increase are unclear, but might include increased discussion and awareness amongst the current generation of women going through it, and also attention in the media and access to safer forms of MHT with updated research. We might also wonder about social factors relating to the pandemic and its impact on menopausal women.

The biopsychosocial model

Moving on to current understanding of the menopause, we will summarise the key biological, psychological and social factors and symptoms that commonly shape the experience of menopause. These are depicted in Figure 8.2.1, which show the main groups of factors – the circles are depicted as overlapping as these factors often interact with one another in complex ways.

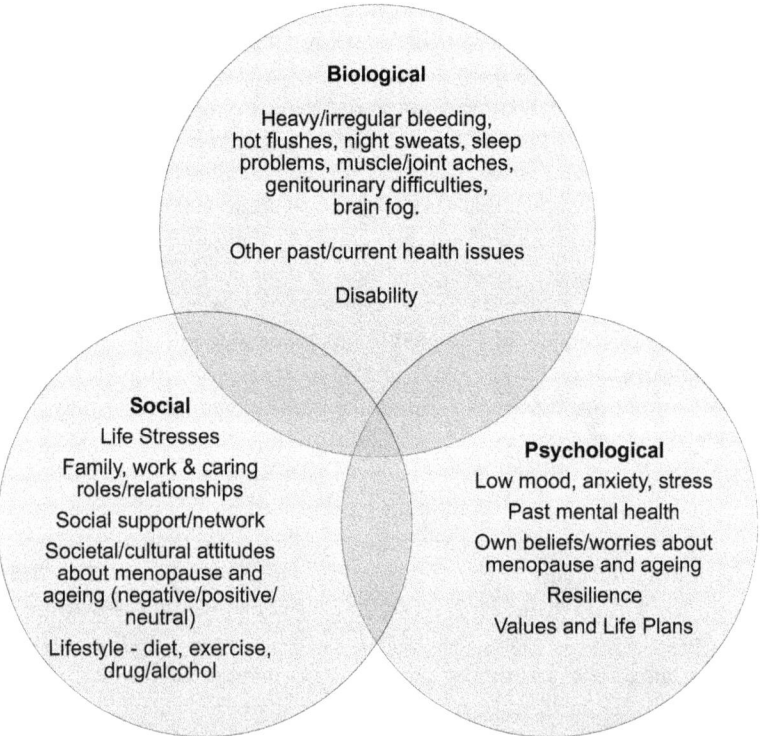

FIGURE 8.2.1 A biopsychosocial model of the menopause (adapted and reproduced from Hunter MS and Smith M. 2021 Living Well through the Menopause, with kind permission of Hachette UK). Note: Hunter MS, Smith M. Living Well through the Menopause. Robinson 2021

Biological factors

Biological mechanisms and symptoms of the menopause and their medical management are discussed in greater detail in other chapters in this book; but the following provides a brief summary of the symptoms most commonly noted;

- Irregular, Heavy or Prolonged Bleeding – changes in the menstrual cycle due to hormone changes mark the beginning of the menopause transition. For women with regular natural cycles, this change can be easy to notice, but others might not be aware due to using hormonal contraception, having conditions with irregular periods (e.g. PCOS, endometriosis) or women who have had a hysterectomy.
- Hot flushes and/or Night Sweats (Vasomotor Symptoms) – these symptoms are the main menopausal symptoms being very commonly experienced, with some variation reported across cultures and countries. They are more likely to be reported in high-income countries than low-and-middle-income countries (however, it is not known whether the actual symptoms, or the degree to which they are reported – perhaps due to stigma and awareness – is what varies). They are also a common trigger for women seeking help, particularly when they are causing significant disruption either in daytime functioning or nighttime sleep disturbance.
- Muscle and Joint Pain – the reduction in hormones during menopause transition may contribute to increased inflammation, lower levels of natural painkillers and reduced bone density. However, it's also the case that general ageing leads to these symptoms in both sexes, and a number of other lifestyle factors also worsen these symptoms (diet, exercise, stress, sleep).
- Sleep Disturbance – difficulties with sleep are generally more common in women than men, and can increase during the menopause. One reason for this is disruption due to night sweats, but other causes of sleep disturbance can also contribute such as depression and stress, which in turn can continue to disrupt sleep in an unhelpful cycle.
- Genitourinary Symptoms – vaginal dryness, irritation and discomfort and pain during intercourse are symptoms which can occur due to hormonal changes. These occur more commonly either later in the menopause transition or following menopause and can persist into older age. Aside from the physical discomfort of having these symptoms, they can have an impact on both new and existing sexual relationships, self-identity and confidence.
- Brain Fog – changes in cognitive functioning are common, with short-term memory, word-finding and concentration difficulties reported. Whilst studies which have tracked cognitive functioning have shown that for most, these changes are temporary and are not an indicator of future decline, for some people they can significantly impact their perceived ability to work and manage

daily functioning. We also know that other life stressors and sleep disturbance can exacerbate these cognitive difficulties.

Other past and present biological factors, while not symptoms of the menopause, are also likely to contribute to and interact with an individual's experience of the menopause transition;

- Past reproductive or fertility issues and trauma which may trigger distress as women come to the end of the reproductive stage of life.

    "I thought I'd come to terms with being childless a few years earlier when we decided not to try other options, but as my periods started to become infrequent the reality of it hit me all over again. People also made thoughtless comments from time to time about me being childless which they hadn't done when I was younger – I guess maybe it had become more obvious to others that I wasn't going to have children but I really didn't need to hear that."

- Coping with other ongoing or new health conditions and disabilities alongside menopausal symptoms. Understanding the interaction of symptoms and conditions can be confusing, and care might feel disjointed between specialisms.

Psychological factors – Does the menopause make me moody?

Most symptom checklists for menopause include one or more common mental health symptoms such as low mood or depression, anxiety, irritability and mood swings. Being able to talk about and get support and treatment for mental health is important; however, the question of whether these symptoms are specifically due to the hormonal changes of the menopause transition is a bit trickier to answer.

We might ask if it matters whether changes in mood are due to hormones or other factors – after all if someone is feeling distressed then we can acknowledge that experience regardless of the reason for it. However, there are specific reasons to try and pick the causal factors apart; different causes will indicate different approaches to treatment and support. It also matters because we know that negative attitudes and beliefs about ageing and menopause are associated with poorer health outcomes and higher rates of mood difficulties, so perpetuating inaccurate stereotypes can contribute to this.

Depression

Rates of depression are at their highest in middle age, but this pattern is found in both men and women[7]. This tells us that while women are more likely to experience symptoms of depression during this time of life, it may not be due to the hormonal changes of the menopause transition. Two recent papers have reviewed the evidence across multiple studies following throughout the menopause transition. One of the papers found that the perimenopausal stage was associated with the greatest increase in levels of depression, and that this increased risk is not found in the postmenopausal stage[8]. The other paper did not find a general relationship between the menopause transition and depressive symptoms or major depression. However, they did find that some specific subgroups of women may be more likely to experience depression during this time[9].

Some of these were menopause-related – women were more likely to experience low mood if they had more severe hot flushes or night sweats that interfered with their lives or caused sleep disturbance, or if they had experienced a longer duration of the menopause transition. These hormone changes and vasomotor symptoms, together with the meaning we might attach to these symptoms and attitudes toward the menopause can combine to trigger low mood. If we think of menopause symptoms as a sign that we are in decline and becoming unattractive, then feeling low in mood and negative about the future is not a surprising reaction[10].

Aside from these factors relating to the menopause, a range of other social and lifestyle factors are also associated with increased risk of depression generally – life stressors which contribute to depression at any time can be part of the cause of low mood during the menopause transition. Of course, these can also interact – coping with menopause symptoms will be understandably more difficult if we are dealing with competing demands which mean we struggle to find time for self-care or positive change.

> *"I'd been depressed when I was younger and got depressed again during my perimenopause. I had a lot going on and I'm often exhausted – we were going through lots of change at work and a teenage daughter to support with school. My husband and I hit a rough patch, he's got his own mental health problems as well. We've talked about separating which we haven't done, but it's still on the cards. Sometimes it does feel like my mood is affected by my cycles, but really it's such a mix of everything all at once getting on top of me."*

Anxiety

In relation to anxiety, some studies have found that women who experience physical symptoms of anxiety are more likely to have hot flushes and night sweats, and also that the reverse is true – having these types of symptoms can increase anxiety. This can become an escalating cycle between the two, where anxiety drives up the symptoms, and these in turn continue to drive up anxiety.

> *"Recently, I had to present in a virtual meeting at work. I've never been very comfortable with public speaking, and so my anxiety set off a hot flush. Being able to see my face on screen go red and sweaty made it worse and I got stuck while I was speaking. It was so obvious that a colleague made a light joke about it – I know that they were trying to break the tension, but it felt awful for me. Since then I hate seeing my face on screen in meetings and I'm always on the lookout for early signs I'm about to have another hot flush."*

Positive coping and beliefs

Factors associated with positive psychological coping have also been the subject of research in the menopause transition. More positive views about ageing and the menopause are associated with a less disruptive experience of the transition. A recent study identified factors which contribute to resilience during the menopause – optimism, emotional stability and regulation, self-compassion and self-esteem. Scoring higher on these was associated with lower stress and depression and milder menopausal complaints[11]. Thinking about how we build these skills and adopt more helpful beliefs can act as a protective factor as we navigate the menopause transition.

Social factors

Experiences of the menopause transition happen within a wider context of family, work or other commitments, social and cultural networks which shape expectations and behaviours. Societal and cultural influences can impact menopause symptoms through common lifestyle factors such as diet, exercise, stress levels, alcohol and drug use. The midlife is also a particularly busy time of life for many women who are often juggling multiple competing demands with menopausal changes in amongst the mix.

Family roles

The availability of reliable contraception in the latter half of the twentieth century resulted in women delaying the age they started having children and having fewer children in many countries and cultures around the world. Current midlife women have been impacted by this with increased gaps between themselves and the generations both above and below. For many people this means simultaneously supporting ageing parents with fewer siblings to share the load, at the same time as supporting children either still at home or in the process of launching to adulthood. We know that women disproportionately carry the load of unpaid caring responsibilities, and during the pandemic, this burden on many midlife women increased further with supporting children doing their schooling from home and providing support for ageing parents during lockdown.

> *"Even though I work longer hours, I'm the one that the kids ring when they have a question or need something. I also organise and attend appointments with mum. I keep track of everyone's schedule, and run the kids to school and their sports and other hobbies. My husband doesn't think he would be able to ask for time off work to do these things, so I end up doing most of it."*

Midlife, menopause and the workplace

Alongside these changes in families in recent decades, women have also been joining the paid workforce in unprecedented numbers, which has brought many challenges with it. There has been considerable discussion of gendered ageism in the workplace, understanding how and why women are viewed and treated differently from men in the workplace as they get older. At the stage when men generally see their careers continuing to progress, many women experience their careers stagnating through being overlooked and not being supported to manage competing demands on their time in inflexible workplace cultures[4].

In the United Kingdom, we've seen a recent focus on the specific issue of menopause in the workplace. As women aged over 50 make up the largest growing demographic group in the workforce, this is an important issue. Women tend to report that menopausal symptoms are particularly difficult to deal with at work; and in surveys some women report making key career decisions due to the impact of their menopause symptoms, such as working less, stepping down to a less demanding role or not going for promotion. Recent research highlights the diversity of women's experience as well as the two-way relationship between menopause and work[12]. For some women, menopausal symptoms have limited impact on their work; for others, however, the picture is very different. Symptoms such as hot flushes can have perceived negative effects on work performance and prompt feelings of shame or embarrassment, while sleep disturbance or fatigue following night sweats, or the unpredictability of menstrual bleeding, may make work more difficult. However, there is strong evidence that the workplace environment has a direct effect on the experience of menopause. Certain physical (e.g. workplace temperature and ventilation), interpersonal (e.g. perceived managerial support and flexibility, formal meetings or high-visibility work like giving presentations) and inhospitable organisational cultural factors (e.g. circulating negative gender- and age-based stereotypes of midlife female workers) can shape women's experience.

Employers' incapacity to support women through menopause can mean that they take their talents elsewhere[12]. Many women also report feeling unable to discuss their symptoms with their manager or organisation, meaning that these decisions are made without an opportunity to consider adjustments. This is a potential loss to individuals, families, organisations and societies, as we miss out on the benefit of this experience and wisdom in workplaces, and occurring at a time when workforce shortages in the United Kingdom are at their highest in decades.

> *"I'm the only woman in my office – I work in management in construction. At this stage of my career, I'm looking to progress into more senior roles, I have a lot to offer and I'm good at what I do. I have endometriosis and adenomyosis and I can have really heavy bleeding which can be difficult to manage working on site. I also have pain which is better if I have a specialised chair. I worry that asking for what I need to make me more comfortable at work might prevent me from progressing – maybe I just need to leave and go elsewhere. I'm also considering a hysterectomy to manage the bleeding but it seems extreme to do something irreversible."*

The reactions and attitudes of others around us in the workplace can have a significant impact on how it feels to be a woman in the menopause transition at work. In some cases, people experience that the menopause is rarely raised, and that when it is, it reinforces negative stereotypes that make people even more reluctant to discuss it.

> *"I'm generally known as a pretty even-tempered person at work, but an issue occurred which I felt was very unfair and I let my feelings be known. I didn't lose my temper, but I didn't hold back on expressing my opinion because I felt it was important. Rather than taking me seriously, another senior female colleague asked me if I thought my hormones might have made me angry. I felt really betrayed and undermined, and I've avoided dealing with her if I can ever since then."*

On the other hand, having supportive relationships with colleagues and managers can help women to think about and manage their challenges constructively.

> *"I work with other women who were suffering in silence about menopausal symptoms. After we spoke with each other, work then made an effort to embrace these issues and the Human Resources department has since caught up."*

> *"I have never been a great sleeper, but it got much worse during my perimenopause. Luckily, I had a supportive manager I felt able to raise this with, and we discussed it during my annual appraisal. She agreed I could take power naps, and arrange to start late if I had to. I didn't need these options very often, but it was a big relief to have it written down, and I hardly took any time off as a result."*

One silver lining of the pandemic has been a general increase in remote working and other flexible arrangements; organisations providing these generally see better outcomes and employees report better work-life balance[13]. For midlife women in the menopause transition this can help to manage symptoms and meet other commitments while still managing their work.

> *"My home office is part of a garage conversion and it has helped me work throughout COVID and beyond. It means I can manage the temperature and I can take breaks when I need to. It is my space, but periodically I get invaded by family – sometimes my son sits in here while he's doing his revision. I travel into the office occasionally if it's needed for something specific, but I'm based at home and it works well for my role."*

At the same time, influence over the work environment and flexible working options are not available in many roles, and women in non-managerial or non-professional roles are more likely to work in these settings. Environmental factors such as control over the workplace temperature, adequate ventilation, access to breaks and toilet facilities, the comfort of uniforms and protective wear can influence how well women feel able to manage menopausal symptoms.

Thankfully, in recent years things are starting to change for the better, with many organisations now adopting various strategies to try and support those experiencing the menopause transition in the workplace. These often include having a specific menopause policy, increased options for flexible working, women and menopause networks, training and awareness for general staff and specifically for managers.

> *"My workplace started an online menopause group . . . we were able to have conversations and discussions in a safe space. This was beneficial to a lot of women at work and there was a strong need to push through policies to help women in our workplace."*

Race and ethnicity

There are differences between biological and hormonal changes experienced by women of different races and ethnicity; cultural beliefs also influence women's attitudes and expectations about the menopause and whether they are likely to seek help. In general, menopause-related symptoms are reported to be less prevalent in countries where menopause is viewed as a normal ageing process rather than a disease or deficiency. Attitudes may also vary depending on whether people are living in their country of origin or if they are part of an ethnic minority in a new country and cultural environment[14]. Increasing representation and inclusion of people from different cultural backgrounds can be very powerful in the process of seeking information, treatment and support.

> *"My mother was married in her country very young and wasn't educated. When I started my periods, she didn't have any way to explain it to me, she told me stories that didn't make any sense. So, I learned at a young age how to find things out for myself. . . . In the menopause it was so exciting for me to find female medical doctor who looked like me and talked about the experience from a South Asian woman's perspective."*

> *"I feel really lucky to be part of a local menopause support group with other women from non-white backgrounds. Even though we are quite different from one another, seeing and supporting other women who look like me feels really important."*

Building your own biopsychosocial model

This section is an opportunity for you to think about your personal experience and build your own biopsychosocial model. We invite you to think through the following questions and make notes, particularly noting those things which you find a challenge or resonate as something important to you.

Biological

- Are you experiencing physical symptoms of the menopause? When and where do they tend to happen, and how are they impacting on your day-to-day life?
- Do you have other current health conditions or symptoms alongside your menopause transition, and how is it managing these together?

Psychological

- Do you have difficult feelings about your specific menopause symptoms, for example feeling down, anxious or embarrassed?
- How do you feel about going through the menopause?
- How is your self-esteem? Has menopause changed the way you see yourself?
- How is your mood in general, and has it changed during the menopause transition? If you experience mood changes, which emotions are you finding the most challenging?
- How do you view your age and your health? Are these views overly negative? What thoughts and feelings do you have about your life in the future beyond the menopause?
- What are your values and plans for the future? Do you feel you've met some of your life goals, and do you have others that you are working toward?

Social

- What would you say are your main roles, for example, nurse, mother, friend, football supporter. . . . Are there any that you want to prioritise or step back from a little?
- How are the key family and social relationships in your life? Are you going through losses, bereavements changes and stresses?
- How are you feeling about work or other roles in your life? Are you finding these rewarding and/or demanding? How are you managing to balance the demands in your life?
- Are you facing challenges and stress due to financial insecurity? Do you have adequate funds and access to nutritious food, stable and appropriate housing and a healthy environment?
- Do you have access to healthcare services that have time and understanding to address your specific needs?

- What messages or beliefs have you noticed about menopause or ageing from your family and friends, your workplace and colleagues, your culture, the media? Have any of these impacted you strongly either negatively or positively?
- Do you feel connected to and supported by others in your life – family and friends? Do you spend time with others who are important to you, do you get to engage in enjoyable activities together?
- Do you have enough time to do the things which are important for you? If not, what do you think gets in the way? Do you know what things you'd like to do more of and less of?
- Are there aspects of your lifestyle that you'd like to change – such as diet, exercise, smoking, alcohol/drugs, sleep, rest/relaxation?

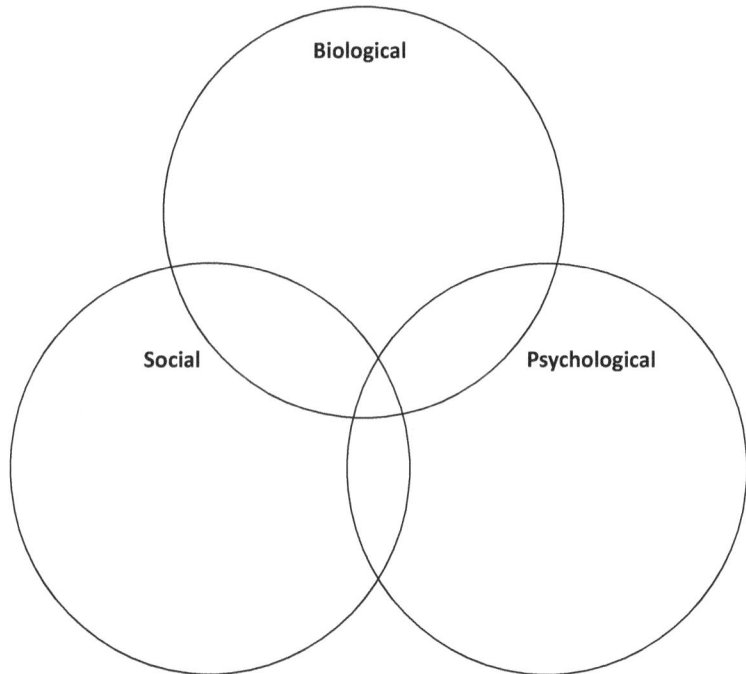

Once you have answered these questions, look through your list and think about whether there are key areas that feel like priorities that you would like to address. It can also be helpful to think about which factors you feel will be easiest for you to do something about (i.e. your 'quick wins'), and whether there are some where you'll need information or support from others.

Making changes and seeking support

A piece of welcome news is that it is common that many menopause symptoms tend to improve after the end of the menopause – including vasomotor symptoms, mood difficulties and brain fog. However, as symptoms during the menopause transition can persist over a number of years (and some of our busiest years) and for some women may continue beyond their menopause transition, having access to helpful strategies and treatments can be vital for minimising and managing symptoms.

Feeling empowered to make informed decisions which takes individual experience and background into account can help us to be more effective in managing ongoing conditions. Although health services may be under pressure and have decreased flexibility, we would encourage you to think about whether you have important preferences, and to ask for these to be met where possible (e.g. clinician gender, cultural background, specialism). Taking adequate time to consider important treatment decisions and having access to unbiased sources of information and opportunities to ask questions is particularly helpful for decisions which involve potential long-term or non-reversible treatment options.

An advantage of the biopsychosocial perspective over a narrower biological model of menopause is that it provides a wider range of potential interventions in addition to the option of MHT (or as an alternative for those women who are either unable or do not wish to pursue a hormonal approach). As other chapters in this book provide information and expertise regarding medical treatments, we focus here on psychological and social treatments and supports.

Psychological approaches

Psychological approaches can be helpful to women in managing physical, psychological and relational factors during the menopause transition. There has been some recent scepticism expressed about the recommendation of psychological therapies for menopause symptoms; some have expressed that this is implying that that the symptoms are "all in the mind". However, psychological approaches are used in a range of physical health conditions, and can be effective not only in changing thoughts and feelings, but also in altering our physiology and neurochemistry.

- Cognitive Behavioural Therapy (CBT) has been shown to help women in specifically managing hot flushes and night sweats, reducing the severity of the experience and the impact on day-to-day life[10].
- CBT is also recommended for depression, anxiety and for sleep disturbance.
- Mindfulness and meditation-based interventions have also been found to help with mood and anxiety difficulties during menopause.
- Compassion-focused approaches may be helpful, as higher self-compassion is associated both with more positive views of ageing, body image and milder menopausal complaints.

These approaches can be sought through formal therapy, and are also available in self-help formats including books and apps.

Health/Well-being

Aside from approaches to treat specific symptoms, it is also helpful to promote and maintain good general health and well-being through lifestyle approaches (e.g. good nutrition, exercise, relaxation and spending time in nature, as well as addressing excessive drug and alcohol use). Making changes to long-term habits can be challenging on your own, so you may wish to ask your GP about programmes available via referral, or join local or online groups to get support with these. Also recognise that changing a lot of things at the same time can be challenging, and so it may be helpful to make changes gradually – starting with those that feel easier or most important to you.

Group support can also help to normalise women's experiences and improve quality of life. In the United Kingdom, Menopause Cafés are available in many areas, and if there isn't one in your area, you may wish to set one up with friends (see www.menopausecafe.net for existing cafés, and information about establishing new cafés). There are online support groups through social media networks which you can find for support and information – with the caveat that it's helpful to identify whether these groups have commercial interests or a particular bias in their group.

Family roles

It is common that roles and responsibilities in families become established without conscious decisions and discussion, and are influenced by factors including our own families of origin and wider society. As we mentioned earlier, women are more likely to carry a heavier burden of family caring and co-ordinating responsibilities in family groups even when also working. If family demands are contributing to your stress, it can be helpful to explain about the menopause – educate those around you – and have a discussion about what can help at home. For example, you might want to reduce or share some roles and responsibilities with your partner/spouse, siblings and older/adult children. We tend to take on more roles/responsibilities during mid-life, so review the demands on you and consider what are the priorities.

In the workplace

With the increase in awareness about menopause in the workplace, many organisations are now providing information and support networks for menopause. By taking part in these, you can benefit from the support your workplace can provide, and it may also be an opportunity to influence your workplace.

Find out if your workplace has a Menopause Policy and see what it offers in terms of your support. If they don't, and you feel able to speak to your manager or someone in HR, let them know about https://helptogrow.campaign.gov.uk/menopause-and-the-workplace/ which has government guidance for employers as well as suggestions for workers.

In relation to the most common menopausal symptoms, there are a number of adjustments which you might wish to discuss or request in your workplace;

- Hot flushes – ventilation, access to fans, discussion with staff about room temperature settings for enclosed spaces, uniforms made from light and breathable fabrics, uniform styles to suit different body shapes and sizes
- Irregular/Heavy Bleeding – adequate access to toilet facilities, available free sanitary products for women who are caught out, 'Black Cardi' initiatives
- Sleep difficulties and fatigue – flexible hours, time and spaces for rest-breaks
- Muscle/joint pain – assessment of workstations to ensure good posture, supportive chairs, sit/stand desks, frequency of breaks

If you are in a workplace that does not have formal networks or support available, think about who else in your workplace might be a supportive ally for you to start having discussions with. You might also connect with women in your industry in other organisations to hear about how others are dealing with the issue, to share support and ideas. If you are in a trade union or can join one, you can ask them to get involved to represent the needs of menopausal people in discussion with workplaces.

Final thoughts

Although the menopause can be a challenging time of life, there is real reason for optimism. We encourage women to challenge overly negative views about mid-aged and older women and instead to focus on the wisdom and experience that age brings. Remember the information about the adaptive function of menopause, the relief of 'No periods!' and studies show that well-being tends to improve after menopause. By reflecting on the range of factors contributing to your experience of menopause and that point to areas for change, you may find not only that you can improve how you cope with your current challenges, but that you transition to the next phase of life with a renewed sense of purpose and opportunity.

References

1. Hunter MS. Psychological aspects of the menopause. In *Managing the Menopause*, Panay N, Briggs P, Kovacs GT, 2nd Edition. Cambridge University Press, 2020.
2. Wood BM, Negrey JD, Brown JL et al. Demographic and hormonal evidence for menopause in wild chimpanzees. *Science* 2023; 382; eadd5473. doi: 10.1126/science.add5473.
3. Mattern S. *The Slow Moon Climbs*. Princeton University Press, Princeton, 2019.
4. Ryan L. *Revolting Women: Why Midlife Women are Walking Out, and What to do About it.* Practical Inspiration Publishing, 2023.

5 Hickey M, LaCroix AZ, Doust J et al. An empowerment model for managing menopause. *The Lancet* 2024; 403; 947–957. doi: 10.1016/S0140-6736(23)02799-X.
6 Wilson RA, Wilson TA. The fate of the nontreated postmenopausal woman: A plea for the maintenance of adequate estrogen from puberty to the grave. *Journal of the American Geriatrics Society* 1963; 11: 347–362.
7 Arias de la Torre J, Vilagut G, Ronaldson A et al. Prevalence and age patterns of depression in the United Kingdom. A population-based study. *Journal of Affective Disorders* 2021; 279: 164–172. doi: 10.1016/j.jad.2020.09.129.
8 Badawy Y, Spector A, Li Z et al. The risk of depression in the menopausal stages: A systematic review and meta-analysis. *Journal of Affective Disorders* 2024; 357: 126–133.
9 Brown L, Hunter MS, Chen R et al. Promoting good mental health over the menopause transition. *The Lancet* 2024; 969–983. doi: 10.1016/S0140-6736(23)02801-5.
10 Hunter MS, Smith M. *Managing Hot Flushes and Night Sweats: A Cognitive Behavioural Self-help Guide to the Menopause*, 2nd Edition. Routledge, 2021.
11 Suss H, Willi J, Grub J et al. Psychosocial factors promoting resilience during the menopausal transition. *Archives of Women's Mental Health* 2021; 24: 231–241. doi: 10.1007/s00737-020-01055-7.
12 Jack G, Riach K, Hickey M et al. Menopause in the workplace: Building evidence, changing workplaces, supporting women. *Maturitas* 2021; 151: 63–64. doi: 10.1016/j.maturitas.2021.07.001.
13 LeanIn.Org and McKinsey & Company. *Women in the Workplace*. 2023. https://womenintheworkplace.com/.
14 The British Menopause Society. *Menopause in Ethnic Minority Women*. 2023. https://thebms.org.uk/wp-content/uploads/2023/06/20-BMS-TfC-Menopause-in-ethnic-minority-women-JUNE2023-A.pdf.

Scene 3 Don't mention the 'M' word!

Dr Meena Khatwa

Exploring taboos shrouding the reality of menopause

> "I love being a woman, but then I think, oh my God, it's just like we do get the bum end of the deal!"
>
> *Belinda*

When I was invited to contribute to this book, I immediately experienced a multitude of emotions. Firstly, the annoying gremlin whispering in my ear: "W*hy you, what's your expertise?"* Once this self-doubt had been quashed, I felt a sense of excitement and humility. Of course, I can write this; I'm one of many living with perimenopause, navigating the highs and lows. My own journey has drawn me to like-minded women, and knowing you are not alone brings comfort. I joined and became fully engaged with the University College London Menopause Network and chaired two events, one of which celebrated World Menopause Day 2024. It was humbling to hear other women's experiences, and now I've been given a platform. Although I'm an academic, by taking a creative non-fiction and auto-ethnographic approach, I can delve deeper and grab more visceral moments and meanings. This method allows the writer to be subjective and reflexive about cultural experiences, as described by Sally Denshire:

> "Auto-ethnographers often blur boundaries, crafting fictions and other ways of being true in the interests of rewriting selves in the social world"[1].

I'm sharing personal reflections of a 50+ South Asian, British-born, perimenopausal woman raising a teenage daughter. These are important signposts to flag as they lay the foundation for what follows. I don't speak for other women; my own views are my own. However, I believe it is also wise to seek other voices alongside my own narrative. Thus, the passages I write are peppered with stories from other women, whose permission I have sought. I also draw on academic and non-academic sources to underpin my ideas on tackling the complexities and myths of menopause. The social world I explore within this context stems from my own reproductive journey. I don't believe you can look at this as an 'isolated' life transition. From the outset, I unravel the mysticism that shrouds our experiences and conversations about menarche (when periods start) and menopause (when periods stop). The contributors' anecdotes will hopefully resonate because what we have in common are our stories. Throughout this chapter, I flit between timelines;

it's not a linear story, but snapshots capturing pertinent milestones. This is a sentiment shared by feminist writer bell hooks: "*The longing to tell one's story and the process of telling is symbolically a gesture of longing to recover the past in such a way that one experiences both a sense of reunion and a sense of release"*[2].

We are book ends: a tale of two generations

> *"You know you're pushed into adulthood when you bleed, and I'd rather have somebody who held my hand and took me along that journey."*
>
> *Anjali*

We begin where the paths of a mother and daughter converge. The year is 2021, and I'm experiencing a mental, physical and emotional test of endurance. Five years prior, my body decided to throw me confusing curveballs concerning my menstrual cycle. Since then, I'd had many blood tests, scans and cervical screenings investigating my heavy bleeding. This was partially due to my request to have the Mirena® coil fitted, but unclear scan results were left unresolved. Though my attempts were well-meaning, like many women, my self-care inevitably got pushed aside as day-to-day priorities took precedence. A study conducted by Bloom UK, a professional network for women in communications, reported a staggering 93% lacked a good work/life balance, which had negatively impacted their mental health[3]. Feelings of spreading ourselves too thin were also expressed by the women I spoke to, such as Lina, who worked as a teacher:

> *"Oh, wow! How am I supposed to deal with this? I was in the class, and I must have gone to the back . . . sat down and got a glass of water. The heat just comes up, you're very aware and it drained me. I had no energy . . . what you need to know about me is I'm the one that does everything. . . . I'm the one that keeps on going."*
>
> *Lina*

While attempting to handle my own work/home challenges, coupled with health-related issues, I now had to grapple with an emerging milestone from another family member. It's a typical weekday morning and it's my turn to do the school run. I'm still half asleep, but the sips of hot tea awaken my taste buds, sending sparks of caffeine to my brain to jolt it from slumber. The tiredness I experienced was of a different kind now, not from the usual work meetings and deadlines, but resembling more a battery leaking energy, depleted of illuminated life.

I had never suffered from insomnia and always slept well to the point of smugness. My partner had described it as *"the gift of sleep."* I had slept through the great storm of 1987, when Michael Fish brushed aside a viewer's warnings of the impending Storm Ciarán and remember feeling shocked at the aftermath, hearing fellow school peers excitedly sharing how they didn't get any sleep! Or when I had to be nudged awake by the midwives when my daughter was crying shortly after she had been born.

I now experienced disrupted sleep and had to contend with night sweats. I was thankful the seasons were cooler and, to my partner's dismay, the open windows offered the comfort of winter breeze. However, living in inner London, we also had to contend with the external soundtrack of occasional sirens and the screeching howls of urban foxes.

The hot flushes and night sweats had sadly meant relinquishing my cosy attire, but I refused to give up my tea, even though my body heat radiated through my clothes. I believe when I began to experience these symptoms, which I now understood to be perimenopausal, I was still in denial. I wanted to go back to the former me before I resembled a damp sponge! This sentiment is also echoed by Ada Calhoun (2020),

> *"One answer is: denial. We have had incentives for a long time to pretend we are the same as men in every way. For decades, women have had to argue that they could still work and function through those messy period, pregnancy and menopause-related symptoms, and as a result we've minimised them, both to others and to ourselves"*[4].

Like clockwork, I felt beads of sweat on my brow, and the clamminess ensued. I frantically fanned myself and thought I'll need to change my clothes again! I glanced over to my daughter who was filling a bowl with cereal. In a fleeting moment, her mood changed from contentment to sadness as she clutched her stomach and let out a little sob. I gave her a knowing hug; the pain is all too familiar to me. As she wrapped her arms around me, she whimpered, *"Oh Mamma, we are bookends!"* Moved by her poetic expression, I immediately experienced an overwhelming feeling of empathy and replied, *"Yes, we are."* I process this moment and contemplate that my daughter and I stood at opposite points of our fertility paths. She is at the beginning – with the burgeoning blossom of youth unfurling its petals – and me slowly shedding what remains of my younger self. Though only 10, her body was signalling signs of puberty, mine navigating the tricky terrain of perimenopause. She asked, *"Is it going to hurt like this every time?"* At first, I was reluctant, and perhaps wanted to shield her, but I stressed how everyone is different. After all, she is still young and not mature enough to handle such realities and as mothers, we have heightened awareness of our daughter's needs. This is in stark contrast to what was maybe lacking in our childhoods, a sentiment shared by Belinda:

> *"I guess it's a generational thing . . . but I wanna make sure that with my girls I talked to them about everything. If they're worried . . . that they shouldn't feel embarrassed. Because I'm kind of aware that I didn't always feel like I could talk to my mum."*

Equally, I was also aware that girls are reaching puberty much earlier, potentially a confusing and frightening time for many. This came to light in the 1980s when Professor Marcia Herman-Giddens, working in a paediatric clinic at Duke University

Medical Center in North Carolina, observed young girls showing early signs of sexual maturation. She went on to collect data from 17,000 girls and found on average, the onset of puberty was between 8 and 9 years. However, Giddens was not prepared for the controversy the published findings stirred with many doctors who refused to accept this, as reported in the *New York Times*:

> "I had no idea it would be so huge, Herman-Giddens told me recently. The Lolita syndrome – the prurient fascination with the sexuality of young girls – created a lot of emotional interest. As a feminist, I wish it didn't"[5].

Grappling with such transitions, particularly for mothers and daughters at the same time, is a delicate balancing act, whereby hormonal collisions are bound to be inevitable. During my own experiences as a teenager, these milestones were shrouded in mystery; there was no open dialogue between my mother and me about any of these impending changes. Perhaps this was a cultural barrier growing up in a South Asian household, as equally there was no knowledge transfer between my mother and her mother. This was also noted by some of the older women I spoke to, who lacked a formal or even informal sex education:

> "When I was about 11, I started [getting] pains in my tummy. I didn't know what was going on. I was in East Africa then, my mum never told us about these things, it was secret to talk about these things, it was shameful in those days [during] the late 60s."
>
> *Devi*

> "I was probably 15 when my mum told me how a baby is born, though I'd had been having periods before then, probably 13 when I bled. I had no idea about the mechanics of how it worked in the human body."
>
> *Madhu*

The taboo nature of body politics is internalised, and therefore, in my case, I sought identification elsewhere. My turning point was discovering Judy Blume's *Are You There God? It's Me, Margaret* (originally published in 1970). I recall reading it secretly, because the content dealt with periods, religion and sexuality, and was frowned upon in a strict Hindu household. Growing up, I was warned of Western influences corrupting young minds. If faced with scenes of romantic kisses in films or TV dramas, the channel was immediately changed. You wouldn't see this kind of behaviour in vintage Bollywood films either; instead, tilting heads and encircled arms implied a passionate embrace. Blume's book was a welcome revelation for a teen British Asian girl growing up in 1980s England, I deeply connected with the fictitious character called Margaret. When the film adaptation was released (2023), I was keen to watch it with my family. It was a nostalgic trip for me as memories flooded back of hiding in my bedroom sneakily reading a few pages. For my daughter, who had started her period by then, this innocent time of self-discovery had passed, as the film images were all too familiar. Had this generation grown up too fast? The prevalence of social media has meant that young people have greater agency, freely seeking out information from a myriad of influencers, TikTokers and Instagrammers. Furthermore, my daughter was privy to my journey of change; she'd seen me at my most vulnerable and, for someone so young, knew how to comfort me: a blanket, a hot drink and a biscuit. How many other mothers and daughters are going through this private but seismic change? This is echoed by Kate Figes (2004):

> *"She wants Radio 1 on in the car; I have developed a chilling preference for Radio 2. She bounds up the stairs with ease, wants to wallow in her new sexuality and go out dancing all night. I am beginning to creak with aching joints as the oestrogen plummets. Most nights, I am so knackered that my new best thing is going to bed"*[6].

The collision of these two hormonal worlds is not an isolated incident as statistical evidence finds women increasingly choosing to have babies in their mid-30s: *"Since menopause typically occurs between ages 45 and 55, that means a whole lot more clashing of reproductive stages in families nationwide"* . It is vital to acknowledge this ever-increasing phenomenon. I take comfort in knowing my daughter will be far more knowledgeable than I am. However, we are not there yet, as the following section reveals the persistent stigma and taboos that still pervade today.

Secrets and taboos: it's a bleeding shame!

> *"It's really fear-based . . . we are told that our bodies are dirty and shameful and wrong . . . because we can't ask questions about periods, because that's the dirty thing that comes out right at the end of every month."*
>
> Sophia

I don't know whether I live in a typically average family household in the United Kingdom, where my daughter, partner and I can talk freely about menstruation and menopause. There have been many occasions where I've asked my partner to buy pads and he has supported me, though a tad reluctant. Not because he is embarrassed, but due to my very specific needs. I'm always taken aback by how our period products are on display in the bathroom. If you are caught short, it isn't always easy to call out to someone to get you a pad. Perhaps it's inevitable living in a house with women, but is this the norm in other households? I was glad to hear this experience was shared by other mothers raising teenagers:

"It was very shut away when I was growing up . . . sanitary products were in [a] knicker drawer, so nobody could see them, and they wouldn't be left around the house. It's quite different in our house, I've always just put them in the bathroom, and you know they're in bags. They're everywhere [laughs]!"

Monica

Academic research has shown varying opinions and experiences from a male viewpoint. An Australian study reported that men often learnt information about menstruation from sexual and romantic partners[8]. Similarly, a U.S. study found that boys would learn about menstruation by overhearing discussions among female friends and class peers[9]. More recently, a UK study (2022) conducted by healthcare experts at an online pharmacy, found amongst 1,500 male participants that 52% stated never purchasing period products for their partners, with 42% thinking it's too embarrassing[10]. Where does this shame stem from and why does it persist today?

The stigma around menstruation is not just confined to male attitudes. History shows generations of women are also subjected to the perpetuation of cultural and social taboos. However, it is imperative we address levels of knowledge transfer from mother to daughter, and from the old to the young. This complex topic is steeped in ritualistic, traditional and societal constructs around menstruation, as Hawkeye (2020) writes: "*Mothers' attitudes toward menstruation shapes the menstrual education girls receive which, if inadequate, might negatively affect daughters' experience of menarche and ongoing perspectives toward menstruation and sexuality*"[11] . What I explore next are the nuances of a global perspective, complemented by the rich accounts of the women I spoke to.

When my daughter started her period just shy of her 12th birthday, she calculated how many years she would bleed for, and the number shocked her. In that moment, I thought "*Welcome to the world of womanhood,*" but I sensitively dealt with the 'period sentence' she had received. If she takes after me, then years of stomach cramps and heavy periods are inevitable. Many of the South Asian women I spoke to mirrored my experiences. Lina had to take days off school and as she described: "*Life just stopped.*" I remember in my teen years being doubled up in pain, my mum and sister looking at me, unsure of how to comfort me as they were fortunate enough not to endure the same symptoms. My coming-of-age story is in stark contrast to my daughter's, and I believe this bodes well for her generation, who talk more openly about periods. Casting my mind back, I remember at age 14, going to my mum and whispering that I had got my period. She nodded and ushered me to the cupboard under the stairs. I wondered what I was about to receive. She handed me a carrier bag which included a packet of sanitary pads and plastic knickers with a pad lining. I remember feeling rather surprised by the preemptive preparation, though the conversation was minimal, practical and devoid of comfort. When I asked the other women to recall first period memories, I was overwhelmed by the outpouring of honesty. As so much was shared, I've grouped them into two themes:

Confusion and fear around starting periods too early or too late

Devi, age 11 recalls: *"I went to school and started bleeding and thought, oh my God, what has happened? My salwar [tunic] was full of blood, oh my God, I have hurt myself somewhere. I was so scared if my mum found out . . . she is going to hit me . . . so I put my salwar in the basket of dirty clothes and hid it in there."*

Jaya's mother was concerned with her daughter's late period, as she started at 15. Her mother blamed her tomboyish behaviour (for example, climbing trees) and recalls her mum saying: *"Girls who play sport, got it late."*

Mothers deferring responsibility for period education to older siblings, neighbours, friends

Both Bhavni and Devi sought help from their older sisters and did not tell their mothers directly. Yasmin was advised to speak to her neighbour's daughter, who was two years older. Similarly, Anjali was encouraged to speak to a girl of a similar age in the same apartment block. In Rani's case, even though her parents were doctors, she recalled: *"I didn't feel that the relationship was there to talk about."* Her father, a gynaecologist, instead drew a biological illustration of the uterus.

In similar taboo behaviour, and although I was raised in the United Kingdom, I was given strict instructions:

1. Don't parade sanitary towels or leave them on display where they are visible to men.
2. Talking about my periods to any male member living in the house was not permitted.
3. I must wash my hair on the fourth or fifth day of my period.
4. If I was menstruating, a visit to the temple meant sitting at the back to avoid polluting others with my impurity! (This last rule was particularly surprising to me.)

There was no clear explanation, but these residual rituals were played out in many British Asian households. For example, Priya explained how her mother-in-law would not allow her to enter the kitchen (considered a religious space where food is prepared) for five days during the menstrual cycle. I did as I was told and never questioned it, however I felt incredibly self-conscious when sitting at the back of the temple, no neon sign was necessary, my private periods had been 'outed' for all the community to see.

Nonetheless, alongside these repressive attitudes, I discovered 'positive' celebratory cultural rituals relating to a girl's first period. For example, African countries such as Benin, Cameroon and Zambia, reported girls receiving special treatment, gifts, perfume, underwear and jewellery[12]. Menarche is considered a marker of womanhood: *"A time of significant psychological and sociocultural adjustment, potentially leading girls to reconceptualize their identity as women within the patriarchal societies they live"*[13]. Similar celebrations (saree parties) are often observed in Tamil families, whereby news is shared with the whole community of a young girl's first period. I was keen to investigate such events further. For example, Anjali received a letter from her grandfather after her mother had shared the news. He praised her for becoming an adult, and Maya was presented with a watch at a small gathering and was made the centre of attention, as she recalls:

> *"You're supposed to wear certain kinds of clothes. So, in Tamil, they would say, 'Periyamanushi' that means, like, 'aged woman'. So, when you're still a child and being called a woman, or almost equivalent of adult. That's just a very bizarre concept."*

This mirrors my own experience of menstrual segregation when both men and women sat in front of me in the temple, knowing about my period, which filled me with shame. In contrast, my experiences of menstruation pale in comparison to those of fellow women across the globe. Some of the older generation shared how they used large pieces of cloth to absorb menstrual blood, resulting in discomfort, and had to wash them every day. Devi recalls that after washing them, her mother would hang them far from the house so they weren't visible. Bhavni used her initiative by swapping rags for cotton wool to absorb the blood and avoid them. However, both women expressed relief when using pads once they arrived in the United Kingdom. While using pads was a marked improvement for women in India, purchasing them was still shrouded in secrecy. As Madhu recalls, a specific shop or pharmacy wrapped the products in newspaper *"so you can't see the packet."* However, this defeated the purpose, as Maya and Anjali both explained, that conspicuous packaging meant that: *"I would be a target . . . people would know that I'm on my period."*

As a transition into womanhood, menstruation was often associated with sexual maturity and marriage. In many cultures, early marriages was seen as preventative for women not to have children out of wedlock[14]. For migrant women living in the West, practices such as these would be legally restricted. When researching studies for this section, I experienced conflicting feelings towards the private and public nuances of having something so personal exposed, as *"even though menarche celebration attempts to promote positive messages such as welcoming into womanhood, it may be confusing to process as girls across cultural contexts are often simultaneously receiving stigmatizing messages about the taboo nature of menstruation, a bodily function to be contained and hidden"*[15].

Centuries-old traditions drawn from religious texts deem menstruation to be *"positioned as negative"*[16]. Furthermore, historically and cross-culturally, menstrual blood has been *"discursively constructed as being poisonous, magical polluting 'monstrous feminine'"*[17]. Women in certain cultures (for example, Sudanese and Indian) are restricted from entering kitchens or carrying out household duties. I was keen to explore this further with the women I spoke to, particularly those from India. As Maya described:

> *"Grandpa is super religious, that means not entering the kitchen, you don't get to sleep in the same room as other people. Or even if you do, you have a teeny tiny corner, where you keep your utensils for eating and drinking."*

Maya was fortunate to at least have a room in the Himalaya's Pindar Valley. Translated as 'land of gods', women are segregated here. The poorer women are confined to a cowshed and not allowed to interact with people. The confinement includes no access to bathing or toilet facilities, and women had to wash outdoors in the river. A study carried out by Joshy et al. (2019) noted these restrictions impacted women's mobility, health, education and self-esteem, and explains: *"Menstruation is not seen as a 'normal' biological process that enables women to give birth, but instead seen as impure, menstruating girls and women are considered untouchable"*[18] . Young women also experienced great anxiety, being led to believe that their proximity to men (including fathers and brothers) whilst menstruating could cause illness in them. Menstrual segregation also meant girls were not allowed to go to school and were instead were homeschooled.

Similar practices are also carried out in rural parts of Nepal where ancient traditions are practised called '*chhaupadi*', translated as 'untouchable being'. Girls are banished, in isolation, to cold mud huts during the duration of their cycle. These practices have led to unfortunate consequences such as viruses, bacterial infections and violent sexual attacks[19]. Although this segregation was outlawed in 2017, the practices persist today.

We may not see such extreme practices in Western culture, but that does not mean repressive social attitudes around menstruation do not exist. In the podcast series *Betwixt the Sheets*, Kate Lister and guest Elissa Stein, co-author of *Flow: The Cultural Story of Menstruation* (2009), presented an episode titled *"The History of Periods"* (aired in March 2023). What struck me was how the notion of impurity can be explicit, as in the cases stated above, or implied ever so subtly, as Stein found in her research around menstrual product packaging. She draws the listeners' attention to the history of language, such as 'feminine hygiene', which implies menstruation is unclean, or that it smells, also offering women scented products. My role as a mother is therefore to ensure that I've not clung onto these residual practices so that my daughter is not shamed by menstruation.

This section ends with tales of two young girls' first period. Firstly, regarding my daughter: it is a cool May evening, and we are in the garden sitting around the fire pit. As my partner and I stare into the glowing embers, we are jolted by a small squeal, only to discover our daughter has started her first period. The full moon is shining bright and after some comforting and celebratory hugs, all three of us dance around the fire in what could be described as an urban celebration of womanhood.

Secondly, from a girl in rural India:

> *"I ran from school towards the jungle and hid myself in a cave. When I didn't return home my parents got worried and started searching for me. I was scared and started crying when my parents found me, they told me to remain there. They sent pooris and sweet rice, I had to stay far away from home in a hut in the jungle for 11 days"*[18].

I'm encouraged that attitudes are changing in parts of the world where menstrual segregation persists and visible in the mainstream media. One example was mentioned by Bhavni and Priya, who praised the film *Pad Man* (2018) directed by R. Balki, based on the true story of Arunachalam Muruganantham. By observing his wife's own menstrual segregation and use of unhygienic rags, he decided to produce low-cost pads despite the shame he faced.

The fear of loss: managing my mid-life menopause identity

"So many of us are starting to dance with perimenopause, but we have no idea" [20].

Our metamorphosis is inevitable but also full of complexities. I stare at myself in the mirror, spotting the crow's feet around my eyes, my energy tank half full and my patience wearing thinner than usual. It all culminates in that fateful day when your body signals menopause transition. I have found how my symptoms, both physical and psychosocial (e.g. social support, coping, emotional intelligence), mirror the experiences of so many other women[21]. Studies show that, *"the global population of postmenopausal women is growing. In 2021, women aged 50 and over accounted for 26% of all women and girls globally"*[22].

Over recent years, we have seen progressive exposure on menopause, and therefore a much-needed focus on *"the female-specific transitional life phases in women's natural ageing process"*[23]. Many high-profile women in the mainstream media have shone a light on menopause, dispelling the myths. For example, Davina McCall's documentary *Sex, Myths and Menopause* (2021); Mariella Frostrup and Alice Smellie's book *Cracking the Menopause: While Keeping Yourself Together* (2022); and more recently, Channel 4's comedy show *The Change*, starring Bridget Christie (2023). However, when I first started experiencing symptoms, media coverage wasn't as prevalent, and I didn't fully understand the changes to my body, and it happened so gradually. Unlike menstruation, where in school, I was taught sex education, it came as a complete shock. Surely, I was too young at 42, but during the summer of 2016, I was about to embark on a *"stormy passage"*[24].

We had just come to the end of a week of festivities, culminating in my younger brother getting married. A cacophony of traditions, from dhol (Indian drum) playing to a flash mob musical rendition of *West Side Story*. A long-awaited holiday to Portugal was in the offing, and while packing I wondered whether I should take some pads. I tended to strategically book trips that didn't coincide with my monthly cycle. At this stage, my periods ran like clockwork; I recognised the monthly signs and my mobile app would notify me when the impending floodgates were about to open. However, this time something was not right; my period was late and it felt disconcerting. I remember feeling a heady mix of trepidation and some joy . . . another baby? I was too old and more importantly, we weren't trying. This delay also triggered memories of my first birth experience. All I could think was, *"I don't want to die!"* A tad over-dramatic, but after my near-death emergency caesarean section and related complications, my partner and I had decided not to have any more children.

The memory of those six traumatic days in hospital reared its ugly head from time to time. Instead of holding my firstborn, I was too weak, having lost two litres of blood during surgery. I was dosed up on morphine and codeine, experienced severe vomiting and struggled to breastfeed my daughter because of tongue tie. I remember how my daughter's godmother was shocked at my demeanour – rather than seeing a glowing mother cradling her baby, she was faced with an ashen husk. This digression is important to note because a missed period dredged up all those associations. The pregnancy test revealed a single pink line indicating it was negative. I was relieved but perplexed. Those feelings were pushed aside and during the holiday, on the eve of my birthday, I started my period. In Carolan's (2000) study of Irish women, she found that women expressed a mix of anxiety and hope when a period was late. It was also described as *"distasteful"* as continued fertility in menopausal women was frowned upon[25]. This confusion was also shared by some women I chatted with, as Bhavni described: *"I was around 46 when my period first stopped, it was a shock and my husband suggested we go to the chemist and get a pregnancy test, the chemist who handed me the test told me not to worry. I tested negative and then went to my GP to find out what was going on."*

Looking back, I had no idea what perimenopause was and was astounded to read that it could last over four years but could also prolong between 10 and 15 years[20]. I was not a conscious witness to my mother's own menopause; there were no conversations about this transition. I recalled curtains being drawn during the day, as my mother tried to sleep in complete darkness. She experienced throbbing migraines and would place a wet flannel on her forehead to ease the pain. Sometimes it was so severe it would induce vomiting. During those occasions, we had to be considerate children, talking in whispers and watching TV on low volume. For me, I did not like adjusting to an unpredictable cycle, and every late period resulted in a negative pregnancy test. Each time I felt relief but also a slight tinge of disappointment. On one occasion, I sobbed uncontrollably and couldn't pinpoint why. My partner comforted me, allowing the emotions to tumble out. What did the sorrow symbolise? It gradually dawned on me that I was grieving for my 'fertile younger self'. Grief expert Lianna Champ provides clarity on honouring the grieving process of menopause:

> *" . . . and so we hit menopause either gradually or sometimes like a runaway train and we mourn for everything that was, as we try to come to terms with mother nature's conveyer belt"*[26].

How do women manage the loss privately as well as outwardly, when for centuries the social and symbolic constructs of womanhood have been intertwined with fertility and *"at menstruation women are using a biological given, that is the loss of menstrual blood, in order not only to express femininity, but also to reaffirm their acceptance of the female social role"*[27]. Veida Skultans further describes how reproductive and non-reproductive roles are central to the public image of the adult female. If our identities evolve around fertility, what does it then mean when your fertility is in decline? You have to contend with irrational and rational feelings and perceptions of attractiveness, youthfulness and what society projects onto us as the definition of woman.

Since the age of 14, my periods were my constant companion. Love or loathe them, they were part of me, and I understood them. I speak from my personal viewpoint, but my hormones would drop me clues, warning of the impending period. The monthly spots would appear around the chin, my hair would become lank and greasy, my stomach bloated and my breasts sensitive. I formed ritualistic habits, and for around 7 days, I hunkered down with my survival period kit: a full stock of pads for different flows, a trusty hot water bottle, painkillers, bars of chocolate, mugs of tea and a stack of go-to comfort movies. Even though every month I endured stomach cramps, the monthly cycle ironically allowed for rest, self-care and positive solitude. I would then reappear every month full of vitality and a youthful glow whereby, *"physical attractiveness is our most valuable asset"*[28]. Now, decades later, I am entering mid-life, uncharted territory, and having to readapt and understand what my body is signalling. I have no shame in admitting I cried with the realisation that something was shifting like the sands of time. I could see the fertile, young part of life slip away, and this was also shared by Belinda, who since her teens has experienced painful ovulation: *"I got sad that I didn't feel that anymore. I was gutted. I'm still gutted, so I'm still at that stage now where I don't know if I'm going to get a period this month, or if there's gonna be another 3- or 4-month break. And I know it happens, but I'm devastated about it."*

Women who are busy juggling work, home and family life are not provided the space to process this seismic shift. In Nosek's (2010) study, women reported fear, shame and embarrassment and described ageing as *"doom,"* and talking about it as *"taboo."* One interviewee from her study described the secrecy of it:

> *"It's a very complex . . . situation. I think it has to do with women seeing themselves as feminine, and . . . when they're no longer fertile . . . women have a long history in this culture of hiding their age. If you're in menopause, you're not a kid . . . some people associate it with the cessation of their feminine attractiveness"* [29].

Alongside tackling emotional and psychosocial symptoms, women have also had to endure physical symptoms. There is a chasm between what is shared between generations. For me, I was struck by the acceptance exuded by older women; there is a stoicism in this generation whereby it is *"part of the natural aging process,"* as stressed by members of a Newfoundland village fishing community, *"it is a hardship that must be endured"*[30]. This sentiment was also echoed by some of the older women I spoke to who didn't choose HRT due to fears at the time of getting cancer and took the more *'natural'* path. However, women of a similar age to myself shared a lack of support from mothers:

> *"So, I think she judges me for taking HRT and for making a big deal about the perimenopause. . . . She'll say, well, I've never had any problems, and you just have to get on with it . . . it's very black and white, so she's, like, 'I was fine, so everyone else is fine!"*
>
> ## *Belinda*

There has been a gradual shift over the years in cultural and social narratives, as women are becoming more vocal. Perhaps it is selective attention, but the stigma around perimenopause seems to be slowly dissipating. In March 2023, Drew Barrymore had her first hot flush live on her TV chat show while interviewing Jennifer Aniston: *"I am so hot, I think I'm having my first perimenopause hot flashes . . . Whoa!"*[31] I've had many conversations with friends and colleagues over tea or at a party, discussing symptoms. Before I eventually went on HRT, which was described to me as a 'game-changer', I was not happy in my own skin. I experienced the same shame and despair as described by many other women.

It was Christmas 2021 and while sitting in my mother's lounge, playing board games and sipping wine, a sudden heat rose up my neck, as if an internal boiler had been activated. Then came the night sweats and hot flushes, constantly mopping my brow and taking clothes to work. I would go to bed dry and wake up soaked; even being hugged by my loved ones was difficult as the heat raged. I used humour to downplay my paranoia that my sweaty presence could be seen by others and called myself *'clammy mammy'*. There is solace in knowing millions of women around the world experience similar symptoms and insecurities, describing them as *'private summers'*[32] or *'bochornos'* (embarrassment)[33] – a common phrase in Ecuador.

It is only through vocalising my symptoms, and not being ashamed, that I have received pearls of wisdom from older women. For someone who channelled 'hygge' every winter, I now slept under a wafer-thin 2.5 tog duvet with the window open in December. Looking back, while I was being prodded and poked to determine a diagnosis, I felt my body had held me hostage, and I was under house arrest. I began to experience flooding to the point of anaemia, and when the slightest cough or sneeze resulted in a deluge, and for the seventh time I had to shower again and change my clothes, I think it is fair to say you start to question your own sanity. I was not alone in experiencing these debilitating symptoms of perimenopause, as Monica recalls:

> *"When my periods became extremely heavy, and I had awful flooding, it was so painful. . . . I could just feel it coming . . . I cried. On one occasion . . . I needed to get to a toilet quickly, because it was running down my legs, it was awful. I found a hairdresser nearby, I just said, I'm sorry I'm in a horrible situation, the ladies were lovely, I changed my sanitary products, but had to leave and go and buy knickers. It really traumatised me . . . and after that I became really sort of fearful that I was not in control."*

Humour was the go-to mechanism to diffuse the trial my body had put me under, referring to the flooding as *"the period that just kept giving."* The toll it takes on your physical and emotional well-being is difficult to put into words, and I was thankful that I had colleagues who were sympathetic and allowed me to work from home. It is ironic how I grieved the end of my menstrual cycle but now I was wishing for it to just end; the only silver lining was discovering period knickers and revisiting my teen rituals again of feel-good films, hot water bottles and bed rest. I am sadly not alone, as it is estimated that one in three women will experience abnormal menstruation, although Georgina Davies goes further, writing that this figure might be underestimated, *"due to stigma that still surrounds menstruation"*[34].

The association between ageing and menopause is prevalent in many cultures – some are ambivalent, some embrace it and some view it as the *"widow's plague"*, as described by mothers in Utz's (2011) study comparing two generations. Similar feelings were also expressed by Sudanese women as *"sin al ya-iss"*, meaning the *"age of despair"*[35]. These fears were compounded by traditional patriarchal societies, whereby fertility is highly regarded, and menopause would lead to *"men leaving their wives"*[36]. However, these hormonal changes are like a double-edged sword, whereby the loss of fertility is also considered a virtue, described by women in Botswana as *"not to lament"*[30]. This is also found in Irish communities raising large families, where menopause provided freedom from repeated pregnancies[25]. These important ageing transitions hold complex meanings for women, differing between generations and ethnic groups.

Acceptance and agency: the shifting sands of menopausal ageing

"It's amazing! It's given me my life back. I never have to think about [my period] . . . it's great, I don't think I miss it at all!"

Madhu

I'm in my eighth year of perimenopause and it's been a rollercoaster! I've had to adopt coping strategies and re-evaluate my identity. My family has seen me at my worst (mood swings, low energy, hot flushes, flooding) and best with perimenopause (changes in HRT management). I count myself lucky that I never reached the point of severe anxiety or suicidal thoughts. I was struck by a powerful account of one woman's story in the *Guardian*, Karen Arthur, who had been signed off with anxiety from her teaching job and had come too close to ending her life, saying, *"I remember thinking how desperate you have to be . . . (and thinking very lucidly) I don't want to die, I don't want to kill myself, that's too real for me."* She ended up going to a pub and proceeded to write in her journal describing that day as the *"lowest but also the highest point"*[37]. Intimate narratives such as these help lift the veil and allow for meaningful discussion on stigma around menopause. I would describe myself now as a 'work in progress', a sentiment also shared by Monica, *"It was nice to be able to make sense of what was happening before."*

The preoccupation with perimenopause had taken precedence, and hovering somewhere in the distance was my next milestone. In September 2023, I turned 50 and spent the evening eating dinner overlooking Tokyo's skyline with my family. The months leading up to the Japan adventure were a mix of excitement but also feelings of reluctance and denial. I was begrudgingly dragging my heels towards this unforeseen path that lay ahead of me; my partner kept telling me, *"fifties are the new forties!"* That may well be, but I really liked my forties; you're straddled between feeling young enough but with a dollop of maturity. When I ponder my 50s, it seems closer to retirement. These feelings were strangely familiar to when I mourned my younger fertile self. I was coming to terms with ageing now, as: *"menopause is regarded as an undeniable end of a woman's ability to procreate, as well as her symbolic entrance into the second half of her life – taking on non-reproductive social roles"*[28].

What would the second half of my life have in store? I was jolted to reality after my 13-hour flight back from Japan, which resulted in swollen ankles and pains shooting up towards my knees. Thankfully, the GP ruled out anything serious but asked whether I had done any strenuous activities. I happily told him about the trip, the places we visited, impressing him with the daily 10,000 step count, and the upcoming 50th birthday party. The GP took a sharp intake of breath, looked me square in the eyes and *said:* "Oh you're 50, that explains it! The pains you are experiencing come with getting old, you've reached that age." I came out feeling, "So is that it? I'm old now!" I was dealing with a multitude of contradictory emotions. I acknowledged I didn't have the same tolerance levels for juggling work and home life, which resulted in longer periods of tiredness, and as Belinda described: *"I don't have the bandwidth."* Alongside this realisation, however, I also discovered the beginnings of a more rebellious side. I understood what it meant to be half a century old and ageing seemed to matter more! I acquired a no-nonsense approach, obtaining a superpower level of chutzpah. It meant I could just say *no*, where previously others' demands superseded my own. In Hvas' (2005) study, the women had become better at prioritising and ignoring trifles, as one woman, who suffered a stroke several years earlier, said, *"You have to stop and ask yourself: what do you really want from the rest of your life?"*[38]

I was intrigued to explore the co-existence between menopause and accepting ageing further, alongside other cultural interpretations. What was striking were the generational attitudes towards ageing, as this mother in a study expressed: *"menopause just happened. We didn't do much about it or discuss it with others. It wasn't something that we worried about"*[28]. Whereas her daughter took a different approach to menopausal experiences and wanted to be heard. This was also observed by Monica who described how menopause seemed to be *"a breeze"* for her mother and had experienced *"one sweat!"* These two viewpoints on menopause fell either into a natural midlife transition or an unpleasant marker of old age. However, perhaps such silent stoicism could be masking feelings of fear or shame. As one woman (in her late 60s), in the same study, described severe bouts of mood swings and depression and was admitted by her physician to a mental hospital. She was diagnosed as suicidal and as she stated, *"I needed support not pills"*[28]. As described previously, hormonal bodily experiences are not openly shared and stem from generations of instilled secrecy. In a study by Ussher et al. (2019), one migrant woman expressed: "*It is shame to talk about sex with anyone in my culture and I feel embarrassed to talk about it*"[39] . Priya provided a more spiritual explanation that she had learnt from her mother: "*Menopause is God's way of saying your womb has had enough, no release of eggs, your vagina has had enough, it is time to shut down.*"

However, what I have learnt is that the ever-shifting associations with menopause vary from denial and ambivalence to acceptance, as described by Margaret Mead as "*post-menopausal zest*"[40] . This is further purported in many studies examining an eastern philosophical lens, where ageing is associated with freedom, in contrast to a more Western notion of *the fear of ageing* because of "*living in a youth orientated culture*"[41] . Many women saw the benefits of menstrual cessation as a form of liberation, where not getting pregnant was considered a relief. This was echoed by Madhu as well:

> "*[Periods have] not gone away completely, but they've reduced significantly, and just the thought of not having to base every decision of your life around when the next period is. The freedom was not external, it was internal. I had sort of imprisoned my mind around those things.*"

This denotes an empowering shift, as also advocated in feminist health discourse, whereby "*menopause is less likely to be anticipated as a negative experience*" [24]. What resonated with me was the societal shifts in female reproductive identity, and how the powerful positioning of older women was enshrined in freedom. This was apparent in many cultures, "*where old women enjoy a high status, hence suffer fewer symptoms, if they notice menopause at all, than women in cultures where old people have less status*"[38]. I saw this in my own Rajasthani community where my grandmother was clearly the elder matriarch of the family. She was amongst a circle of wise, older women who made the decisions concerning family matters, such as suitors for their children, domestic issues and finances. My gran was married at 16, had nine children and passed away at the age of 92. Her role, like many Indian women, shifted from menstrual segregation to reaching an elevated status level in old age. Flint's research in Rajput, North India (1990), highlighted this cultural and societal power shift. Menopause actually resulted in greater freedom for Indian women, as "*she can emerge from the purdah*"[42] . A similar phenomenon is also found in Chandigarh, where "*women reported that with menopause, they attained manhood*"[43] . Comparable cultural changes are seen in South Cameroon, Africa, where "*women are liberated from the submission to the man, she becomes his equal, she is like a man*"[44] . This is also mirrored in other developing countries such as Thailand, Zimbabwe and, more specifically, Nigeria, Togo, Ghana and Benin, where menopausal women are considered to hold supernatural voodoo powers, increasing their autonomy as they get older[45] . How does this then compare to the attitudes and perceptions of women and menopause in the West? Flint argues that, while not being subjected to menstrual segregation, women in America experience menopausal change more negatively than those in Rajput[42]. There is no simplistic answer to menopause and ageing – the journey is full of subjective contradictions and is steeped in generations of historical and cultural stigma.

Conclusion

> *"The dread and the secrecy around menopause is because, as a society, we're terrified of aging."*
>
> Sophia

The catalyst for writing this chapter was my daughter's reference to us as 'bookends'. The journeys my daughter and I are currently on are different, yet relatable. I have provided an honest and personal account of my menopause transition so far, which I hope will resonate. Although I draw on a South Asian background to frame my auto-ethnographic approach, the trials and tribulations I have experienced at each reproductive stage are universal. I wanted to avoid a navel-gazing exercise and am so grateful to the other South Asian women from diverse backgrounds and generations. I did not anticipate the sheer generosity of time and the intimacy of the stories each has shared. Their honesty and openness have shone a light on past and present social and cultural taboos. As Maya said, *"it's very interesting how society constructs an identity of who a woman is, and who a woman isn't, for that matter."*

These encounters were informal conversations, women just talking, sharing knowledge and stories on menarche and menopause. Our experiences are often perplexing contradictions: menstruation is deemed impure, but also celebrated. We mourn our youth, but also embrace some of the advantages we gain when attaining our 'infertile cloak of invisibility'. Progression is evident from what I have observed so far, but we must continue to equip future generations in dismantling negative social constructs and taboos, starting with the very first drop of menstrual blood. The most surprising revelation for me is learning how some cultures celebrate ageing, and that menopause can also be a symbol of liberation: a milestone rather than a millstone. However, liberation starts at the very beginning of a young woman's journey, when menstrual segregation is no more, and we readdress notions around impurity. *It also begins with small and simple changes which can make all the difference.* This positive account from Anjali encapsulates this:

> *"There's definitely a sense of liberation . . . because of the way things have moved on. A couple of weeks ago, I was buying some sanitary products from Superdrug, pop music was on . . . and they wanna make you feel happy. . . . I was thinking that's an amazing thing to be able to walk to this counter and be served by a male cashier, I bought some sanitary pads. . . . I feel very good about this, we've really moved on quite a lot from that . . . hostility, it's quite a nice kind of journey to have made!"*

Many thanks to the women who so generously shared their time and experiences and permitted their stories to be shared. All the names have been changed to protect identities.

Thank you to Lionel Openshaw for helping with editing.

References

1. Denshire S. On auto-ethnography. *Current Sociology* 2014; 62 (6): 831–850.
2. Hooks B. *Talking Back: Thinking Feminist, Thinking Black.* South End Press, 1989.
3. Brand A. 93% of women say their work-life balance has negatively impacted their mental health. *Diversity News* 2024 [cited 2024 21 April 2024]. https://hrreview.co.uk/hr-news/diversity-news/93-of-women-say-their-work-life-balance-has-negatively-impacted-their-mental-health/374421.
4. Calhoun A. Surviving perimenopause: 'I was overwhelmed and full of rage. Why was I so badly prepared?'. *Guardian*, 2020.
5. Well E. Puberty before age 10: A new normal. *The New York Times Magazine*, 2012, New York.
6. Figes K. *What About Me: The Diaries and E-mails of a Menopausal Mother and Teenage Daughter.* Pan Books, London, 2004.
7. Tillotson K. Extra hormones in the house with mom in menopause and kids in puberty. *The Seattle Times*, US, 2012.
8. Peranovic T, Bentley B. Men and menstruation: A qualitative exploration of beliefs, attitudes and experiences. *Sex Roles* 2017; 77: 113–124.
9. Fingerson L. Agency and the body in adolescent menstrual talk. *Childhood* 2005; 12 (1): 91–110.
10. Katsa H. Men are still too 'Embarrassed' to buy period products, apparently. *HUFFPOST*, 2022.
11. Hawkey AJ, Ussher JM, Perz J. "I Treat My Daughters Not Like My Mother Treated Me": Migrant and refugee women's constructions and experiences of menarche and menstruation. *The Palgrave Handbook of Critical Menstruation Studies* 2020: 99–113.
12. Uskul AK. Women's menarche stories from a multicultural sample. *Social Science & Medicine* 2004; 59 (4): 667–679.
13. Jackson TE, Falmagne RJ. Women wearing white: Discourses of menstruation and the experience of menarche. *Feminism & Psychology* 2013; 23 (3): 379–398.
14. Hawkey AJ, Ussher JM, Perz J. Regulation and resistance: Negotiation of premarital sexuality in the context of migrant and refugee women. *The Journal of Sex Research* 2018; 55 (9): 1116–1133.
15. Johnston-Robledo I, Chrisler JC. The menstrual mark: Menstruation as social stigma. *The Palgrave Handbook of Critical Menstruation Studies* 2020: 181–199.
16. Bramwell R. Blood and milk: Constructions of female bodily fluids in Western society. *Women & Health* 2001; 34 (4): 85–96.
17. Ussher JM. *Managing the Monstrous Feminine: Regulating the Reproductive Body.* Routledge, 2006.
18. Joshy N, Prakash K, Ramdey K. Social taboos and menstrual practices in the Pindar Valley. *Indian Journal of Gender Studies* 2019; 26 (1–2): 79–95.
19. BBC NEWS. Nepal woman suffocates in banned 'menstruation hut'. 2019 [cited 2023 05 May 2023]. https://www.bbc.co.uk/news/world-asia-47112769.
20. Hill M. *Perimenopause Power: Navigating Your Hormones on the Journey to Menopause.* Bloomsbury Publishing, 2021.
21. Bauld R, Brown RF. Stress, psychological distress, psychosocial factors, menopause symptoms and physical health in women. *Maturitas* 2009; 62 (2): 160–165.
22. WHO. Menopause. 2022 [cited 2024 07 April]. https://www.who.int/news-room/fact-sheets/detail/menopause.

23 Ballard KD, Kuh DJ, Wadsworth ME. The role of the menopause in women's experiences of the 'change of life'. *Sociology of Health & Illness* 2001; 23 (4): 397–424.
24 Coupland J, Williams A. Conflicting discourses, shifting ideologies: Pharmaceutical, alternative' and feminist emancipatory texts on the menopause. *Discourse & Society* 2002; 13 (4): 419–445.
25 Carolan M. Menopause: Irish women's voices. *Journal of Obstetric, Gynecologic, & Neonatal Nursing* 2000; 29 (4): 397–404.
26 Champ L. Is the menopause a grieving process. 2021 [cited 2024 28 March 2024]. https://welldoing.org/article/is-menopause-grieving-process.
27 Skultans V. The symbolic significance of menstruation and the menopause. *Man* 1970; 5 (4): 639–651.
28 Utz RL. Like mother,(not) like daughter: The social construction of menopause and aging. *Journal of Aging Studies* 2011; 25 (2): 143–154.
29 Nosek M, Kennedy HP, Gudmundsdottir M. Silence, stigma, and shame: A postmodern analysis of distress during menopause. *Advances in Nursing Science* 2010; 33 (3): E24–E36.
30 Shea JL. Menopause and midlife aging in cross-cultural perspective: Findings from ethnographic research in China. *Journal of Cross-Cultural Gerontology* 2020; 35 (4): 367–388.
31 Etienne V. Drew Barrymore has first hot flash — with Jennifer Aniston by her side: 'So Glad This Is Documented'. 2023 [cited 2023 13 April]. https://people.com/health/drew-barrymore-has-first-hot-flash-with-jennifer-aniston-menopause/#:~:text=%22I%20realized%20that%20I%20was,it%2010%20years%20like%20this!%22.
32 Dillaway H, Byrnes M, Miller S et al. Talking "among us": How women from different racial–ethnic groups define and discuss menopause. *Health Care for Women International* 2008; 29 (7): 766–781.
33 Guardian. 'Me and my menopause': A view from women around the world 2024 [cited 2024 20 February]. https://www.theguardian.com/global-development/2024/feb/07/menopause-reproductive-health-stigma-medical-treatment-information-mood-anxiety-support.
34 Davies G. Perimenopause periods left me needing a transfusion. 2023 [cited 2024 19 April]. https://www.bbc.co.uk/news/uk-scotland-65532730.
35 Hall L, Callister LC, Berry JA et al. Meanings of menopause: Cultural influences on perception and management of menopause. *Journal of Holistic Nursing* 2007; 25 (2): 106–118.
36 Im E-O, Meleis AI. Meanings of menopause to Korean immigrant women. *Western Journal of Nursing Research* 2000; 22 (1): 84–102.
37 Hinsliff G. Not just hot flushes: How menopause can destroy mental health. *Guardian*, 2023.
38 Hvas L. Menopausal women's positive experience of growing older. *Maturitas* 2006; 54 (3): 245–251.
39 Ussher JM, Hawkey AJ, Perz J. 'Age of despair', or 'when life starts': Migrant and refugee women negotiate constructions of menopause. *Culture, Health & Sexuality* 2019; 21 (7): 741–756.
40 Mead M. *On Freud's View of Female Psychology*. éditeur non identifié, 1974.
41 Logan JR, Ward R, Spitze G. As old as you feel: Age identity in middle and later life. *Social Forces* 1992; 71 (2): 451–467.
42 Flint M, Samil RS. Cultural and subcultural meanings of the menopause. *Annals of the New York Academy of Sciences* 1990; 592 (1): 134–147.
43 Kaur S, Walia I, Singh A. How menopause affects the lives of women in suburban Chandigarh, India. *Climacteric* 2004; 7 (2): 175–180.
44 Vincent J-F. La ménopause, chemin de la liberté selon les femmes beti du Sud-Cameroun. *Journal des africanistes* 2003; 73 (2): 121–136.
45 Alidou S, Verpoorten M. Only women can whisper to gods: Voodoo, menopause and women's autonomy. *World Development* 2019; 119: 40–54.

Scene 4 Can we pass the baton from sport?

Anna Allerton

Myth: Menopause stops my career ambitions

Reality: This can be a time in your life when you can thrive professionally – harnessing all your experience, wisdom and strengths to stay current and find joy in your profession.

How? By working smarter, *not* harder

The reality for many women experiencing perimenopause or menopause is that the symptoms can become disruptors to careers. Where on the scale these are impacting women is very individual, but there are steps you can take to build toolkits that support your bespoke management of your personal needs.

There are two fundamental pillars of executive coaching that I want to invite you to hold close throughout this chapter – challenge and accountability. While it may feel really tough and overwhelming to get on top of your symptoms at work, the aim here is to present inspiration that can help you face the challenge with action that will see you do something to shift the dial. To feel empowered, to use this time in our lives to deepen our self-awareness and find the confidence to move forward professionally in a more considered way. In a way that serves you and your needs best.

To help do this, I'm going to lean into the world of professional women's sport and performance for inspiration. There is much we can learn from female athletes to positively impact careers during our menopause journeys. In fact, there are several parallels between the evolution of professional women's sport and the current menopause movement.

Some background for context. Before qualifying as a certified executive coach, I was a journalist and producer for the best part of two decades at Sky Sports. In 2012, I founded, produced and led the *Sportswomen* programme with a small but mighty team. We were the first production that dedicated coverage solely to women's sports news and were purpose-led in disrupting the media landscape to put women's sport on the agenda. Back when it was barely spoken about, we were determined that this would not become a box-ticking exercise and worked tirelessly to play our part in making sure the voices of women were heard and respected.

Then perimenopause came along when I was 38 while on maternity leave with a newborn and a 2-year-old. It was when I began the return to work that things imploded for me and my career. Unheard by my GP for 10 months, live TV alongside anxiety, pain, bloating, low mood, loss of joy, insomnia and brain fog were a terrible combination. My debilitating symptoms called time on that chapter in my life.

But life throws twists and turns at us, and my experience led me to do what I am doing now – supporting women to maintain their midlife careers through my executive coaching. Honouring many of the same values that saw me champion women's sport when very few were, I have spent years studying and building a model that tackles a lot of the issues women face professionally during menopause.

Let's first begin by looking at the changing face of the workplace that presents challenge for many. An environment that promotes doing more, with urgency, with a lack of regard for boundaries and life balance in order to get the win, the title or the goal. We are seeing the emergence of cultures that promote always being available and accessible in a fast-paced world. There's been a huge increase in remote working, evolving technology amongst an expanding intergenerational workforce.

We know that navigating menopause is not a one-size-fits-all approach. This can be overwhelming for some, while others lean into it with a renewed sense of purpose. Some may find this time freeing to enjoy careers on their own terms, whereas others may feel buried and burnt out. Casting aside the need to conform and bend around a system or political structure contrasts with increasing levels of stress or self-doubt. Or a renewed sense of purpose and energy in some may not be mirrored by those who feel unsupported and unheard.

If professional athletes worked in this pressure cooker environment over time, they would likely burnout before they even got a chance at seeing the podium. This isn't to say that pressure and stress don't exist for them – they do in abundance. But it is their mindset and how they operate in that space that sets them apart.

To succeed over the longer term, athletes adopt a strategy and a winning mindset that is authentic to their individual strengths and biology. They tap into toolkits designed to help them push through adversity or immense challenges. They do it step by step, day by day. They are meticulous, selfish almost – but always goal-focused.

While in the short term, harder and faster may fuel the workplace demand for instant results, it doesn't support female retention – or the bottom line. It's a mindset that supports the few, not the majority.

Much like working with our hormones rather than against them, it is possible to be successful and thrive in your job if you take steps to explore how to work *smarter* during menopause. For a long time, I have believed that the missing piece of the corporate puzzle in understanding the 'glass ceiling' is full awareness of menopause and the implementation of a robust long-term strategy to successfully navigate it. When business leaders question why women are not progressing into leadership roles despite the resources and commitment to quotas and diversity targets, they need to ask themselves how they are breaking down barriers and becoming menopause-supportive cultures.

While a menopause policy is a great starting block, what is required is better management to provide a more individualised approach. Services that offer support with an open mind to working differently but as productively as possible during this time should also be considered by the business community.

A menopause rebrand is required in the workplace.

Evidence is building that paints a concerning picture of the impact of menopause in the workplace. While some women cruise through this time of life, others have to navigate symptoms that create a deep impact on their ability to do their job.

Women's careers are paying the price for poor support and care during menopause.

Women make up nearly half of the UK working population, and menopausal women are the fastest-growing demographic of the UK workforce[1]. By 2030, there will be 1.2 billion women in menopause globally.

It is impossible to ignore menopause at work when it impacts individuals and businesses at this scale. And with over 13 million in menopause in the United Kingdom – it will be a stretch to find workplaces where this is not being experienced, particularly when 8 out of 10 menopausal people are currently in work [2].

Research from the Fawcett Society in 2022 found that 1 in 10 women quit work because of menopause symptoms[3].

While there are a growing number of progressive employers recognising that this is a very real concern for the future success of business, the reality is that for many women this is not something openly discussed and supported in the workplace.

The same survey found that "8 in 10 menopausal women say their workplace has no basic support in place for them – no support networks (79%), no absence policies (81%) and no information sharing with staff (79%)".

Once believed to only impact a small demographic of the workforce, a deeper understanding is required on how to best support women's health from when they first enter the workplace and for every decade until they retire.

Intergeneration considerations: "You're too young"

Often overlooked are the intergenerational considerations of menopause. Fuelled by stereotypes and myths that this is about women in their fifties getting hot and angry, for a long while the conversation has centred around women between 45 and 55.

But what about women in each decade of their life cycle, including the intersectional and cultural considerations?

Women can experience menopause under the age of 40, which means perimenopause could have started in their thirties.

There are a variety of reasons women will go through this under 40. For some, it will be a natural transition. Other reasons can be premature ovarian insufficiency (POI), or it being triggered by surgery or certain treatments, such as chemotherapy. Raising these voices and stories will support creating workplace systems that best support women in all stages of their lives.

Opening up the intergenerational discussion offers insight and expertise through lived experiences. It also ensures that all demographics are served in ongoing menopause awareness and education. Menopause is not a one-size-fits-all issue and it shouldn't be treated as such in the workplace.

The same applies to the medical profession. Women reading this who have been told by their GP that they are "too young" for menopause will likely relate to it feeling like a door slamming in their face. Dismissing women who present with symptoms can have long-term implications and impact.

Just when your hormones are tricking you into believing you are going mad, being regularly dismissed and unheard by your GP does start to make you think that you indeed are losing it.

It's a deeply troubling and challenging moment in any woman's life if she is being denied access to basic care and treatment that could transform her quality of life. And the longer she remains untreated, the harder it will become to manage symptoms at work.

While there will always be averages and those in the majority, failure to understand and integrate intergenerational menopause risks creates a siloed community of women who remain unheard, underserved and misunderstood.

The individualised approach

It is possible to feel empowered, to embrace growth and find individualised ways to perform in careers if we take steps to *Work Smarter in Menopause®*. This is a coaching model I developed over many years to support midlife women.

Some are being forced to make changes that conflict with how they've always shown up at work. Many are exploring steps to address the negative impact symptoms are having on their careers. In doing so, they are putting in huge work and time into this. For others, it's the realisation that something needs to change, and the desire to be strategic about the path ahead.

In my executive coaching practice, I witness the impact menopause can have on careers, varying from:

- Increased people-pleasing.
- The self-doubt is being dialled right up.
- Working longer days with nothing to show for it.
- Conflicting values.
- Reputation and personal brand concerns.
- Low confidence.
- Burnout.
- A lack of ambition and focus.
- Loss of joy.
- A time to pivot.
- A recognition of an opportunity to take back control.

- A deeper clarity on what works and what doesn't.
- A desire not to settle and to push on in a sustainable way.
- A time when we can focus on self and explore ways that make us happier and ready to embrace the second spring.

These are just some of the themes that women are navigating. It's not all negative, either.

There are many factors that are forcing us to confront our reality, alongside our health: childcare, caring responsibilities and financial considerations, to name a few.

Women will typically spend decades building confidence, experience, wisdom and ability and then along comes perimenopause and menopause – and bam: it feels like a derailment, often when careers are entering the senior stages.

Performance: The shared learning between women's sport and menopause

Gone are the days when women leave the workplace once they become mothers; ovary retirement does not mean a retirement from work. It's a new phase and a new chapter that needs to be navigated in a different way.

The ongoing development and growth of professional women's sport is affording us insight into our own performance across the female life cycle that transcends the elite.

The London Olympic Games (2012) triggered a turning point for women's sport in the United Kingdom. It was the moment that I founded and launched the *Sportswomen* programme on Sky Sports. There was an appetite for storytelling and an opportunity to pull women's sport into the mainstream. Public awareness and appreciation for the athletes of Team GB created an opportunity for sports to build and develop bespoke women's strategies for growth. After all, it was the women of Team GB who won the majority of medals for the country in London[4].

Much like the Davina McCall Menopause programme on Channel 4 in 2021, *Sex, Myths and the Menopause* became the opportunity for midlife health to hit the mainstream and, fortunately, it has stayed at the forefront of public awareness ever since, thanks to a mighty group of women using their voices. It is often a moment in time, like the London Games, that creates opportunities to change.

What followed London saw some athletes beginning to turn professional and selected sport paying female players full-time for the first time. In May 2014, the ECB offered the first professional contracts for their female cricketers. By 2019, England Rugby was paying every female member of their squad. No longer were some athletes having to juggle full-time jobs alongside evening training, weekend fixtures and unpaid international travel.

An increase in exposure created new audiences and there has been a swell in media coverage ever since. A similar pattern has followed in the menopause space.

A report published by the House of Commons Women's and Equalities Committee in February 2024 concluded that "the increased attention (in women's sport) has brought into the spotlight the inequality of support for, and lack of understanding of, the health and physiological needs of women and girls across sport".

The report cites the specific example of anterior cruciate ligament (ACL) knee injuries for female athletes, arguing that *"it has shown a systemic gender inequality in sports and exercise research."* Much like there is for women's health during menopause, the report calls for action for women's midlife health.

While there is still a long way to go, the impact of certain investments in sport has led to many professional athletes benefiting from impactful science and research. This has fuelled deepening awareness and debate about equal pay, maternity leave, motherhood and menstruation. Investment in science and women's health interventions can be adapted for use by women not just in elite sport.

One area of focus has been on better understanding athletes' menstrual cycles. In 2020, a BBC Elite British Sportswomen's Survey found that "60% of respondents said their performance had been affected by their period, and they had missed training or competitions because of it". This data increased to 88% in 2024. The analysis of the findings concludes that the impact menstrual cycles have on athletes is largely misunderstood.

This has seen the evolution of individualised approaches to training. Monitoring and understanding hormonal fluctuations allow coaches to better calculate how to operate precision training in tune with an athlete's individual cycle. Chelsea FC began bespoke training programmes in 2020 around players' menstrual cycles in an attempt to boost performance and reduce injuries.

Allowing individualised data to inform how hormones affect physiological and psychological behaviours can support women to tune into their hormones. This can inform and empower women to deepen their own awareness of symptoms, use it to support them in speaking with their GP, feel validated and take ownership during menopause. In the workplace, it provides information about:

- The presence of symptoms
- Trigger points
- Where you are at your best
- Where you are at your most vulnerable.
- Specific days, moments or times that are noticeable
- Best use of flexible hours
- What interventions you may need?

In the same way that athletes now train smarter around their hormones, women in work can adapt how they are operating alongside their hormones and symptom logs. Individualised data can create patterns of behaviour that then inform the actions taken.

Athlete story: Michelle Dillon

What role does mindset play in this? Michelle Dillon is a former World and European Triathlon champion and two-time Olympian. She now competes as a masters athlete and works as an Olympic coach with athletes from the beginner level to the elite.

Reflecting on a significant moment in her life ahead of an Age Group World Championships, Michelle offers a story that many of us can relate to. Not necessarily in terms of competing in a world championship, but when you have been preparing for an important sport/work/social event, then something out of your control happens which could derail your plan. How are you going to react? You could throw in the towel, or you could explore how you can overcome this challenge and draw on your resilience. This is what happened to Michelle and how she reacted, shared here to offer insight into a mindset that can be adopted by women in their careers.

> *"I had a cyst on my ovary in 2023 which exploded one night in bed. I started bleeding and I had the World Championships coming up and I had been training really hard for that. I couldn't sit on my bike with the pain. A week before, I explored pulling out but something inside me said 'don't'."*

> *"I was swimming and biking really well. I hadn't run for three months. But I still went and won the bloody thing."*

How did she overcome this enormous life hurdle? *"I believed in my ability."*

Michelle was able to reconnect with her 'why', her strength and her values in that moment. Michelle dug deep to overcome adversity.

So, what can professional women in their careers learn from this example?

"It all comes from the mind. I believed in my ability as an athlete – that's what I held on to. Not that I feel like this, look like that or have this symptom. I believed I could win!" says Michelle.

> *"In your career, if you believe in your ability in your role, you are good at that, then you know you can deliver it, you must (find a way to) back yourself."*

Not always easy during menopause to believe in yourself – especially when brain fog and other symptoms create so much uncertainty. But this is all about small steps. You could begin by reconnecting and reaffirming your values as a great starting point.

What are the elements that guide and inform how you show up in the world? They are the beliefs and principles unique to how you live your life. The objective of this exercise is to start the work to reconnect with who you are, so you can create an anchor point to lean into, so you can also get back on that bike in the face of adversity, much like Michelle.

Menopause can pull us so far away from who we are and what makes us so unique. This shows up in different ways at work. Many of us struggle to recognise ourselves during perimenopause and beyond, so considering the big question of "who am I" can start to take you back to your core. You could start this work by drawing up a list of your strengths or your superpowers. However, this sits with you – it's about owning what makes you so fantastic in your role.

> *"I like to think back to when I was doing really well and being successful,"* says Michelle. *"Draw on experiences and moments in your career. Think back to what your best speech was, that winning pitch, for example. Whatever you've done before; if you've done it once – you can do it again,"* she says.

This is where we revisit my invitation to you to consider what is showing up as a challenge and how you can take action to hold yourself accountable to that work. Going through menopause can leave us feeling lower than ever. It makes us feel like managing our symptoms and exercising self-compassion is a full-time job on its own. Sling in the GP lottery, isolating feelings, being unheard, exercise, self-care, reading and education – the list is endless. It can deepen the pressure and sap the joy. Alongside all this, we have to show up in our jobs and perform.

> *"One of the most powerful things to help you connect back is visualisation,"* says Dillon. *"It's a hugely valuable tool for me – I saw myself win that Age Group World Championships. If you visualise it hard enough and think about it deep enough you can take yourself back to that. The problem is the symptoms puts a dampener on this. Anxiety is very real. How do you overcome that when you are in front of people, and you are trying to perform. It's not easy."*

That's where we need menopause-supportive cultures. Women can't do this on their own. They are already working incredibly hard trying to hold up all this whilst empowering themselves to move forwards. We've explored the impact this is having on the workplace and why I support calls for a menopause rebrand in the workplace.

Conclusions

There are many pillars explored in this book about well-being, nutrition, exercise, gut health and other holistic interventions that have a huge role in how we manage all this. Absorb them and take them in. They are vital tools for how we show up as the best versions of ourselves in our careers.

For individuals looking to make their working life easier during menopause, I want to end with some thoughts for you to reflect on with the hope they can support you in taking small steps forwards:

- Revisit your values – what is this telling you about yourself right now?
- Reaffirm your strengths – you are not here by luck, so dive back into what makes you so brilliant at your job.
- Where are you now and where do you want to get to?

- What do you need to support you in achieving that?
- How do you plan to hold yourself to account?
- How can you define your anchor points?
- Could you tune into and track your symptoms?
- What is that data telling you?
- Breathe
- Allow space for reflection each week – a few moments spent considering the wins (great or small).
- Who can you think all through this with trust and safety?
- Consider how you speak to yourself with love and kindness.
- Journaling, note-taking, affirmations – all tools to help you navigate these areas of work.
- Technology – note-taking apps, AI assistants (like Alexa), dictation tools.
- Get comfortable exploring how to say 'no' more often.
- Delegate more.
- What are your non-negotiables?
- Push out interference that is not serving you well.
- Nature – soak it up.
- Morning light – take it in.
- Find your tribe – supportive and authentic people who value you.
- Mentoring – find someone who has walked this path. How are you harnessing their wisdom?

One step at a time

- Give yourself grace.

References

1 Source: "No Time To Step Back" report. Produced by Helen Tomlinson with Mims Davies MP for the UK Government. March 2023.
2 Source: NHS England & NHS Improvement: Internal Menopause in the Workplace questionnaire for NHS organisations. March 2022.
3 Source: "Menopause and the Workplace" survey, Fawcett Society, June 2022.
4 Team GB website.

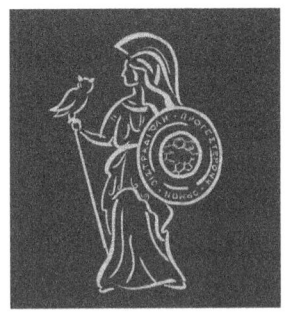

Act 9

Towards Positive Ageing

Collaboratively removing barriers for sustainable person-centred system support

Act 8 Towards Positive Ageing

Collaboratively removing barriers for sustainable person-centred system support

*Dr Marzena Nieroda, Dr Abdul Seckam,
Dr Dania Posso, Dr Rodrigo Rodriguez-Fernandez,
Dr Orlanda Allen, Professor André Coutinho,
Thalia Anagnostopoulou, Professor Joyce Harper,
Dr Nicky Keay*

Menopause, a natural biological phase typically occurring at the average age of 52, marks the end of women's reproductive years as menstruation ceases[1]. The symptoms associated with menopause, such as mood swings, night sweats, hot flushes, sleep disturbances and cognitive challenges, can significantly impact a woman's well-being, confidence and her performance at work.

A recent study conducted by the Institute of Fiscal Studies[2] utilising data from Norway and Sweden sheds light on the diverse effects of menopause on women's lives. The study indicates a sudden but temporary surge in both primary care and specialist doctor visits during the menopausal transition, alongside a sustained increase in the use of medications. This rise is primarily driven by the uptake of Hormone Replacement Therapy (HRT) and antidepressants aimed at managing menopausal symptoms. From an economic standpoint, the study highlights substantial and enduring declines in employment rates and earnings among menopausal women, accompanied by a greater reliance on social welfare assistance. These adverse economic consequences are particularly notable among women without a college education, as well as those working in larger workplaces or with fewer female coworkers aged 45 or older.

The notable challenges associated with this natural process contribute to emergence and existence of menopause stereotypes, influencing societal perceptions and support for women undergoing this natural transition. Stigmatisation portrays menopause as a symbol of ageing and decline, potentially leading to shame and reluctance to seek help, especially among those who might need it most. Stigma can impede understanding and support, affecting well-being, confidence, work performance or relationships, potentially further deepening negative impact of this process on health, quality of life and overall happiness. Misinformation and false beliefs surrounding menopause, coupled with cultural taboos and societal norms that discourage open discussion, contribute to stigma and create barriers.

Efforts to challenge stereotypes, foster acceptance and shift perceptions regarding ageing and menopause necessitate a holistic approach encompassing education, enhanced support services, and social, familial and workplace backing. However, achieving these objectives demands a systemic transformation driven by mission-oriented innovation, characterised by clear, ambitious and time-bound goals capable of effecting transformative change. Inspired by the Observatory of Public Sector Innovation and supported by the OECD[3] mission-driven innovation encompasses the development or enhancement of technological, social or organisational solutions aimed at addressing significant societal challenges and generating public value. We view the need to overcome the prevailing stereotypes and barriers surrounding positive ageing and menopause as a mission, prompting collaborative efforts to confront this issue. The removal of existing stigma can serve as an initial step needed to support menopausal females, ensuring that they do not perceive themselves as lesser or less valuable. This can encourage more open discussions, facilitate the search for support and inform and propel the broader adaptation process that females undergo.

Furthermore, as this form of systemic innovation is likely to involve engagement with commercial entities to support females (e.g. at their workplaces), these endeavours are closely aligned with the Environmental, Social and Governance (ESG) sustainability objectives[4,5]. This alignment is particularly evident in relation to environmental and social impacts. Beginning in 2024, the Corporate Sustainability Reporting Directive (CSRD) mandates companies to disclose a broader spectrum of ESG impacts over short, medium and long-term horizons[6]. This encompasses a comprehensive assessment of the environmental and social ramifications of their operations across their value chain.

Of notable significance in these new regulations is the heightened focus on social factors, including aspects such as working conditions, community impacts or product safety and quality. It is imperative for commercial enterprises to comprehend the origins of these social impacts across diverse stakeholder groups to garner support from investors. As highlighted by George Serafen in his publication in the *Harvard Business Review*[7] companies must effectively engage in various ESG practices to secure backing from investors and other pertinent stakeholders. Central to this endeavour is the integration of ESG efforts into both strategic planning and operational activities.

Given the extensive nature of the challenge and the potential avenues of assistance for menopausal individuals, our team of authors, representing diverse backgrounds, coordinated and participated in a knowledge exchange workshop centred on Workplace Equity to Support Healthy Ageing and Women's Health. This workshop was convened at UCL Global Business School for Health on 20 March 2024. During the workshop, we delved into various hurdles that must be addressed to offer support to women and subsequently proposed potential solutions. Within this chapter, we consolidate the diverse discussions held during the event and advocate for a cultural shift that acknowledges menopause as a natural stage of life, thereby fostering holistic well-being. An illustration of the identified barriers and solutions is listed in Figure 9.1.1. We trust that our reflections and

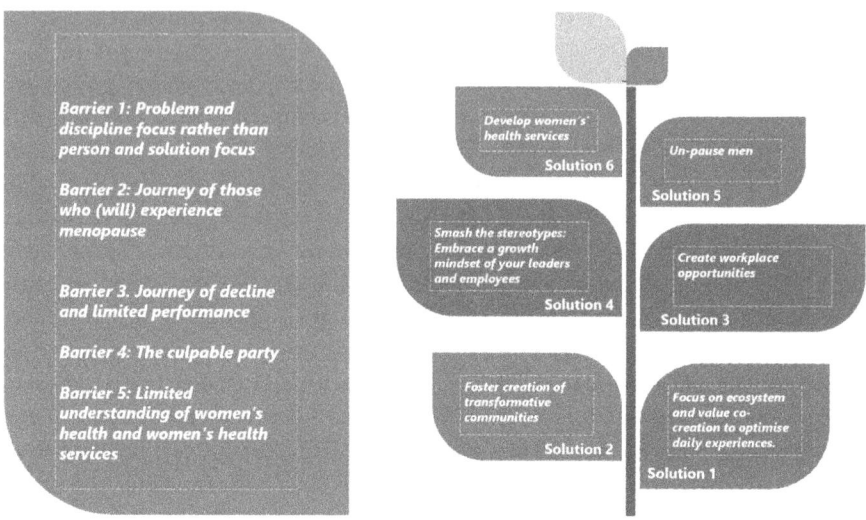

FIGURE 9.1.1 Barriers and solutions to positive ageing

ideas will serve as food for thought for various stakeholders capable of influencing and contributing to women's well-being.

Barrier 1 Problem and discipline focus rather than person and solution focus

Menopause is frequently examined through singular disciplinary lenses, resulting in a fragmented understanding of the topic. Discourse typically revolves around different facets of menopause, such as symptoms, their understanding, processes, treatments and associated experiences. As a result, various fields of science and expertise, including medicine, education, digital health, policy and specific therapies like HRT, are pivotal in addressing perimenopause symptoms. However, the lack of integration and coordination among these disciplines can perpetuate stigma by framing menopause solely as a medical issue. Despite recent efforts to combat stigmatisation and overmedicalisation associated with menopause, the persistent use of terms like "patients"[8] and the focus on the role of health services may inadvertently reinforce a medicalised perspective. Additionally, framing menopause in terms of economic challenges posed by an ageing population can further stigmatise it, overlooking its broader societal and individual impacts as a natural life transition[9].

However, in a research study carried out at University College London we found out that individuals often find themselves and their daily experiences at the centre of this contemporary problem framing, only to encounter stigma as a result. Paradoxically, they are the ones most in need of assistance and support during this transitional phase. However, the challenges they often experience are outside of the medical and healthcare sectors, and voiced by Anna (all names used throughout this chapter are pseudonyms allocated to each research participant), 53 years old:

> *"I think society needs to take responsibility for breaking down some of those stereotypes. But building that into the systems that we have, whether that's education or whether it's social care or whatever but we should be normalising ageing and not seeing this as a barrier to people getting something out of their life."*

Therefore, a viable solution may involve reframing the issue from the perspective of their needs. Interestingly, in our research about their perceptions and experiences of menopause, many women revealed challenges stemming from broader societal perspectives and emphasised the need for a range of solutions, including medical, natural or social resources to support this transition. Many of them noted that their experiences, symptoms and subsequent feelings of shame or embarrassment occur either at home or in the workplace. Helen, 62 years old, said to us:

> *"No one had ever told me about the menopause. That moment, I just think. Ohh embarrassing. Yeah, embarrassing. I don't like to use the word shameful. Shame. Yeah, yeah, I think I felt ashamed. Yeah. And embarrassed."*

Consequently, effective solutions should adopt a multidisciplinary approach, placing women and their daily experiences at the core of all activities and interventions. Josephine, 54 years old, reflected:

> *"I think from my perspective, it's the physical. It's the emotional, it's the mental, maybe even the spiritual as well. It's about a combination of all those factors and how they inform each other, but also how they support us to live to our maximum as individuals who are ageing."*

This necessitates facilitating cross-disciplinary collaboration to dismantle silos and offer support to women.

Barrier 2 Journey of those who (will) experience menopause

In contemporary approaches to supporting women through hormonal changes, the focus is often segmented based on the stage of their journey. This segmentation typically includes females who have not yet reached menopause, those experiencing perimenopause, those who have reached menopause and those who have moved beyond it. However, such labelling can evoke feelings of worry among women, as indicated by Sandra, 52 years old:

> *"I'd be seen as being lesser if I did that (admitted she is peri-menopausal), and I'm not that."*

Younger females may be reluctant to confront the idea of ageing, while older females may feel ashamed or uncomfortable when labelled, particularly if they experience symptoms in professional settings. Lily, 30 years old female, says *"I'm not a huge fan of ageing, to be honest. So yeah. Like, I'm not ready,"* pointing to the thirst for maintaining youth also voiced by Zoe, 41 years old: *"I think we're all trying to maintain the youth for longer."*

The emphasis on distinct groups and stages of menopause within various research areas such as healthcare, public health or education can perpetuate stereotypes and hinder efforts to challenge them. To overcome this barrier and confront existing stereotypes effectively, it's imperative to view the challenge through the lens of an ecosystem that supports transition, and position different groups as part of that ecosystem.

The journey of ageing and menopause involves behavioural changes that require adaptation from a young age and support from the broader environment. It's essential to acknowledge that ageing begins from conception, and lifestyle behaviours related to exercise, nutrition, sleep and stress management play crucial roles in promoting healthy ageing and menopause. Research from Yale School of Public Health highlights the significant impact of lifestyle factors on chronic health conditions such as cancer, diabetes, obesity and cardiovascular disease. Unhealthy body weight, sedentary behaviour and poor diets have been associated with increased incidence and mortality rates for various cancers and metabolic diseases. Additionally, lifestyle factors can influence hormone levels, energy metabolism, cellular growth, inflammatory responses, DNA repair and immune function[10]. Many women we spoke to in our research emphasise the importance of lifestyle choices for managing menopause symptoms, a sentiment supported by health and menopause centres like the Australian Menopause Society, which recognises that lifestyle modifications can improve well-being and symptom tolerance[11]. Therefore, as stressed by these women, lifestyle changes should be introduced early in life. One of our research participants, Rona, 50 years old, stated:

> *"I think you can be healthy, but I think it needs to be healthy at the beginning is what I'm saying. I think you need to be healthy throughout. I think if you're abusing your body when you're in your teens and you're 20s, that won't help you. When your menopause, I think personally think it will mock up your metabolism and your you know, your functioning of your body and also your habits and the way that you behave."*

Furthermore, understanding, support and adaptation strategies should be available throughout the lifespan from various stakeholders within the surrounding ecosystem.

In our research, we've recognised that ageing transitions necessitate support from one's social circles, including partners, family members and colleagues in the workplace. It's crucial to challenge myths surrounding gender and age in the context of menopause support. Engaging with males is relevant to combat the misconception that menopause is solely a female concern.

What is "Man-On-Pause" – *A male perspective*

Too often we hear the following labels about our female colleagues and counterparts:

"Ageing lady, unhealthy lady, all flushed and flustered Jane, weighty Betty" and the list is endless! Misogynistic, lack of understanding, lack of empathy, rude . . . Yes to all these! Contrary, to the lack of support, supportive language and phrases, males need to educate, empower and embed an empathetic approach. We need to understand the woman who is fulfilling her life potential and going through natural processes and stages in life. Understanding menopause is crucial for everyone, regardless of gender, as it impacts not only women but also their partners, families and communities. Whilst males do not experience menopause themselves, having knowledge and empathy about this natural transition can greatly benefit relationships and support ecosystems. Jane, 68 years old, mentioned:

> *"It's back to that education I mentioned earlier both for men and women and not being embarrassed about talking about it. This is a natural thing that women go through, and how can men support them?"*

There is plenty of work to be done in that department. A qualitative study by Hidiroglu and colleagues[12] explored menopause among males in Istanbul, Turkey. They provided a better understanding of this phase to improve the care delivered to menopausal women. Thirty-three (n=33) married men took part in in-depth one-to-one interviews. It was suggested that the males lacked knowledge about both menstruation and menopause and defined menopause as loss of fecundity, increased weight and loss of beauty. These experiences and views were from an age range of 40- to 77-year-old men. Moreover, these sorts of findings are seen among males from various backgrounds and cultures. In our study involving women, similar sentiments were noted, from their perspectives on males in line with knowledge, culture and religious beliefs on menopause, exacerbating the misconceptions and myths around this topic. Such findings only add to the misuse and inappropriate language, increased cultural taboos and lack of education and support around menopause. As Jane, 68 years old, elaborates:

> *"In my home I'm really proud of the fact, actually, that the way we've brought the boys up mean they've got a really positive attitude to women. But, in general there are more things that perhaps could be done in the home to get that balance and to support the women, particularly menopause shouldn't be seen as an illness. Menopause should be seen as a phase of the life cycle."*

Barrier 3 Journey of decline and limited performance

The emphasis on menopause as a health condition often leads to the use of specific medical terminology that shapes the narrative surrounding this natural transition. This focus can result in discussions about menopause centred on concepts such as hormone deficiency, loss of ovarian function, disability or cognitive decline[13]. The language used to describe symptoms and their impact on daily life and work performance tends to be negative, reinforcing a sense of limitation and fixed capabilities. This use of limiting language may act as a barrier to the development of dynamic and adaptive coping ageing strategies[14]. It has the potential to activate a fixed mindset in how people approach ageing and how women approach menopause. Of note is that menopause can occur relatively early in a woman's life, compared to perceived ageing in men.

The framework of mindset was developed by world-renowned Stanford University psychologist Carol Dweck. Mindsets are beliefs about oneself and the world that influence perceptions, thoughts, feelings and actions. Dweck[15,16] identified mindsets, or implicit theories, about the malleability of abilities as significant drivers of responses to challenges and learning. In fixed mindsets, individuals believe abilities are static, while growth mindsets view abilities as malleable. Most people hold a combination of both mindsets about different aspects of themselves. Holding a growth mindset is associated with adaptive self-regulatory strategies. There are various strategies, including rituals that promote a growth mindset, recommended for the context of ageing, although these were initially developed based on research with children, which is the most common application of this learning framework[17]. Those strategies include rituals eliciting positive memories, perceptions and goals. The way individuals and others perceive, write about and speak about ageing can influence the development of a fixed mindset, potentially making adaptation through the menopausal transition and ageing more challenging if the framing implies decline.

In the context of ageing, individuals with a fixed mindset may perceive ageing as an inevitable decline, believing that their abilities and health will inevitably deteriorate as they grow older. They may be more prone to adopting passive coping strategies and avoiding challenges related to ageing, leading to decreased engagement in activities that promote physical and mental well-being. Fixed mindset individuals may also be less likely to seek out opportunities for personal growth and development as they age, potentially leading to feelings of helplessness or resignation.

On the other hand, individuals with a growth mindset may view ageing as a dynamic process with opportunities for continued learning, growth and adaptation. They are more likely to adopt proactive adaptation strategies and embrace challenges associated with ageing, such as adopting healthy lifestyle habits, engaging in lifelong learning and seeking out new experiences. A growth mindset can lead to greater resilience in the face of age-related changes and a more positive outlook on the ageing process overall.

To facilitate better adaptation to ageing and menopause, fostering a more growth-oriented perspective through language and communication can be vital in promoting resilience and well-being during this life stage. Similarly, a growth mindset can also be beneficial in supporting men during andropause, the male equivalent of menopause. By adopting a growth mindset, men experiencing "andropause" (slight gradual decline, rather than cessation of testosterone production[18]) can view this transitional phase as an opportunity for personal growth and development rather than a decline in vitality, well-being and masculinity.

Although unlike men, women experience a dramatic drop in reproductive hormones[19] it is crucial to recognise the similarities in coping mechanisms needed to positively adapt to naturally declining levels of sex steroid hormones occurring at both menopause and andropause. The disproportionate focus on menopause and women in media, research and public attention may inadvertently reinforce perceptions of fixed or diminishing abilities in women, while men's experiences during andropause receive less visibility. An example of such initiatives and negative language includes recent UK policy changes posing a risk for employers to be sued for disability discrimination if they fail to make 'reasonable adjustments' for menopausal women, in accordance with Equality and Human Rights Commision[20]. While such considerations are very important and women's needs should be accommodated, the language linking menopause with disability is likely to create certain perceptions of ability, which might further impact how women perceive their capabilities and ageing. This discrepancy in attention and negative language could potentially influence employee perceptions and opportunities, leading to disparities in how menopause and andropause are perceived and supported in the workplace. Therefore, it is essential to foster inclusive dialogue and support systems that acknowledge the unique experiences of individuals of all genders navigating hormonal transitions associated with ageing.

Barrier 4 The culpable party

The absence of a multidisciplinary approach to address challenges related to ageing and menopause, coupled with limited consideration of the potential impacts of addressing these issues, contributes to the development of narratives that may not effectively address the problem holistically. This approach can create perceptions of blame for certain stakeholders within the ecosystem and hinder collaborative efforts that could support the positive change from coming to fruition.

Currently, it is not uncommon to encounter research or popular media articles highlighting pressing issues reported by women and other stakeholders related to menopause. Some narratives point to uninformed general practitioners who struggle to recognise menopause symptoms or are hesitant to prescribe HRT treatments. Others highlight the profit-driven motives of commercial companies that capitalise on the mediatisation of menopause for financial gain. There is also significant attention on the marketing of health claims, which is perceived as contributing to uninformed decisions.

While each of these findings contains elements of truth, it's essential to consider whether they represent objective or slightly partial perceptions influenced by the visible aspects of the broader system. Let's elaborate with an example: the surge in health and wellness supplements, accompanied by growing criticism of false claims. Undeniably, there are many instances where such criticism is valid. However, solely focusing on these claims represents only a partial problem within the wider system.

The Supplement Research Programme, led by Dr Pieter Cohen, an associate professor at Harvard Medical School and an internist at Cambridge Health Alliance, has uncovered alarming discrepancies in supplement contents[21]. For instance, melatonin gummies, marketed for sleep and stress relief, were found to contain up to 347% more of the stated ingredient[22]. Furthermore, combining dietary supplements with medications can pose serious risks, including life-threatening effects. For instance, St John's wort, an herbal supplement, can reduce the effectiveness of drugs for HIV/AIDS, heart disease, depression, organ transplants and birth control pills. Depending on the medication, the consequences can be severe. Additionally, substances like warfarin, *Ginkgo biloba*, aspirin and vitamin E can all thin the blood. Mixing any of these products together may elevate the risk of internal bleeding or stroke[23]. Dr Cohen advises against weight loss, sexual performance and cognitive enhancement supplements due to insufficient evidence of efficacy, as supplements are not required to be tested for efficacy in human trials[24]. Crucially, he urges consumers to opt for supplements from reputable brands with third-party certification, such as the National Institutes of Health, U.S. Pharmacopeia or NSF International, to ensure safety and efficacy.

As this example alone illustrates, the existence of any health solution on the market is enabled by a range of different stakeholders (e.g. regulatory bodies, policymakers, manufacturers, marketers, healthcare providers), each responsible for and impacting the final product or solution available on the market. If we consider the existence of these solutions from a systemic perspective, rather than an individual stakeholder perspective, it could be more likely that transparency in relation to all these processes could be enhanced. This, in turn, hopefully leads to collaborative efforts to address any existing problems and barriers to safe and effective solutions. Additionally, considering the quickly evolving space of ESG sustainable practices, many commercial companies might realise that they could face reputational and financial damage if rating low on various social impact measures – which relate to well-being outcomes or product quality and safety.

Barrier 5 Limited understanding of women's health and women's health services

Defining women's health, understanding its scientific underpinnings and translating this knowledge into comprehensive and inclusive healthcare services for women pose significant and persistent challenges. While certain health issues, such as those related to reproductive organs like contraception, fertility, maternal health, menopause, gynaecology and women's oncology, are well-recognised, there remains a gap in support and care for women facing conditions beyond reproductive health concerns[25]. This includes conditions like cardiovascular disease, diabetes and Alzheimer's disease[26], which affect women differently than men, as well as those such as migraines, autoimmune diseases, osteoporosis, anxiety, depression, urinary tract infections and lung cancer, which disproportionately impact women[27]. Moreover, it's crucial to acknowledge and address racial disparities and inequalities in women's healthcare and services[28]. Women of colour often experience unique health challenges due to unequal access to care, disparities in the quality of care, a shortage of culturally competent healthcare providers and systemic biases within the healthcare system.

The study, conducted by one of the authors with physicians in leadership roles, aimed to explore gender bias in healthcare and organisational settings and find ways to address challenges in women's healthcare services. The findings revealed several barriers that require attention.

While women's health was defined as encompassing all bodily systems affecting women, men participating in the study tended to focus on maternity and conditions related to the female reproductive system and menopause. This discrepancy was evident in the reluctance of women, especially those with young children, to seek healthcare unless in emergencies, due to the lack of integration in services. Moreover, healthcare services in England are not adequately tailored for pregnant women, leading to delays in accessing specialised care for non-pregnancy-related issues during pregnancy. Many clinicians felt the gender of the patient didn't affect their clinical decision making with patients and treated them based on symptoms regardless of the gender.

Towards sustainable solutions

To effectively address all the aforementioned challenges, it is crucial to adopt a comprehensive, interdisciplinary perspective that acknowledges the complex interplay of biological, psychological, social and environmental factors impacting individuals' experiences of ageing and menopause. This inclusive approach can help foster understanding, promote collaboration and facilitate the development of effective solutions that support the well-being of individuals across the lifespan. Grounded in this principle, our efforts have focused on identifying and addressing the root causes of challenges faced by females, as illustrated in the barriers section above. Through research, we have identified that a significant portion of these challenges arises within the spheres of work and home, influenced by broader environmental factors. As a result, we have prioritised initiatives within the workplace and the wider ecosystem, recognising their potential to catalyse systemic innovation and positively impact the experiences of females. In the sections below, we present an ecosystem approach to developing support, which connects different elements of the ecosystem for support.

Solution 1 Focus on ecosystem and value co-creation to optimise daily experiences

While many health transformations have very complex biology, processes and solutions, the key to recognise is that those transformations take place during daily experiences, where the health sector and services do not always reach. That is why it is important to understand the ecosystem that can either support or hinder how people progress

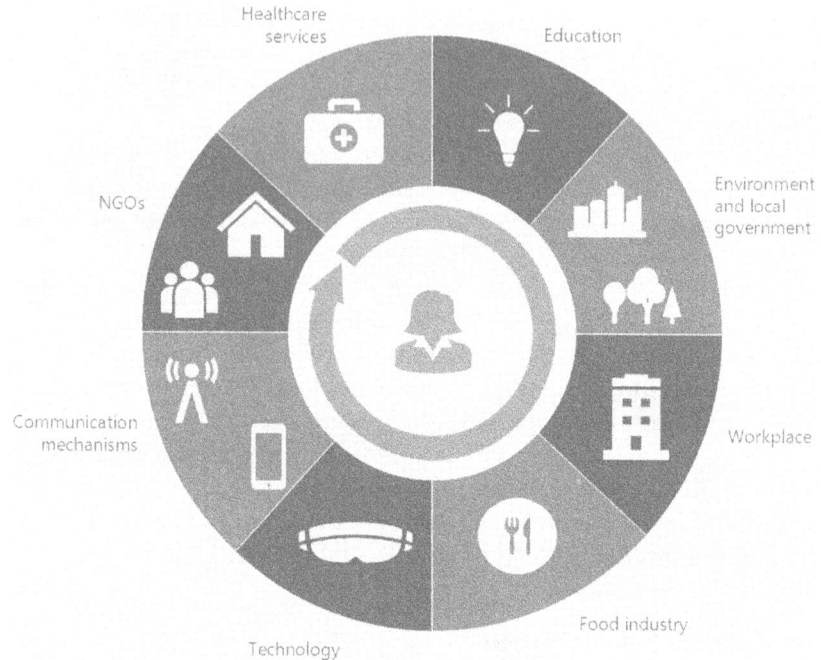

FIGURE 9.1.2 Systems approach to wellbeing

towards health behaviours. This type of system solutions have been recognised in the context of other complex societal challenges, like obesity for example[29]. Systems approaches to societal challenges focus on understanding those challenges as a complex problem influenced by multiple interacting factors within various systems, including individual, social, environmental, economic and policy domains, as illustrated in Figure 9.1.2. At its core, systems approaches recognise that health problems are not simply a result of individual choices or behaviours but is instead influenced by a wide range of interconnected factors, coming from different stakeholders like workplace, home, family, social groups and technology.

Consequently, understanding the menopausal transition as an ageing and behavioural change journey is crucial for women navigating this period, as this journey approach recognises needs and processes that lead to adapting lifestyles and choices to cope effectively. In order to change behaviours, we need to be aware that a change is needed and could be beneficial, we need to understand different options and choices we have to support our behaviour, we need to have an opportunity to interact with different elements of the system that could support our efforts and we need system support to reward the changes we managed to introduce, support ongoing efforts and habit formation. This journey doesn't happen in isolation; it's influenced by social circles, such as those at home or work.

Service research offers valuable insights into utilising the ecosystem's structure and dynamics to support behavioural change[30]. By considering service design and the wider support ecosystem, akin to diverse societal groups collaborating, we can create value and collectively facilitate behavioural change[31]. When individuals find value in certain actions (e.g. physical activity), they're more likely to sustain them. This body of research emphasises the importance of leveraging resources from various sources within the ecosystem to make activities and behaviours more accessible and achievable. For example, cancer patients often collaborate with healthcare providers, explore complementary therapies, educate themselves about their condition and involve loved ones in their care[32]. These strategies help patients navigate cancer treatments and enhance their quality of life. By tapping into a range of resources, individuals can better cope with health challenges and improve their overall well-being.

Supporting menopausal transition as part of an ecosystem can enable organisations to fulfil social impact objectives outlined by ESG standards. By viewing menopause as a journey of behavioural change and drawing from service research, organisations can design interventions that effectively leverage the ecosystem's structure and dynamics. In evaluating the social impact of such initiatives, potential ESG measures include improvements in physical and mental health outcomes, gender equality promotion, community engagement levels, enhancement of employee satisfaction and productivity and ensuring inclusivity and diversity in organisational policies and practices. Through a concerted focus on these measures, organisations demonstrate their commitment to supporting women through the menopausal transition while fostering holistic well-being within their ecosystems.

Solution 2 Foster creation of transformative communities

Transformational communities are groups of people who gather together to bring about positive and sustainable change in society. By generating flows of engagement and activating ecosystems, community members challenge existing models to lead social, economic, cultural, regulatory or environmental impact through collaboration and coordination, or by enacting each respective institution they represent like businesses, social organisations, governments or universities. Transformational communities are driven by the desire to create and foster inclusive, empowered and marked shift in the current state of things. Transformational communities by design can activate the collective agency for the good, amplify culturally rooted experiences, generate dynamic capabilities and deploy effective governance systems. Here are some examples of such communities addressing healthy ageing and female health ageing:

Ageing@Coimbra[33]: Situated in the Centro Region of Portugal, Ageing@Coimbra is a consortium led by the University of Coimbra. It aims to enhance the well-being of elderly individuals through improved social services and healthcare. By fostering quadruple helix collaboration involving academia, government, healthcare institutions and the private sector, it promotes active and healthy ageing. The consortium initiates innovative projects and supports young entrepreneurship in health services, with action groups focusing on areas like prescription adherence and falls prevention.

Healthy Ageing Community of Practice[34]: This collaborative learning community brings together businesses, researchers, investors and policymakers to advance knowledge and innovation in healthy ageing. With over 1,000 members, it offers workshops, networking opportunities and informative sessions to drive impactful projects and insights. Part of the UK Research and Innovation's Healthy Ageing Challenge, it strives to empower older adults to remain active, independent and socially connected as they age.

AGE Platform Europe[35]: As the largest European network representing older people, AGE Platform Europe advocates for the diverse needs and aspirations of the older population in the European Union. Through projects addressing age-friendly cities, urban exploration for seniors, combating violence against older women and promoting awareness against ageism, it ensures that older adults' voices are heard in policymaking at the European level. AGE Platform Europe emphasises a rights-based and life-course approach to ageing, advocating for policies that support older individuals throughout their lives.

Solution 3 Create workplace opportunities

The pursuit of workplace wellness for healthy ageing demands a strategic blend of awareness building, resources and planning, which can support the behaviour change journey. By anchoring interventions in evidence-based practices and leveraging insights from academic research, organisations can cultivate environments that promote holistic well-being and empower employees to thrive. As we navigate the complex landscape of modern workplaces, let us remain steadfast in our commitment to fostering health, vitality and resilience among all members of the workforce.

The first pillar: Creating awareness and support

Understand the importance of awareness and mitigate the challenge of undiagnosed conditions: In the domain of workplace wellness, fostering awareness assumes a crucial role in both preventing and managing health adversities, particularly those linked with menopause. Evidence consistently reveals that timely recognition and intervention substantially improve health outcomes across various health conditions. For instance, Mosca et al. (2004)[36] underscored the profound impact of awareness campaigns in reducing the prevalence of undiagnosed hypertension in women, thus preventing potential complications like stroke and heart attack. Given that postmenopausal women are already susceptible to conditions such as osteoporosis and cardiovascular disease, it becomes imperative to address modifiable physical and cognitive factors that could exacerbate medical complexities[37]. The complexities associated with undiagnosed conditions underscore the urgent necessity for proactive strategies in tackling menopause-related health challenges in the workplace promptly. This underscores the critical significance of early intervention in safeguarding the health and overall well-being of employees, accentuating the interconnectedness of menopausal symptoms with other diseases and long-term health outcomes.

Deploy strategies for raising awareness: Effective initiatives within the workplace must encompass multifaceted strategies to engage and support individuals experiencing menopause. Drawing from behavioural science principles, interventions may leverage various channels, such as interactive workshops, targeted messaging campaigns and incentives for participation[38]. Furthermore, integrating digital health technologies, such as mobile applications and wearable devices, enhances accessibility and engagement among tech-savvy employees[39]. By adopting a comprehensive approach, organisations can foster a culture of health literacy and empower employees to take proactive steps towards wellness.

Second pillar: Providing adequate resources and skills

Provide holistic wellness support: Beyond raising awareness, workplace wellness programs must offer comprehensive support mechanisms to address the multifaceted needs of employees. This entails not only access to medical services but also resources for mental and emotional well-being. Research underscores the interconnectedness of physical and mental health, emphasising the importance of integrated approaches to wellness[40]. Thus, organisations must prioritise initiatives that promote stress management, resilience-building and work-life balance alongside traditional healthcare services.

Empower through education and training: Empowerment lies at the heart of effective wellness programming. By equipping employees with knowledge and skills, organisations empower individuals to take ownership of their health journeys. Educational workshops, skill-building sessions and personalised coaching foster a culture of self-efficacy and proactive health management[41]. Moreover, investing in employee training programs enhances organisational capacity for promoting health and wellness, creating a ripple effect that extends beyond individual empowerment to organisational culture transformation.

Third pillar: The role of strategic planning

Move from vision to action and sustainable impact: The planning imperative: Strategic planning forms the bedrock of successful workplace wellness initiatives, guiding organisations from vision to action. Goetzel et al (2014) emphasise the importance of systematic planning in achieving sustainable outcomes. Central to this approach is the articulation of clear goals, objectives and performance metrics, which serve as guiding beacons for program implementation and evaluation. A well-crafted strategy encompasses not only the initial rollout of interventions but also long-term sustainability and impact. This necessitates careful consideration of resource allocation, stakeholder engagement and scalability[42]. By integrating feedback loops and iterative processes into the planning framework, organisations can adapt to evolving needs and maximise the effectiveness of their wellness initiatives.

Solution 4 Smash the stereotypes: embrace a growth mindset of your leaders and employees

In terms of a growth mindset during the menopause it is important that this is not just an individual responsibility but a collective one. The attitude towards people ageing in the workplace and women is deeply ingrained in society as one of stagnation and often referred to as "going into cruise-control". This is quite a dangerous assumption and one that negates the idea of ageing as an asset and contribution which it is. In order to thrive, organisations should be looking to widen the range of employees and strive for a wide range of employees that represent the fabric of society and not reinforce the notions of a "sell buy date" when it comes to age and also age and intersection. This of course is an attitude that is deeply ingrained in society and we can try to change it by taking recruitment actions that challenge this notion.

Institutional data from one of the author's employers, shows that when it comes to women, in particular the highest representation at a senior level is between the ages of 25 to 34 at 75%. Women over 55 only occupy 27%, which is concerning but also validating in terms of backing up anecdotal evidence that age has an impact on the professional trajectory of women. If we take said UK organisation as an example, the majority of over 55 are concentrated in the middle and junior roles. There is of course the school of thought that some women due to child-rearing and caring responsibilities choose to remain in these roles but what about those who haven't and who in this contributor's opinion are the majority. Interestingly, are organisations looking closely enough at their employment and performance data by age and gender groups?

In a sense it is the line manager's responsibility, if not institutional responsibility, to celebrate and support the development of older women who have hit a glass ceiling. We propose that positive action extends to age and that some senior role interviews plus a place on Leadership Programmes for high-potential individuals are ringfenced for those women who have been trying to progress for several years. Diagnostics and focus groups should be made available to women over 55 in junior grades to assess whether they are there by choice or because of institutional and societal barriers. In the build-up to these interviews, coaching and workshops to identify gaps should be provided. This is by no means a novel idea in terms of positive action; what is novel is that the focus is usually on other protected characteristics.

We are not arguing that there is no representation of women over 55s in senior roles, we are saying that progression is stunted so if you are already not senior therein lies the challenge. It is about acknowledging that there is room for growth, evolution and learning during and post menopause and that organisations should not shy away from what can be seen as an awkward challenge for those who do not share the experience.

Solution 5 Un-Pause men

As mentioned earlier menopause is a multifaceted, natural process women will endure in their lifetime. Males have a pivotal role in educating themselves and using evidence-based supportive literature and interventions to increase awareness regarding menopause to help and to be able to better support their female counterparts; so that all counterparts can have a smooth transition into postmenopausal years.

In a study by Koyuncu et al[43] to evaluate the effectiveness of health education, the efficacy of a training program, information about menopausal symptoms, knowledge and attitude towards menopause was collected before and after health education. It was suggested that there was a decrease in the somatic and psychological subdimensions of the menopausal symptom evaluation scale and the total score. Positive changes were observed in the levels of knowledge about menopause, and positive and negative emotional subscales of the menopause attitude assessment scale. This study highlighted that health education is an effective method to positively change the perceived severity of menopausal symptoms and menopause-related levels of knowledge and attitude.

Education resources and materials are available and can be used to help men understand menopause better; including books, reputable online sources, articles and attending seminars, workshops and engaging with health professionals around this topic. Another supportive measure for heterosexual men attending medical consultations with their partners or asking questions during visits with healthcare providers. Understanding the medical aspects of menopause, such as symptoms, hormonal changes and associated health risks, can enhance empathy and supportive dialogue with males. This could be translated into the workplace and community settings.

Other solutions include better open and honest communication between men and women, and women with other women, to foster and engender better relationships. Support groups in the workplace and among partners can offer a safer space to share experiences, seek advice and break down the barriers and taboos around menopause. Additionally, an empathetic approach will then develop, enabling the understanding and supportive strategies for men, especially if it starts early in life. This was also voiced by research participants in our study, with Jackie, 62 years old, mentioning:

> *"For example, my partner, I don't think that he would like to sit down and watch a program about the menopause, whereas I think younger men would, yeah."*

As men we need to do better in understanding menopause; it is not just about the physical changes women go through, but the psychosocial implications and aspects of this transition. Furthermore, being engaged, empowered, informed and supportive can play a significant role in helping us navigate the menopause journey with empathy and dignity. Jackie, 62 years old, mentioned:

> *". . I'm wondering if it needs to be touched on in schools. When people are older . . . , I think young people need to know about it, but not . . . just females. Men need to know. Young men need to know about it as well."*

While ageing discussions often centre on women due to menopause, it's crucial to recognise that men also undergo significant changes with age. Andropause, the gradual decline in testosterone levels in men, is one such change, yet it's often overlooked or under-discussed compared to menopause. Societal expectations of masculinity can hinder men from openly addressing their experiences with andropause and seeking support.

By acknowledging the impact of ageing on both genders and promoting open dialogue and support, we can diminish the stigma surrounding ageing. This inclusive approach not only benefits women but also creates a supportive environment where men feel more comfortable discussing their ageing-related challenges and seeking help. Ultimately, fostering support for both men and women in navigating the ageing process can enhance the well-being and quality of life for everyone involved.

Solution 6 Develop women's health services

There is also the need to focus on creating health services for women that are focused on biological, emotional and social needs of females. The proposed solution could focus on a life course approach, which acknowledges that the rate of decline in function is influenced by the highest level of function achieved earlier in life, shaped by developmental processes and early environmental influences[44].

Therefore, for women's health services to align with a life course approach, they must recognise (and be able to capture for a better understanding of health history) reproductive health needs as well as other general health needs that are likely to affect females at different stages of their lives. As a result, either through a questionnaire, existing healthcare records or healthcare practitioner inquiries, informed decisions and support should be enabled based on (1) reproductive health needs including prior HPV vaccination, menstrual health, gynaecological conditions, cervical screening, gynaecological cancers, sexual health and well-being, contraception, pregnancy, fertility, pregnancy loss, abortion care, postnatal support, pelvic floor health, perimenopause and menopause, as well as breast cancer screening; and (2) general health needs, including well-being and lifestyle, weight, exercise and smoking, mental health, long-term conditions, the health impact of violence against women and girls, osteoporosis and bone health, as well as dementia and Alzheimer's.

> *To exemplify the life course approaches in integrated health services, we'll delve into a case study from a hypothetical women's health hub. A 46-year-old woman sought help at the clinic, presenting a constellation of symptoms. These included dry mouth, jaw pain and a swollen right ankle, along with discomfort in her sole and heel, hindering her mobility. She had two children aged 9 months and 2 years. Juggling the responsibilities of a working mother, fatigue weighed heavily on her, exacerbated by disrupted sleep due to her young children's needs. She also reported feeling mentally less sharp, attributing this decline to her exhaustion. Additionally, she had a medical history of premenstrual syndrome (PMS) and autoimmune hypothyroidism. During her pregnancies, she experienced hand joint swelling*

and carpal tunnel syndrome, believed to be linked to pregnancy-related changes. Despite still experiencing menstrual cycles, these were gradually becoming irregular, occurring every 3 to 6 weeks and her PMS was a lot worse. She thought that all her symptoms were due to being a working mother with young children. Upon attending the women's health hub, after listening carefully to her story, the medical doctor explained that given her age and symptoms, most likely she was experiencing perimenopause. Irregular menstrual cycles and exacerbation of PMS are recognised as being suggestive of perimenopause. Although musculoskeletal issues can be a symptom associated with perimenopause, in view of her history of autoimmune hypothyroidism and worsening of joint issues during pregnancy, blood tests were conducted to check on thyroid function, autoantibodies and inflammatory markers. Although thyroid function was fine, the other findings, in the context of her clinical history were very suggestive of rheumatoid arthritis. In addition to advice around lifestyle in terms of exercise, nutrition and stress management, treatment for rheumatoid arthritis was started, together with sequential hormone replacement therapy (HRT) patches. Advice was given about contraception. Her mouth symptoms ameliorated, and she noticed improvements in her sleep, energy levels and cognitive function. Morning stiffness ceased to be an issue, marking a significant improvement in her overall well-being.

A way forward

Removing stigma surrounding menopause and ageing, and promoting equality, could foster a more inclusive and supportive environment for all individuals navigating the challenges of ageing and menopause. Moving forward to ensure person-centred systems, sustainability and social impact involves recognising and addressing barriers individuals face during menopause and ageing. Solutions including ecosystem-focused approaches, engaging men, creating workplace opportunities and enhancing women's health services offer a glimpse into a system of holistic support. Collaboration and knowledge exchange among stakeholders are crucial for effective implementation, while monitoring impact ensures interventions make a meaningful difference. While collaboration in this case will not always be easy, focusing on initiatives that foster a culture of continuous improvement ensures long-term success. By taking these steps, we can create supportive systems that prioritise individual well-being, contribute to sustainability and drive positive social change.

This challenge and the process of addressing it as described in this chapter highlights the relevance of research and universities in ensuring that the various types of knowledge that traditionally come from disciplinary and narrow areas are actually connected into a meaningful whole, where social impact is likely to realise. While there are various challenges with knowledge exchange and mobilising different stakeholders and resources, adopting person-centred approaches to identify the root of the needs shaping social impact is the key to knowledge exchange. Considering the fact that universities often operate within their own ecosystems, and co-create knowledge within those ecosystems, it is critical for those institutions to facilitate multidisciplinary teams which could connect the depth and breadth of knowledge for greatest impact.

References

1. Faubion SS, Enders F, Hedges MS et al. Impact of menopause symptoms on women in the workplace. *Mayo Clinic Proceedings* 2023; 98 (6): 833–845. doi: 10.1016/j.mayocp.2023.02.025.
2. Conti G, Ginja R, Persson P et al. The menopause "penalty". *Institute for Fiscal Studies* 2024 [Preprint]. https://ifs.org.uk/sites/default/files/2024-03/WP202405-The-menopause-penalty_0.pdf. Accessed April 2024.
3. Observatory of Public Sector Innovation, Organisation for Economic Co-operation and Development. Setting clear outcomes for ambitious missions 2021. https://oecd-opsi.org/work-areas/mission-oriented-innovation/#:~:text=Mission%2Doriented%20innovation%20refers%20to,%2C%20climate%20mitigation%2C%20clean%20oceans%2C. Accessed April 2024.
4. Henisz W, Koller T, Nuttal R. Five ways that ESG creates value. *McKinsey Quarterly* 2019. https://www.mckinsey.com/~/media/McKinsey/Business%20Functions/Strategy%20and%20Corporate%20Finance/Our%20Insights/Five%20ways%20that%20ESG%20creates%20value/Five-ways-that-ESG-creates-value.ashx. Accessed April 2024.
5. Philip Morris International. Integrated report 2023. https://www.pmi.com/sustainability/reporting-on-sustainability. Accessed April 2024.
6. Farzam R, Bartels W, Stanley K et al. Beyond environmental impact: The case of social in ESG. *Deloitte* 2024. https://www2.deloitte.com/nl/nl/pages/sustainability/articles/beyond-environmental-impact-the-case-of-social-in-esg.html. Accessed April 2024.
7. Serafeim G. Social-impact efforts that create real value. *Harvard Business Review* 2020; 98 (5): 38–48. https://hbr.org/2020/09/social-impact-efforts-that-create-real-value. Accessed April 2024.
8. Hickey M, LaCroix AS, Doust J et al. An empowerment model for managing menopause. *The Lancet* 2024; 403 (10430): 947–957. doi: 10.1016/S0140-6736(23)02799-X.
9. Ferguson B, Belloni A. Ageing and health expenditure. *Health Profile for England* 2018. https://ukhsa.blog.gov.uk/2019/01/29/ageing-and-health-expenditure/. Accessed April 2024.
10. Yale School of Public Health. Lifestyle factors: Tobacco and alcohol, obesity and physical activity, nutrition and diabetes. https://ysph.yale.edu/public-health-research-and-practice/interdepartmental-foci/lifestyle-factors/. Accessed April 2024.
11. Australian Menopause Society. Lyfestyle and behavioural modifications for menopausal symptoms. 2019. https://www.menopause.org.au/hp/information-sheets/lifestyle-and-behavioural-modifications-for-menopausal-symptoms. Accessed April 2024.
12. Hidiroglu S, Tanriover O, Ay P et al. A qualitative study on menopause described from the man's perspective. *Journal of the Pakistan Medical Association* 2014; 64 (9): 1031–1036. PMID: 25823183.
13. Jaspers L, Daan NMP, van Dijk GM et al. Health in middle-aged and elderly women: A conceptual framework for healthy menopause. *Maturitas* 2015; 81 (1): 93–98. doi: 10.1016/j.maturitas.2015.02.010.
14. What is health? The ability to adapt. *The Lancet* 2009; 373 (9666): 781. https://www.thelancet.com/journals/lancet/article/PIIS0140-6736(09)60456-6/fulltext.
15. Dweck CS. Motivational processes affecting learning. *American Psychologist* 1986; 14: 1040–1048. doi: 10.1037/0003-066X.41.10.1040.
16. Dweck CS. *Self-theories: Their Role in Motivation, Personality, and Development*. Psychology Press, Philadelphia, PA, 2000.

17 Haslin PA, Burnette J, Ryu NG. Does a growth mindset enable successful aging? *Work, Aging and Retirement* 2021; 7 (2): 79–89. doi: 10.1093/workar/waaa029.
18 Vermeulen A. Andropause. *Maturitas* 2000; 34 (1): 5–15.
19 Male menopause: Myth vs. fact. *The Journal of Clinical Endocrinology and Metabolism* 2014; 99 (10): 49A–50A. doi: 10.1210/jc.2014-v99i10-49A.
20 The Guardian. Employers must male 'reasonable adjustments' for women going through the menopause 2024. https://www.theguardian.com/society/2024/feb/22/employers-must-make-reasonable-adjustments-for-women-going-through-menopause. Accessed April 2024.
21 Challiance Organisation Supplement Research Program 2024. https://www.challiance.org/academics/research/supplements/about-our-work. Accessed April 2024.
22 Cohen PA, Avula B, Wang YH et al. Quantity of melatonin and CBD in melatonin gummies sold in the US. *JAMA* 2023; 329 (16): 1401–1402. doi: 10.1001/jama.2023.2296.
23 U.S. Food and Drug Administration. Mixing medications and dietary supplements can endanger your health. https://www.fda.gov/consumers/consumer-updates/mixing-medications-and-dietary-supplements-can-endanger-your-health. Accessed April 2024.
24 American Medical Association. Pieter Cohen, MD, explains dietary supplements and regulations 2014. https://www.ama-assn.org/delivering-care/public-health/pieter-cohen-md-explains-dietary-supplements-regulations. Accessed April 2024.
25 Weisman CS. Changing definitions of women's health: Implications for health care and policy. *Maternal and Child Health Journal* 1997; 1 (3): 179–189. doi: 10.1023/a:1026225513674.
26 Merone L, Tsey K, Russell D et al. Mind the gap: Reporting and analysis of sex and gender in health research in Australia, a cross-sectional study. *Women's Health Reports* 2022; 3 (1): 759–767. doi: 10.1089/whr.2022.0033.
27 Kmietowicz Z. Health inequality: "Women's Health Ambassador" will help deliver strategy to close gender gap in England. *BMJ* 2021; 375: n3142–n3142. doi: 10.1136/bmj.n3142.
28 Department of Health and Social Care UK. Women's health strategy 2021. https://assets.publishing.service.gov.uk/media/62d93c65d3bf7f2862f26a48/Womens-Health-Strategy-easy-read.pdf. Accessed April 2024.
29 Public Health England. Whole systems approach to obesity 2019. https://www.gov.uk/government/publications/whole-systems-approach-to-obesity. Accessed April 2024.
30 Gallan AS, McColl-Kennedy JR, Barakshina T et al. Transforming community well-being through patients' lived experiences. *Journal of Business Research* 2019; 100: 376–391. doi: 10.1016/j.jbusres.2018.12.029.
31 Patrício L, Fisk R, Cunha JC et al. Multilevel service design: From customer value constellation to service experience blueprinting. *Journal of Service Research* 2011; 14 (2): 180–200.
32 McColl-Kennedy JR, Vargo SL, Dagger TS et al. Health care customer value cocreation practice styles. *Journal of Service Research* 2021; 15 (4): 370–389. doi: 10.1177/1094670512442806.
33 https://ageingcoimbra.pt/en/best-practices.
34 https://iuk.ktn-uk.org/programme/healthy-ageing-community/.
35 https://www.age-platform.eu/about/our-vision-and-mission/.
36 Mosca L, Ferris A, Fabunmi R et al. Tracking women's awareness of heart disease: An American Heart Association national study. *Circulation* 2004; 109 (5): 573–579. doi: 10.1161/CIR.0b013e318287cf2f.
37 Santoro N, Epperson CN, Mathews SB. Menopausal symptoms and their management. *Endocrinology and Metabolism Clinics* 2015; 44 (3): 497–515. doi: 10.1016/j.ecl.2015.05.001.
38 Huang H, Mattke S, Batorsky B et al. Incentives, program configuration, and employee uptake of workplace wellness programs. *Journal of Occupational and Environmental Medicine* 2016; 58 (1): 30–34. https://www.jstor.org/stable/48500833. Accessed April 2024.
39 Howarth A, Quesada J, Silva J et al. The impact of digital health interventions on health-related outcomes in the workplace: A systematic review. *Digital Health* 2018: 4. doi: 10.1177/2055207618770861.

40 Goetzel RZ, Roemer EC, Kent KB et al. Integration of workplace prevention programs and organizational effectiveness. *American Psychological Association* 2019: 279–294. doi: 10.1037/0000149-017.
41 Goetzel RZ, Henke RM, Tabrizi M et al. Do workplace health promotion (wellness) programs work? *Journal of Occupational and Environmental Medicine* 2014; 56 (9): 927–934. doi: 10.1097/JOM.0000000000000276.
42 Goetzel Z. Designing and implementing successful workplace health and well-being initiatives. *American Journal of Health Promotion* 2020; 34 (1): 112–112. doi: 10.1177/0890117119887785.
43 Koyuncu T, Unsal A, Arslantas D. Evaluation of the effectiveness of health education on menopause symptoms and knowledge and attitude in terms of menopause. *Journal of Epidemiology and Global Health* 2018; 8 (1): 8–12. doi: 10.2991/j.jegh.2018.08.103.
44 Dodds RM, Syddall HE, Cooper R et al. Gripstrength across the life course: Normative data from twelve British studies. *PLoS One* 2014; 9 (12): e113637. doi: 10.1371/journal.pone.0113637.

Coda

The wisdom of Athena

Dr Nicky Keay and Dr Tamara Dragadze

Athena guided Odysseus through trials and obstacles. Navigating the female hormone odyssey presents many challenges, culminating in graduation to menopause and beyond. Every woman's experience is different, but each of us must draw on our own inner Athena to progress through the hormone dance of life.

Terpsichore: the ancient Greek muse of dance

Dancing is my inspiration. Taking a ballet class enables me to engage my physical and mental faculties and share the experience with my close circle of friends. Tamara is a shining example for all of us in the class. At nearly 80 years, Tamara regularly takes class, up to four times a week. I am determined to be still taking class in the future like Tamara.

Tamara immediately came to mind for the coda to this book. I am delighted and grateful that she agreed to share her personal story to inspire others.

> "The older one gets, the more one feels that the present moment must be enjoyed, comparable to a state of grace."
>
> *Marie Curie*

Coda

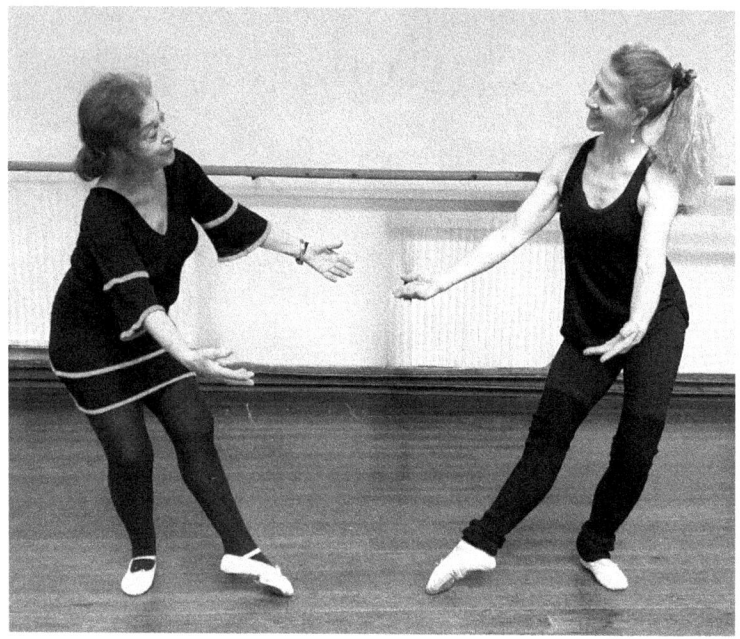

Dr Nicky Keay and Dr Tamrara Dragadze dancing together at Dance Attic.

Terpsichore and Menopause

Dr Tamara Dragadze

It started with my friend and colleague in Georgia, Academician Professor Lia Melikishvili, with whom I have written many papers and recently edited a book together. Almost eerily, she in Tbilisi and I thousands of miles away in London, found ourselves writing about the same subjects. But more impressively, we always seemed to get the same illnesses. So, when she got unbearable pains in her joints and then all her bones, she was finally diagnosed with problems related to do with the menopause and was put on hormone replacement therapy (HRT).

Therefore, as soon as I myself started to get pain in my bones, I knew what to do: I immediately got myself referred to the gynaecologist at the local Chelsea and Westminster Hospital. Of course, I was offered HRT, but when I said that I'd like to try something natural, he replied: "*Well, go natural and die aged 55 like your mother did, or else take hormone replacement therapy and have a good chance of living to a good old age.*"

I replied that with what he had just said, I was left with no choice! So, I went on HRT and never looked back. Until, still on it 18 years later, I developed breast cancer. I was operated on while it was still *in situ* and told to stop HRT immediately. By that time, aged 67, the menopause was well over and so I had avoided all its symptoms.

A postmenopause age blip came when I lost my temper in my late 50s. I had an ovarian cyst, but when I was brought the consent form for the operation in Hammersmith Hospital, I read that it was to remove both my ovaries. I did not want the healthy one to be removed for the sake of NHS convenience, and so I asked the young intern, "*What role do ovaries play?*"

"An ovary is for having babies," she replied, "*but as you are over 50, you don't need that.*" I agreed. "*And it is also for having a sex drive, but as you are over 50, you don't need that either.*"

' "What! My sex drive! Go away!" I shouted and threw the paper back at her.

Soon the surgeon herself came to see me. "*I will help you with your sex drive,*" she declared, "*'by doing an incision low down, below the bikini line. And I will do beaded stitches so the scar will be minimum.*" And I duly signed the consent form for just the one ovary to be removed and apologised for having shouted at the intern, however wrong she had been.

A few weeks after my 70th birthday, I had a near-drowning accident in the South of France. The lack of oxygen, until I got a regular heartbeat back, caused a part of my brain to die. I was in a coma for nine days and on a life-support machine.

My two adult children were told they were unlikely to find the mother they had known because I would either be in a vegetative state or unable even to recognise them. When I was brought out of the coma, I hallucinated about there being a fireplace by my bed and that a cat had come into my room with her kittens. My children asked me if I knew who they were and I told them what a stupid question and said their names. They went out to tell the doctor who said that they had told him I spoke several languages. Between them they were able to ask me questions in all six and I replied perfectly in each of the languages. However, we soon discovered that I had lost the link between my brain and my movement. Even my voice was in a whisper. I soon was able to move my head and then my hands. The part of my brain which had died had been linked to movement, to memory and partly to self-control.

The brain, however, is amazing because it allows different pathways to reach the same destinations as the ones you have lost.

After three weeks in France and nearly two months in a general hospital in London, I was moved to the Royal Hospital for Neuro-disability. The staff there worked with me, and I received extra help during the weekly visits of my ballet teacher, who is also a physiotherapist. They performed repeated movements with my lifeless limbs until my brain reconnected with them. The longest task was to regain sensation below my waist. It was not because I wasn't trying; the greatest nightmare was that I was completely incontinent. With extra advice from my ballet teacher, I worked tirelessly to strengthen my muscles. Seven months after my accident, I walked away from my wheelchair and up the stairs to my first-floor flat.

I had to wait a while until I really came back to being alive. That happened when my ballet teacher tested me in a private ballet lesson — her gift, including studio hire — to see if I could return to classes without harming the other students as well as myself.

I had trained in ballet since I was a child. Unfortunately, I peaked when I was only 15. I could do anything, it seemed. Losing the need for new challenges, I then did more Spanish dancing than before and ended up in a company doing both. After that, deciding what I would do next, I realised that with my shape I was unlikely to get very far as a classical dancer, mainly because my brother told me so, as he was a ballet dancer himself. And best to do something else. From doing drama to becoming a student of Anthropology and Sociology, I put ballet behind me. For thirty years I didn't touch it. I bored myself silly doing Keep Fit classes but no ballet. Once, for a time in Leeds, I gave ballet classes at the United Caribbean Association because their members' children had wanted to do ballet in a tutu and not be pushed into jazz dancing by the prejudiced dance schools downtown. I did that for a while and even put on a production of Coppélia. But that came to an end when I left Leeds and I never touched ballet again. Though my mother had composed music for ballets and had played for classes regularly, and one of my brothers and his wife were professional ballet dancers, except for that brief return, I amputated ballet completely out of my life. Until, on my 50th birthday, I decided it was stupid to boycott what had been so much a part of my existence and had stood over me like a shadow. So, I went back to doing a few Silver Swans classes and very soon was doing regular classes with various teachers until finally I found my teacher Josephine Bell who since then has seen me through thick and thin and breathed life into my every day.

After the careful test described above, she told me I could return to class, the standard session first and the advanced next. Given that, when I miss classes, I get cramps and my back seizes up, I try not to miss them. I had a car accident in 1987 and my strong muscles kept my two damaged vertebrae in place. The immobility after my drowning accident caused me to take morphine-based painkillers for nearly two years until I had built up my back muscles again. And so now, I am condemned to exercise, or else I pay for it! I also try to walk 5 kilometres a day but do not always succeed, so ballet classes are my mainstay.

I am a woman of faith and I recite set prayers daily, but sometimes in ballet class, I can pray for what I cannot say in words. Sometimes I dedicate my dancing in the class to someone, often to my late brother who had been a dancer. But on Saturdays, I occasionally dance for the Fulham Football Team, where I make that extra effort for their sake, for them to carry it on to the pitch later in the day.

My memory has been seriously harmed by my accident, but when I am able to give a quick glance at what another dancer is doing, who is usually faultless and who is usually Nicola, I have been able to do full classes four times a week, even now in my 81st year.

I know that taking HRT, once the right one was found, minimised the effects of menopause. And although my life before it was momentous, especially having two children, my life since then has been virtually unmarked by it. I am so fortunate to live near my grandchildren and to participate in their care, and also to be able to work full-time, although freelance and mostly from home. My ambition, of course, is to live as many years after menopause as before it and be a talkative centenarian who also dances.

Navigating Menopause Myths

- Menopause is a physical/mental illness.
  Distractions of social media Sirens
  Act 1 Misunderstandings around Menopause
  Scene 1 What is menopause?

- Menopause is only about the capacity to reproduce.
  Distractions of social media Sirens
  Act 1 Misunderstandings around Menopause
  Scene 1 What is menopause?

- Menopause happens quickly.
  Distractions of social media Sirens
  Act 1 Misunderstandings around Menopause
  Scene 1 What is menopause?

- Menopause only happens in middle-aged women.
  Distractions of social media Sirens
  Act 1 Misunderstandings around Menopause
  Scene 1 What is menopause?

- Menopause is only about hot flushes.
  Pandora's box
  Act 2 Challenges of Menopause
  Scene 1 Myths of menopausal 'symptoms'

- Weight gain is inevitable with menopause.
  Pandora's box
  Act 2 Challenges of Menopause
  Scene 1 Myths of menopausal 'symptoms'

- Having sex is not possible after menopause.
  Metamorphosis of Aphrodite
  Act 3 Menopause, Sex and Pelvic Health
  Scene 1 No sex after menopause?!

- Menopause means you resign yourself to poor quality of life and health: there is nothing you can do.
  Hippocrates
  Act 4 Mastering Menopause

- There are specific "diets" and supplements for menopause.
  Hippocrates
  Act 4 Mastering Menopause
  Scene 1 The menopause diet?

- There is a particular exercise or type of exercise for menopause.
  Hippocrates
  Act 4 Mastering Menopause
  Scene 2 Where do I start with exercise?
  Scene 3 Demystifying the myths of exercise

- Hormone replacement therapy (HRT) causes breast cancer.
  Scylla and Charybdis
  Act 5 Treatment Options
  Hormone replacement therapy (HRT)

- All women should take HRT.
  Scylla and Charybdis
  Act 5 Treatment Options
  Hormone replacement therapy (HRT)

- No woman needs HRT.
  Scylla and Charybdis
  Act 5 Treatment Options
  Hormone replacement therapy (HRT)

- Menopause means you can no longer be active.
  Terpsichore
  Act 6 Active Women and the Hormone Dance

- Menopause prevents athletes and dancers from training and performing.
  Orpheus and Eurydice
  Act 7 Age Group Athletes

- All women experience menopause in the same way.
  Discord and harmony
  Act 8 Experiencing Menopause

- Menopause is a taboo topic and it is difficult to talk about.
  Discord and harmony
  Act 8 Experiencing Menopause

- When the ovaries retire, it is time to retire from work and life.
  Discord and harmony
  Act 8 Experiencing Menopause

- Embracing menopause as part of ageing.
  Act 9 Towards Positive Ageing
  Collaboratively removing barriers for sustainable person-centred system support

- Navigating the female hormone odyssey.
  Wisdom of Athena
  Coda

Contributor Backgrounds

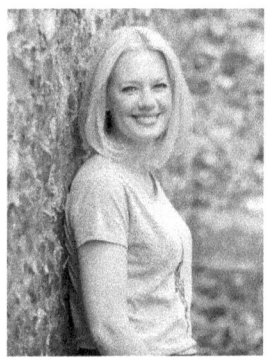

Anna Allerton is a former sports journalist and TV producer of 17 years. She founded and produced the *Sportswomen* programme for Sky and was a pioneer and campaigner for women in sport. She now runs an Executive Coaching & Consultancy business that specialises in supporting professional women to grow and thrive in careers during midlife. She developed her own *Work Smarter in Menopause®* coaching model following her own experience of perimenopause at the age of 38 and campaigns to elevate the voices of women under 40 experiencing menopause.

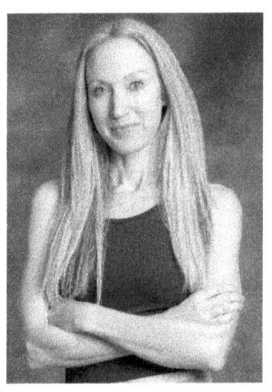

Ally (Alexander) Atkins is a personal trainer and functional mobility specialist and is passionate about the benefits of exercise for women's health. Having overcome her own health challenges in her late 30s, Ally has a deep understanding of the huge potential for change that is available with the right direction. Ally brings a fresh perspective to the fitness world, championing the importance of exercise and strength for women whilst being understanding and supportive. Whether it's conquering health hurdles or unlocking newfound strength, the routines Ally puts together help guide women towards a healthier and more vibrant future.

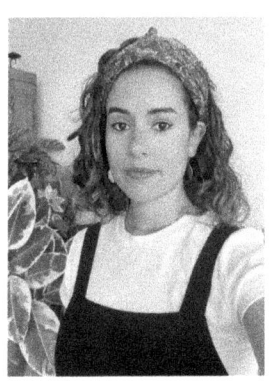

Nora Bahhar is a trainee clinical psychologist at University College London and Camden and Islington NHS Foundation Trust, set to complete her training in 2025. With experience in various NHS settings and research collaborations with London universities, she is also a member of the 'Menopause Mind Lab' at UCL. Nora's clinical and research interests centre on policy and the mental health of women, particularly those who are marginalised and facing systemic barriers. Her doctoral thesis explores the predictors of psychological symptoms in midlife women, aiming to enhance understanding of mental health during menopause. Nora aspires to specialise in women's and sexual health, continuing her engagement with the community through both research and clinical practice.

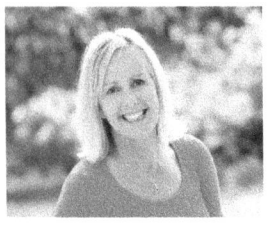 **Christien Bird** After training in the Netherlands, Christien Bird worked with musculoskeletal and women's health outpatients at Central Middlesex Hospital, London, until 1995. She also worked with the clinical research team at Brunel University London. After gaining her master's degree in research methods at King's College London, Christien founded the White Hart Clinic in Barnes in 1995, a busy multidisciplinary practice that offers musculoskeletal, pelvic health, psychological and medical services. Christien is the co-founder of the Menopause Movement online certified training and community platform for health and fitness professionals. She loves everything about movement, continues to compete as an age-group triathlete representing Great Britain. Much of her drive is supporting women in enjoying movement and staying strong.

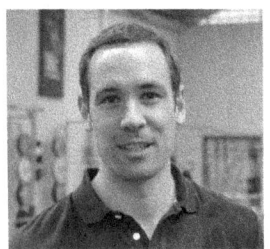 **Dr Richard Blagrove** is a senior lecturer in Physiology and Programme Leader of the MSc Strength and Conditioning (S&C) at Loughborough University. Richard is a UKSCA Accredited S&C Coach and Certified S&C Specialist with the NSCA. He has provided coaching support to athletes of all ages for almost 20 years, including Olympic and Paralympic finalists. Richard's current research investigates issues relating to performance and health in endurance runners, including physiological determinants of performance, the use of strength-based exercise, prevention of injury and recovery from the Relative Energy Deficiency in Sport syndrome.

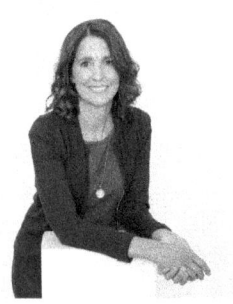 **Lara Briden** is a naturopathic doctor with a focus on women's health. She has consulting rooms in Christchurch, New Zealand and is the author of the popular books *Period Repair Manual*, *Hormone Repair Manual*, and *Metabolism Repair for Women*.

Contributor Backgrounds

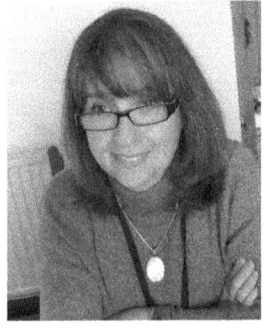

Dr Gillian Campbell After qualifying in 1995 from University College London, Gillian Campbell moved to Derbyshire. She completed her PhD investigating strain in tendons at the University of Nottingham in 2011 and is currently employed there as a postdoctoral research fellow funded by the School of Primary Care Research. Her research interests are pelvic floor disorders in athletic women and barriers to seeking help for pelvic floor symptoms for all women. She has continued to work clinically throughout her academic career, treating both musculoskeletal and pelvic health patients at Ashbourne Physiotherapy & Sports Injuries Centre, where she sees both private patients and NHS referrals. She is the current vice-chair of the Pelvic Obstetric and Gynaecological Physiotherapy group (a professional network for physiotherapist in pelvic health). Her passion for sport and exercise began at university, competing for Scotland as a lightweight rower and sculler. More recently she has moved on land and onto her bike where she still competes regularly in veteran time trials.

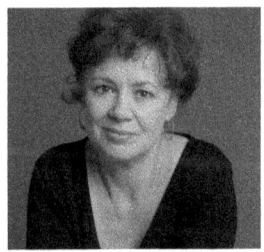

Nikki Crane with a background in dance, Nikki has over 30 years' experience working in the arts, combining experience as a practitioner with leadership roles in strategy and funding. Nikki led the development of Arts Council England's first national strategies for Arts & Criminal Justice and Arts & Health and as Head of Arts Strategy at Guy's & St Thomas' Charity, developed an evidence-based portfolio of arts and health programmes building partnerships between clinicians, academics, arts organisations and local health commissioners. Nikki is now lead for Creative Health at King's College London including supporting the development and delivery of 'SHAPER' (Scaling-up Health-Arts Programmes: Implementation and Effectiveness Research), the world's largest study into the impact of the arts on physical and mental health, supported by a £2.5 million award from Wellcome Trust.

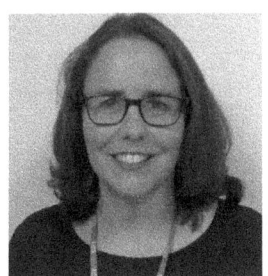

Dr Helen Donovan is a Consultant Clinical Psychologist with over 30 years of experience working in NHS and other public-sector services, including developing and leading adult and older adult psychological services and combining roles as a clinician, trainer, manager, supervisor and researcher. In recent years, Helen's own challenges of the perimenopause led her to become interested in psychological adjustment and approaches to support well-being during the menopause transition, with a particular interest in adapting compassion-based approaches for this life stage. She now works primarily in private practice and is also working in partnership with University College London in the 'Menopause Mind Lab'.

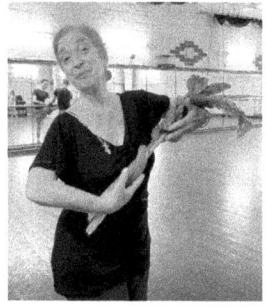

Tamara Dragadze is a British-born anthropologist with Georgian ancestry. Tamara completed her DPhil at Oxford University and is the author of more than 50 academic publications and taught and researched in several British universities. She has also published fiction. Starting ballet at the age of 3, she left it for 30 years after the age of 20 when she learnt she was not in the right shape to be a professional dancer. For her 50th birthday, however, she took up classical ballet again and has never looked back and takes class four times a week.

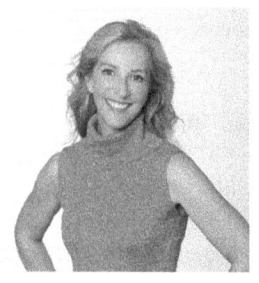

Dinah Hampson is a physiotherapist who is passionate about enjoying life and using her knowledge to promote high performance in others. Dinah holds many certifications including the Sport Physio Diploma and International Sports Physiotherapist qualification, the Diploma of Manual & Manipulative Therapy and Pelvic Health Physiotherapy. Dinah is the founder of Pivot Sport Medicine, a multidisciplinary clinic in Toronto, Canada and Pivot Dancer, a virtual dance injury prevention platform with worldwide membership. Dinah has been on the Canadian medical team for over 15 multisport games, including the Olympics, Youth Olympics, Paralympic, Pan American, World University and Commonwealth Games. Dinah trained in classical ballet and brings a technical eye to her treatment of dancers and artistic athletes. Dinah works regularly with professional dancers from companies such as the National Ballet of Canada, Joffrey Ballet, Dutch National Ballet, Canadian Contemporary Dance Theatre, Singapore Ballet and Cirque du Soleil. Dinah is active in dance science research and is a regular conference presenter.

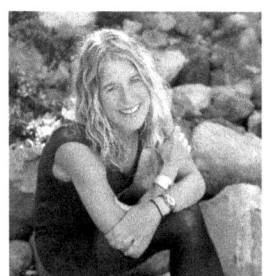

Tenille Hoogland's mission is to transform how female athletes experience sport and reach life-long health and athletic excellence. Her life has centred around sport. She began elite sport as a synchronised swimmer, then in her late 20s became a professional triathlete, representing Canada in various championships. Professionally, Tenille was a senior planner at the 2010 Olympic and Paralympic Winter Games Federal Secretariat, managed numerous IRONMAN events, held a management position at Triathlon Canada and was recognised by her national federation and Canadian Olympic Committee as a Future Sport Leader. Collectively the challenges she faced in sport personally and professionally led her to create the *Mindset, Nutrition, Training, and Recovery Integrated Training System* (MNTR-ITS). Using this system, she now coaches female athletes in perimenopause and beyond to thrive in sport for life and achieve personal excellence.

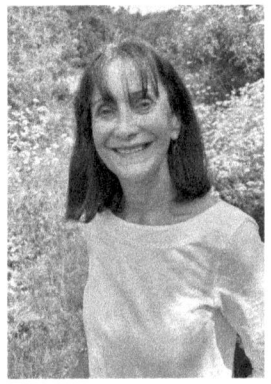

Professor Myra Hunter is Emeritus Professor of Clinical Health Psychology at King's College London, has worked as a clinician and researcher in the area of women's health for over 30 years. She has developed and evaluated cognitive behavioural therapy (CBT) interventions for physical and emotional problems, in women's health, oncology and cardiology. Her work has shown that CBT can effectively reduce the impact of menopausal symptoms on women's lives. She has published over 200 journal articles and 10 books and her research on menopause has established her as an international expert in the field.

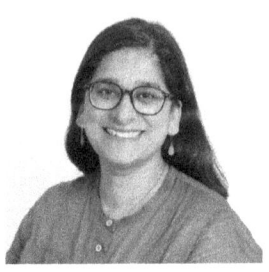

Dr Meena Khatwa is a Senior Research Fellow based at the UCL Social Research Institute, University College, London. Her research interests are in social and health inequalities amongst marginalised communities, and she also teaches at postgraduate level on qualitative methods. She is a well-being champion and one of the co-leads for the UCL Menopause Network. Meena has been awarded grants to explore how women cope with menopause while juggling work and caring responsibilities, and a UCL Public Policy Fellowship with Newham London Borough Council that focuses on South Asian women's mental health. In her spare time, she writes creative non-fiction and sings in an a cappella choir.

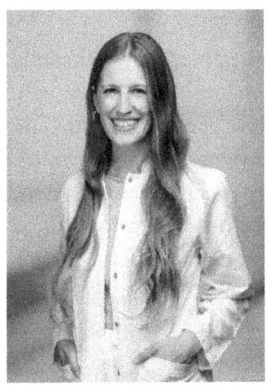

Dr Anne Latz is a physician with a MSc in Business Administration and a doctoral degree in Neuroscience. Certified in Lifestyle Medicine and in Safety Quality Informatics and Leadership at Harvard Medical School, and with professional experience in the private and public sectors, she is an entrepreneur in health tech and health communication, in addition to her active medical practice in psychosomatic medicine and psychotherapy. Engaged in numerous networks, she advocates for personalised prevention, health promotion and communication, and equitable and smart use of new technologies.

Contributor Backgrounds

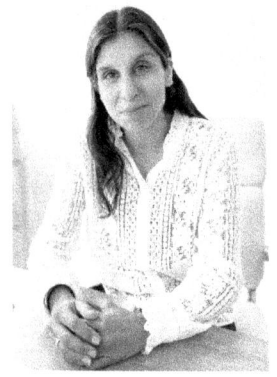

Renee McGregor is a leading sports dietitian and eating disorder specialist with over 20 years of experience, working in clinical and performance nutrition. Renee is passionate about working with individuals and athletes of all levels and ages and is the founder of Team Renee McGregor, managing a team of practitioners, in supporting health, sports performance and managing eating disorders and relative energy deficiency in sport. Renee is also a best-selling author, and her most recent book is *More Fuel You*. When not working, Renee can be found running the mountains and chasing the trails. In 2022, she became British Trail Running Champion in her age group over the short course and 3rd female at The Spine Sprint. Last year she came 4th female and had a top 10 finish, racing in Upper Mustang, Nepal.

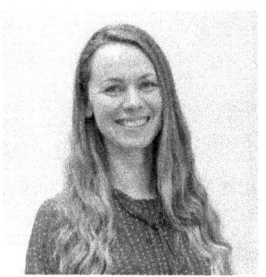

Dr Marzena Nieroda is Assistant Professor of Marketing and Commercialisation for Healthcare and Deputy Director for Partnerships & Enterprise at UCL Global Business School for Health (GBSH). GBSH is a new institute at UCL established in 2021 to bring together business and health to facilitate health innovation and health system strengthening. Marzena explores person-centred co-creation approaches within health and well-being services and systems. Specifically, she explores well-being journeys people experience and co-create within a system, the role and acceptance of technology and mission-oriented innovation in well-being journeys and the role of partnerships and collaboration co-creation within health and well-being systems. She has contributed to research projects funded by Cancer Research UK, Greater Manchester Cancer Vanguard, the European Commission, Digitally Enhanced Advanced Services (DEAS), EPSRC, University College London and the University of Manchester, working within the wider context of health promotion, digital inclusion and addressing health inequalities.

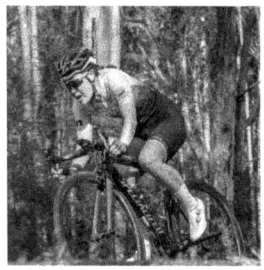

Nicole Oh is a Sydney-born and trained physiotherapist with 25 years of experience, spending 18 of those years working in the United Kingdom. For the past decade, Nicole has specialised in the treatment of cyclists, runners and triathletes. She combines her cycling knowledge and physiotherapy skills to offer bike-fitting services for all levels of riders. Nicole has also written articles for the UK publication *Cycling Weekly* on topics in physiotherapy, bike fitting, cycling injuries, performance and athlete health. Nicole has been a competitive cyclist since 2012, having made the switch from Triathlon. She has won National Masters titles in both the United Kingdom and Australia in a variety of disciplines. She continues to race at Elite level in Australia.

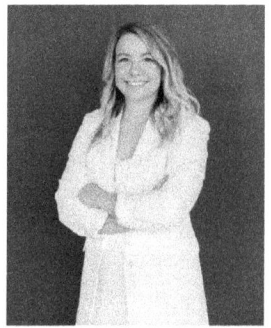

Dr Alyssa Olenick holds a PhD in Exercise Physiology. She is a certified sports nutritionist and CrossFit Level 2 Trainer. Alyssa completed her doctoral training in exercise and human metabolism, sex differences and menstrual cycle physiology. She is currently a postdoctoral research fellow researching the areas of menopause and metabolism. As a coach she specialises in the areas of endurance, strength and hybrid training. She runs her online business 'Doc Lyss Fitness' and is a strength athlete, ultra-marathon runner and all-around fitness lover who is passionate about educating people on science-based fitness to get them into the gyms and on the roads/trails – or often, doing both at the same time!

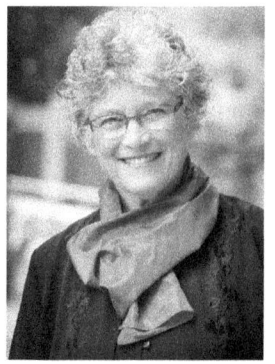

Professor Jerilynn C. Prior has been working for more than 45 years at the University of British Columbia Endocrinology as a healthcare provider, scientist and teacher. An award-winning clinician-scientist, she is known for her innovative concepts that value oestrogen-progesterone interplay as having the potential to transform and improve understanding and treatment of women's reproductive-related issues. She founded the UBC Centre for Menstrual Cycle and Ovulation Research, CeMCOR, in 2002 and launched its informative website in 2003. Prior is an internationally recognised thought-leader on menstrual cycles, ovulation, perimenopause, menopause and osteoporosis prevention. Dr Prior grew up in Alaskan fishing villages, gained an honours MD from Boston University (in 1969) and became Canadian (in 1983) due to her belief in universal health care.

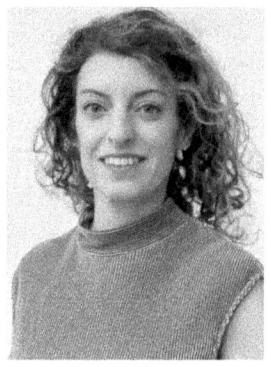

Rebekah Rotstein is a leader for Pilates, bone health and movement education. She is the founder of Buff Bones®, a medically endorsed exercise method for bone and joint health with on-demand programming, online coaching, free public education webinars with UCLA Health and professional training for instructors worldwide. A former ballet dancer, Rebekah worked as a student athletic trainer, before certifying in the Pilates method. Rebekah has presented at Pilates conferences, the International Osteoporosis Foundation Worldwide Conference and the International Association for Dance Medicine and

Science. Rebekah is a member of the Ambassador Leadership Council for the Bone Health and Osteoporosis Foundation and worked as a partner of the U.S. Department of Health and Human Services Office of Women's Health. She serves on the Bone Health Working Group for the Society for Women's Health Research, contributing to the 2021 recommendations published in the *Journal of Women's Health*, and is a member of the Medical Advisory Committee for the National Menopause Foundation.

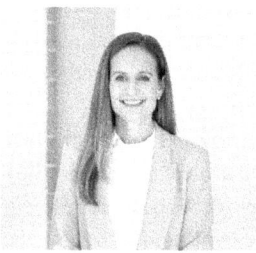

Dr Zoe Schaedel has 17 years' experience as an NHS GP with additional expertise in both sleep medicine and women's health, which she combines into a special interest in sleep during the menopause transition. Dr Schaedel lectures widely on sleep, giving talks to organisations and clinical teams to improve understanding of healthy sleep and how to get it. She also teaches on the International Sleep Medicine Course and sits on the British Sleep Society Education Committee. Dr Schaedel is an accredited British Menopause Society Menopause Specialist and is the co-director of Myla Health, a private women's health clinic as well as being the co-founder of The Good Sleep Clinic, which delivers personalised treatment programmes for insomnia. Dr Schaedel also leads the Brighton and Hove Community NHS Menopause Clinic.

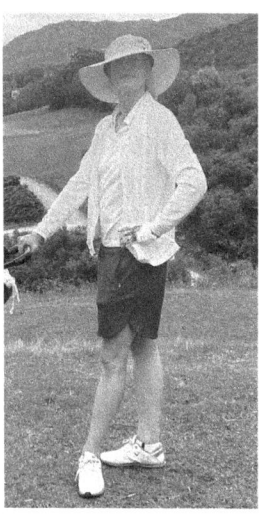

Astrid Sherman is currently the Imperial Society of Teachers of Dancing (ISTD) International Representative for the Americas' and guest teaching between Los Angeles, Vancouver and Spain. After dancing professionally with the Natal Performing Arts Council in South Africa, she immigrated to Canada. There she was artistic director of a large ISTD-based professional training school in Vancouver for 16 years, with many graduates being accepted into companies and postgraduate programs internationally. She has a Fellowship teaching qualification from the ISTD in Imperial Classical Ballet. Her BSc focused in Kinesiology and Gerontology from SFU in Canada and her MA in Dance Pedagogy was from Middlesex University in the UK. She is on the International Association for Dance Medicine & Science (IADMS) Dance Educators' Committee where she is involved in organising Regional and Outreach Virtual Dance Science events. Astrid has presented dance research at many IADMS & Healthy Dancer Canada conferences. She also acts as the *Dancer Wellness Advisor* for Ballet Beyond Borders.

Contributor Backgrounds

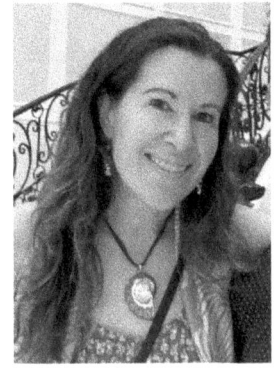

Professor Aimee Spector is Professor of Clinical Psychology of Ageing. Her own experience of cognitive problems in perimenopause led to a research interest in the relationship between menopause, perimenopause and the brain. This has resulted in the development of the UCL 'Menopause Mind Lab'; a team of researchers and clinicians dedicated to understand more about the impact of menopause and perimenopause on both cognition and well-being. Current research studies focus on the impact of biopsychosocial-cultural factors experienced during this transition, and the development and evaluation of interventions to improve cognition, mood and overall quality of life. She is Director of the International Cognitive Stimulation Therapy (CST) centre at UCL and the UCL Dementia Training Academy. Her research to date primarily focuses on the development and evaluation of psychosocial interventions for dementia, with a particular interest in global health. She has published over 165 peer-reviewed papers, 7 book chapters and 12 books and is international lead for University College London's Clinical Psychology doctorate course.

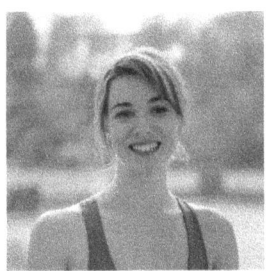

Tiffany Stott is the Dance Health Programmes Manager at Scottish Ballet. She trained as a dancer at London Studio Centre and holds an MSc in Dance Science from Trinity Laban. Her thesis, titled *The effects of rehearsal and performance on salivary cortisol, immunoglobulin and upper respiratory tract infection in professional female ballet dancers*, explored parameters of immune function in dancers. Tiffany is a personal trainer and sports masseuse specialising in corrective exercise; in addition, she ran a dance school for many years. Her current role at Scottish Ballet involves delivering and developing neurological dance programmes for Parkinson's, dementia and multiple sclerosis. She played a major role in developing the 'Health at Hand' resource for health and social care staff, 'Bedside Ballet' for people with reduced mobility as well as resources for people living with long COVID. Her role also involves developing training programmes for health professionals, artists and dance students.

Contributor Backgrounds

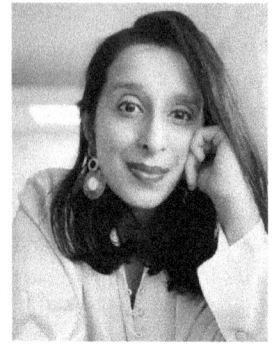

Dr Shema Tariq is a Principal Research Fellow at University College London's Institute for Global Health, and an NHS consultant in Sexual Health and HIV at the Mortimer Market Centre in London, where she set up and runs one of the UK's leading menopause services for women living with HIV. Shema is recognised as an international expert in HIV and menopause, leading a programme of research in this area since 2015, and authoring UK and international clinical guidelines. She is also part of the UCL team developing the UK's first national menopause education and support programme InTune.

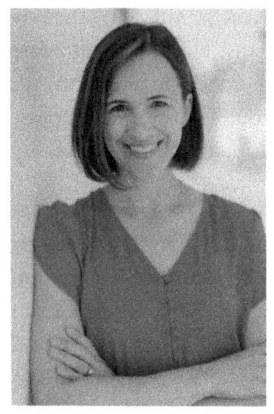

Dr Brooke Winder is a licensed physical therapist and an associate professor at California State University, Long Beach. In her clinical practice she specialises in orthopaedics, pelvic health and dance medicine and her clients include recreational athletes and performing artists as well as university-level and professional dancers. She is an active, published researcher on pelvic health in performing artists throughout the lifespan and presenter at many national and international conferences. Dr Winder earned a Doctor of Physical Therapy degree from the University of Southern California and a BFA in Dance from Chapman University. She is also a Board-Certified Specialist in Orthopaedic Physical Therapy and a BASI-Certified Pilates instructor. Prior to her entry into the world of physical therapy and academia, she trained as a competitive gymnast and later performed as a professional dancer for Southern-California based *Backhausdance*. She is passionate about combining her perspectives as an athlete, clinician, educator and researcher to advocate for improved understanding and optimal care for women and their pelvic health concerns.

www.ingramcontent.com/pod-product-compliance
Lightning Source LLC
Chambersburg PA
CBHW051523020426
42333CB00016B/1754